VARIORUM COLLECTED STUDIES SERIES

Health and Healing
in Early Modern England

Andrew Wear

Health and Healing
in Early Modern England

Studies in Social and Intellectual History

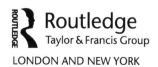

Routledge
Taylor & Francis Group

LONDON AND NEW YORK

First published 1998 in the Variorum Collected Studies Series by Ashgate Publishing

Published 2017 by Routledge
2 Park Square, Milton Park, Abingdon, Oxon OX14 4RN
605 Third Avenue, New York, NY 10017

Routledge is an imprint of the Taylor & Francis Group, an informa business

British Library Cataloguing-in-Publication Data
Wear, A. (Andrew)
    Health and Healing in Early Modern England: Studies in Social
    and Intellectual History.
    (Variorum Collected Studies Series: CS613)
    1. Medicine–England–History–16th century. 2. Medicine–
    England–History–17th century. 3. Healing–England–History–
    16th century. 4. Healing–England–History–17th century.
    I. Title.
    610 . 9' 42' 0903

US Library of Congress Cataloging-in-Publication Data
Wear, A. (Andrew).
    Health and Healing in Early Modern England: Studies in Social and Intellectual
    History/Andrew Wear.
    p. cm. – (Variorum Collected Studies Series: 613).
    1. Medicine–England–History–16th century. 2. Medicine–England–History–
    17th century. 3. Social medicine–England–History–16th century. 4. Social
    medicine–England–History–17th century.
    I. Wear, A. (Andrew), 1946–   . II. Series: Variorum Collected Studies: CS613.
    R487. H395   1998   98–6523
    610' .942' 09031–dc21   CIP

ISBN 13: 978-0-86078-690-0 (hbk)

VARIORUM COLLECTED STUDIES SERIES CS613

CONTENTS

This volume contains x + 332 pages

PUBLISHER'S NOTE

The articles in this volume, as in all others in the Collected Studies Series, have not been given a new, continuous pagination. In order to avoid confusion, and to facilitate their use where these same studies have been referred to elsewhere, the original pagination has been maintained wherever possible.

Each article has been given a Roman number in order of appearance, as listed in the Contents. This number is repeated on each page and quoted in the index entries.

PREFACE

The papers in this volume explore some of the major intellectual and social aspects of early modern medicine. Over the past twenty years, it has become clear that the history of medicine consists not of charting the progress of medicine conceived narrowly, as whatever leads to the knowledge, professions and institutions of the present. Such a Whig view of progress, reflecting the culture and driving ideologies of the newly industrialised countries of the nineteenth and early twentieth centuries, has largely disappeared from academic history. Instead, there is a new openness amongst historians to people, groups, topics and sources which had before been ignored, suppressed, or condemned as wrong, superstitious or just unimportant.

This volume reflects some of these changes in historical perspective. For instance, groups such as the sick poor and patients which are discussed in chapters VIII and VI were largely ignored in older histories of medicine, whilst topics such as the relationship of medicine and religion as discussed in chapters V and VI might well have been viewed as irrational and hence irrelevant. These newer areas of study illustrate the richness and diversity of early modern medicine. Underlying the more open approach of recent histories of medicine, has been the concept of the medical market place, first enunciated by Harold Cook, which has helped to structure the thinking of many early modern historians. It has brought into view the huge number and variety of practitioners, ranging from family members, neighbours, charitable gentlewomen, midwives, wise women, quacks, empirics, herbalists, specialists such as lithotomists and tooth-drawers, apothecaries and surgeons. It has also given a context to the physicians, the élite of the medical practitioners in terms of education and expense, by showing how few their numbers were in relation to the other members of the market place.

The medical market place model has influenced a number of the papers in this volume, but a note of caution is also necessary. The model was conceived and taken up by historians at the time of Reagan and Thatcher and reflects their ruthless free market ideology, which, as is the nature of such things, influenced the thinking and behaviour of even the most left wing of historians. Such 'presentist' history has made the history of medicine a popular and flourishing subject, many of the topics selected for study such as patient-doctor interactions being matters of concern today. Obviously, there are dangers in such an approach as historical understanding may be distorted in the search for present day relevance. The stress on economics can make one blind, for instance, to the healing that was offered not for money but for charity. At a more fundamental level the drive to apply the social sciences of today to the past, and to see their explanations as normative not only distorts the past but contradicts the whole thrust of post-modern deconstructionism which stresses that no system of explanation has explanatory priority over any other. On the other hand, history that does not speak at all to the present can result in mere antiquarianism. My study of ideas of health and the environment (see chapter IV) was initiated by the current interest in the environment, but I hope that I have captured how the topic was conceived of at the time, though, ironically, my conclusion indicated underlying continuities in attitudes that reached to the present.

The volume shows that I do not reject the importance of learned medicine, the medicine taught in the universities and based on Galen, despite the influence of the medical market place model. The learned physicians brought medical thinking, such as metaphors of health and illness, into literate culture. They were the 'grit' around which grew debates about the nature of medicine, medical ethics and the professional and institutional aspects of medicine. In the early sixteenth century they attempted a Galenic revival of medicine which would reform and make it safer. The first two papers discuss aspects of the new Galenic medicine in Continental Europe, and they provide a context for the main focus of this volume which is England. It was an English physician, William Harvey, influenced by the Continental revival of ancient anatomy who made the discovery of the circulation of the blood, which was to be celebrated as emblematic of the 'new science' of the later seventeenth century. As chapter III shows Harvey would not have agreed.

However, it is not extraordinary discoveries which dominate this volume, but the underlying aspects of health and medicine, such as the strong link that was perceived to exist between health and the environment. Chapters V and VI focus upon the relationship between medicine and the most important belief system of the time, religion, which helped to determine the place of medical practice in the world of early modern England as well as shaping a sense of ethical medical behaviour (see chapter VII). Religious charity, which was referred to in calls for better ethical behaviour in medicine, also to some extent underpinned the secular provision for the sick poor under the Poor Laws. How this occurred in practice is studied in detail in chapter VIII in the London parish of St. Bartholomew's Exchange.

The sense of a unified medical culture bridging both lay and élite medical knowledge owed a great deal to the publication of vernacular medical texts. The enterprise of disseminating medical knowledge into easily accessible forms to the literate section of the population was characteristic of much of English medical publishing, though as is discussed in chapter IX the medical-political aims of the authors often differed. Medical practice, which is still largely unexplored by historians, is referred to in many of the papers, and more specifically, in addition to the discussion of sixteenth century continental writings in the *practica* tradition in chapter II, the question of continuity or radical change in medical practice at the time of the 'new science' is considered in chapter X.

In conclusion, the epistemological nature of learned English medicine is discussed from a philosophical and social point of view. Neither approach, should in my view, exclude the other; when they do our ability to understand the thoughts and actions of people in the past is impoverished.

My debts to others are many. I have learned a great deal that I value from Rupert and Marie Hall who sparked my interest in the history of medicine. Together with the members of Aberdeen University they also provided examples of decent and honourable behaviour, of collegiality and a concern with the freedom of expression. My greatest debt of gratitude is to my wife who has given me immense and loving support.

Welcome Institute, London
January 1998

ANDREW WEAR

ACKNOWLEDGEMENTS

Grateful acknowledgement is made to the following persons, institutions , and publishers for their kind permission to reproduce the studies included in this volume: The Trustee, The Wellcome Trust, London (for studies I and VIII); Cambridge University Press, Cambridge (II, IV, VI, X, and XI); Science History Publications Limited, Chalfont St Giles, Bucks (III); Erasmus Publishing B.V., Rotterdam (V); Editions Rodopi B.V., Amsterdam (VII); Routledge, London (IX).

My thanks also go to Jean Runciman who compiled the Index and to Sue Chapman who sorted out the problems of bringing the volume together.

I

Galen in the Renaissance

Preface

Galen in the Renaissance is a very large topic; at the moment our only guide is Owsei Temkin's book *Galenism*[1], and we are fortunate that it is a very good one. There is little need to repeat in detail Temkin's conclusions, so what I have done is to write a short introduction in which some general matters are discussed. There then follow sections on particular topics. These are not specifically related to each other, but describe some problem areas of current research which involve the Galenic tradition. Finally I consider Sanctorius, whose work reflects many of the issues in the rest of the paper.

I have concentrated on certain conceptual issues and have largely omitted discussion of the appearance of new editions (such as that of Aldus of 1525) and translations of Galen which flooded the Renaissance. The linguistic scholarship of the Renaissance was the necessary backcloth against which the great explosion of Galenic studies took place. However, neither skill nor time have allowed me to consider this topic, but fortunately the researches of Richard Durling[2] have done much to illuminate the subject.

Introductory Essay

It is not possible to reach a synthetic and coherent view of Galen's position in the Renaissance. There are other reasons for this apart from the superficial difficulty of dating the Renaissance, and the usual practice of historians of science of extending the scientific Renaissance to 1630 which places the young humanist Leoniceno in the same period as a polished product of the Paduan school like William Harvey.[3]

Another obvious but much more fundamental factor is that the range of Galen's writings means that it is sometimes difficult to find connections between developments in the various specialities within medicine, and also between such disparate subjects as the philosophy of medicine and surgery which lie outside medicine.

I

The question of progress is especially difficult. Often the historian can report that certain writers felt that they were being innovative and progressive yet he notes at the same time the threads of tradition and continuity. At the beginning of the medical Renaissance the retrieval of new Galenic texts (especially in areas like anatomy and physiology) and, more generally, the fresh rendering of Galenic texts gave to early sixteenth century writers the feeling that they could go beyond the Arabs and the mediaeval Latin writers. In anatomy the vehicle for this sense of progress was Galen's newly discovered *Anatomical Procedures* which seems to have been the starting point for Vesalius, though as Durling points out it was not frequently printed in the sixteenth century.[4] Again, as Andrew Cunningham's researches will show, the newly translated *Methodus Medendi* was at the forefront of the attempt by Linacre and others to get the 'new' Galen accepted in Europe. Apart from the question of the impact of new Galenic works we have to consider the pervasive concern of humanist medical writers to have accurate texts and translations. Out of this concern there arose the development of a uniform medical terminology and the frequently reiterated condemnation of the Arabic and mediaeval legacy.

Manardi, the student of Leoniceno and his successor at Ferrara, wrote that the study of terminology was far more necessary for present day writers than for Galen, as Galen partly discovered medicine and partly learned it from authors writing in his own tongue. The problem of translation had been made more difficult by the intermediaries between the time of Galen and the present, Manardi wrote:

> If only they had not been ignorant of both languages, both the one from which they received medicine and the one into which they translated it, then they would not have made medicine to be not only polluted, uncultured and punic and barbarous rather than Latin, but (also) maimed and in many parts mutilated and interpolated.[5]

The condemnation of the preceding period was not unanimous, Nicholas Massa wrote in his *Anatomiae Liber Introductorius* (1536), "I am sorry that I have promised to write for you in these times when the very wise Arabs and many others have been pursued with gratuitous insults, for I do not wish to appear guilty of the same offence".[6]

Nevertheless, a strong case can be made out that there was a definite feeling of progress due to the presentation of a new Galen. This means that we should not automatically contrast the 'new' Paracelsus with the 'old' Galen. However, the sense of progress shared by the humanists did not mean that all threads with the immediate past were cut. The continuity with the mediaeval period is exemplified by the university curricula, where

Arabic writers such as Avicenna are prescribed and in which modern writers rarely feature,[7] thus making it difficult to assess the influence of renaissance writers of medical text-books upon what was actually taught. There was continuity not only in teaching but also in the rehearsal and extension of old debates, of which the most important was that between the 'philosophers' who were the followers of Aristotle and the 'physicians' who followed Galen. This debate probably had its origins in Alexandria[8] (though one can equally say that Galen himself started it) and continued in the mediaeval west.[9] In the Renaissance it was most significant in the latter part of the sixteenth century. However, even in the first half of the sixteenth century Manardi identified himself as a follower of Galen and not of Aristotle. On the question of the suitability of roast or boiled meat for quartan fever Manardi wrote to his correspondent:

> But you have as a champion of your view Aristotle whom everyone regards as an oracle and venerates deservedly. I, however, protected by the shield of Galen especially in these questions which concern a physician rather than a philosopher, do not fear Aristotle at all.[10]

Another factor which tended to diminish the novelty, and in this case the authority, of Galen for the Renaissance, despite the humanists' retrieval of new texts and their refurbishing of old ones, was the fact that Galen *was* second to Hippocrates, despite being 'Prince of Physicians'.[11] Leonhard Fuchs (1501–1566), writing as a humanist, in his resumé of the history of medicine called Galen 'doctissimus Hippocratis interpres', and praised him as "a man most excellent not only in medicine but indeed in all other disciplines".[12] Galen presented himself as a follower of Hippocrates, and Fuchs is being true to Galen's vision of himself. Fuchs gave the highest praise to Hippocrates, writing that he brought back medicine from the darkness to the light and to near perfection.[13] To emphasise his point Fuchs quoted the preface of the *Isagoge* of Soranus, "Medicine, he (Soranus) says, was invented by Apollo in fact, enlarged by Aesculapius and perfected by Hippocrates".[14]

Galen's position as the interpreter of an almost *prisca medicina* is reflected in Fuchs' assertion that God led Galen to medicine in order that he could refute the errors of men like Erasistratus, Asclepiades and Themison. If Galen had not opposed the mendacity of these men then, Fuchs wrote, we would now have a contaminated form of medicine.[15] For Fuchs then, Galen was an interpreter and defender of Hippocratic medicine, but he was not the fount of medicine. Thus Galen was not unchallengeable in the way that Hippocrates might be.

This reiteration in the sixteenth century of Galen's own view of himself may help to explain the fact that even the most Galenic of sixteenth

I

century writers, such as Andreas Laurentius (1558–1609), did not limit himself to Galen alone. The underlying explanation of a particular problem might be broadly Galenic but other authorities would frequently be cited. Galen's role as commentator on Hippocrates meant that he could always be contrasted with other commentators as well as being treated as an authoritative source in his own right. This tended to prevent a full-blooded Galenism being developed, though of course there were always men like Sylvius ready to defend Galen's views, if not to develop them any further.

Humanists were not only concerned to retrieve Galen and one might expect that some of the humanist translators who were influenced by neoplatonism would use Plato to oppose Galen. Whether such a case can be made out is problematic. It is true that Leoniceno called Galen 'homo Platonicus' and pushed him into Plato's camp – not too difficult a thing to do.[16] As to criticism of Galen, Antonioli has argued that Symphorien Champier, a faithful follower of Ficino was critical of Galen and especially opposed the Galenic doctrine of the origin of the veins in the liver with the Platonic view of the heart as the source of life and origin of veins.[17] Temkin, on the other hand, has pointed out that Champier was generally pro-Galen[18] and a cursory reading of Champier's *Practica Nova* (1517)[19] does nothing to dispel that view. More generally, Pagel has pointed out how Paracelsus criticised Galen but praised Hippocrates and Ficino, the latter because he shared his neoplatonic vision.[20] To what extent anti-Galenic feeling existed amongst neoplatonists who were not Paracelsians could be an area for further research.

The idea of progress is also involved in anatomy. Much has been written on sixteenth century anatomy, but as I point out in my study of the *rete mirabile* below (in Section II) the fact that Galen was contradicted on observational detail does not mean that Galen's overall conception of the functioning of the body was challenged by the anatomists. This lack of challenge is only seen by the historian looking back. What sense of progress was held at the time by the anatomists themselves is difficult to grasp. Pagel and Rattansi[21] have written that Vesalius' motive for criticising Galen was his desire to return to a *prisca anatomia*, existing in Alexandrian times, they also add that Vesalius felt that medicine had declined badly after the 'Gothic invasions'.[22] However, when one comes to late sixteenth century writers the humanist paradox of progress by means of regress is not so apparent.[23] Instead of a mythical pristine knowledge it is the teachings of Aristotle which act as the focus of opposition to Galen.

A lot of good historical research has been done on the Aristotelian-Galenic debates, and for the purposes of this conference it would not be useful to go through old material. Pagel,[24] Temkin,[25] Roger[26] and Bylebyl[27] have all contributed to our understanding of how the Aristotelian philosophers and physicians – writers such as Argenterius, Cremonini, Cesalpino, Zabarella, Fabricius, Bauhin, Hofmann and Harvey – were developing an Aristotelian approach to medical issues. The problems ranged over a wide spectrum and included the question of the primacy of the heart or the brain, whether there are three spirits or one, the nature of semen and of generation in general. These disputes all challenged the authority of Galen but as it turned out the overthrow of Galen did not come from the 'progressive' Aristotelians. Temkin puts it well when he writes that in the seventeenth century "Aristotelians and Galenists (a crude antithesis by 1600 already) together were then to appear as traditionalists, and their differences as negligible in the eyes of defenders and enemies alike".[28] However, Argenterius, Cesalpino and the rest did not have the benefit of hindsight, they felt that they were discussing important issues and their work deserves study.

Finally, there must be mentioned the work of Paracelsus, in the Renaissance the radical alternative to Galenic medicine. Although it is not discussed as such in this paper, it must always be kept in mind as bounding and contextualising much of orthodox medicine, whether of an Aristotelian or Galenic bias.

In the sections that follow I have concentrated not on the challenge to Galen, but on the continuation of the Galenic tradition, as in the case of the animal spirits and the *rete mirabile* where Galen's thoughts was preserved under challenge. In the section on astrology where Galen's general tenor of thought was interpreted by renaissance writers, and in my discussion of medical method, when Galen's thought may be said to be both restored and then extended. In the final section I have written about another proponent of Galenic teaching, Sanctorius, rather than about any Aristotelian challenge and this is in keeping with my emphasis on studying the Galenic side of renaissance medicine.

II

Anatomy, Physiology and the Rete Mirabile

From Benedetti to Vesalius and to Harvey the Paduan anatomists lie in wait enticing the historian with visions of progress and of the scientific revolution. However it is extremely doubtful if any of these anatomists, including Harvey, would have been happy with the mechanical picture of the world which Galileo, Descartes and Newton produced. Certainly, independent observation as examplified by Vesalius was to be a part of the

I

new science of the seventeenth century. The teleological Aristotelian or Galenic thought in which the sixteenth century anatomists were immersed was not.

To illustrate my point that the anatomists could not get away from the ancients when it came to theory I will look at the famous case of the *rete mirabile*. The denial of the *rete mirabile* first by Berengario and then by Vesalius is taken by historians as an example of the challenge to Galen's authority.[29] I want to show, however, that the theory behind the *rete mirabile* was not challenged. Galen had stated that the *rete mirabile* produced animal spirits. But despite the denial of the *rete mirabile*, the existence of the animal spirits which formed a lynchpin of Galen's physiology was not denied except by Argenterius.

As the *rete mirabile* could not be observed the anatomists had to decide how the animal spirits were generated – for they were unwilling to deny their existence. Galen had admittedly given them some leeway; as the animal spirits were given only their first alteration in the *rete mirabile* and were finally concocted by the substance of the brain when they entered the ventricles.[30] Thus the sojourn of the spirits in the *rete mirabile* was but a stage in their production, and perhaps not absolutely essential.

Vesalius made a straightforward replacement of the *rete mirabile* by the cerebral arteries:

> ... the Maker of the Universe has used far greater ingenuity than Galen imagined. For He has contrived for the great soporal artery a tortuous channel with a long passage (= carotid canal) in the bone, and he has willed for this passage the very thing for which Galen imagined that the plexus had been built, to wit, that the vital spirit be thoroughly concocted in the many turnings and twistings of the artery, and its matter be so prepared for producing animal spirit.[31]

The final production of the animal spirit was:

> From the air which has entered the brain, and from that vital spirit which, by its devious course, becomes progressively more assimilated in the ventricles to the action of the brain, the animal spirit is elaborated by the cerebral power ('virtus'). We believe that this power depends on the opportune balancing of the elements of the brain substance.[32]

Vesalius' replacement of the *rete mirabile* by a similarly convoluted and tortuous arterial structure set the pattern for some of the anatomists who followed him. Realdo Colombo in the *De Re Anatomica* replaced the *rete mirabile* with the choroid plexus, which, unlike the *rete mirabile*, did exist in man:

> Through these frontal ventricles of the brain the choriform plexuses (choroid

plexus) are led, which we have called reticular. Their use is, in fact, the generation of animal spirits. And what I now relate, since it is my invention, I implore you to attend carefully...[33]

Colombo went on to describe how the air drawn in from the nose passed through the ethmoid bone and was mixed with the vital spirits in the reticular (choroid) plexus and so the animal spirits were produced. He concluded with characteristic pride:

Which matter was observed by no one before me.[34]

When Archangelo Piccolomini (1526–1605) came to discuss the problem in his *Anatomicae Praelectiones* he tried to have the best of both worlds: in the *rete mirabile* the animal spirits were inchoate, and received their full character only in the choroid plexus. Similarly, animal spirits were only conserved in the ventricles, their perfection occurring in the substance of the brain.[35] Piccolomini appealed to other step by step processes that were said to take place in the body to justify this new scheme, citing the way in which venous and arterial blood was made.[36] Whatever Piccolomini's rationalization, the fact remains that he accepted both the *rete mirabile* and the choroid plexus. There is not an iota of doubt or of critical insight to be found in his writings, since all he was interested in was to reconcile different points of view.

The writings of Andreas Laurentius on the subject are similar to those of Piccolomini. In chapter ten of the tenth book of the *Historia Anatomica* he wrote that for the preparation of animal spirits plexuses had been constructed which had a labyrinthine structure of little veins and arteries.[37] A little later in the same chapter, however, he wrote that he preferred to name the plexus which Galen had called *rete mirabile*, the choroid plexus, as the 'neoterics' had done.[38] Rather than assert that Galen was wrong, Laurentius tried to hide Galen's fallibility and stated that what was involved here was a mere change in terminology.

The prevarications did not stop there. In his reply to the question 'What is the Nature of the animal spirit, what is the manner of his generation and the place thereof', Laurentius asserted, (in the rendering of Helkiah Crooke):

... there is stored up a supply (of animal spirits) against time of need in those two complications or textures called Plexus Choroides and Rete mirabile...

The preparation of this spirit is made in those Labyrinths of the small arteries, their coction or elaboration (as some think) in the ventricles...

They therefore are in error who do conceive that this spirit attaineth his proper forme and specifically difference in those textures. For all the complications of

I

vessels as well in the braine as in the testicles and other parts are ordained onely for preparation, but the forme and difference of a thing is supplied by the substance of the part, both to the Aliment and to the spirit.

Wherefore we conclude, that in those complications (choroid plexus and rete mirabile) the spirits are prepared, that in the ventricles they are boyled and labored, but receive their uttermost perfection in the substance of the Braine.[39]

Thus Laurentius accepted, like Piccolomini, the existence in man of both the *rete mirable* and choroid plexus. Apart from their difference over the action of the ventricles (for Piccolomini stated that the animal spirits were only stored there), the views of the two men were identical and both shared the same confidence in the truth of their conclusions.

Because of his Aristotelian bias, Caspar Bauhin might have been expected to exert his critical abilities on the problem. Unfortunately it is impossible to know what his attitude would have been for he stated categorically that he had seen the *rete mirabile* in man:

Vesalius affirmeth that this wonderful Net is onely found in the heads of beasts, but we ... have beene able to make demonstration of it in all the mens heads we have hitherto cut up, although we confesse that in Calves and Oxen it is much greater and more conspicuous. (hominum capitibus hactenus demonstrauimus; non tamen negamus in vitulorum et boum capitibus multo et maius et manifestius conspici.)[40]

Bauhin did not arrive at any conclusion of his own but merely contented himself with repeating the opinions of other people. As he had observed the *rete mirabile* to his own satisfaction, for him there was no problem and so, like the good text-book writer that he was, he gave the views of other authorities.

Harvey's opinions of the *rete mirabile* were taken from Bauhin, as the following shows:

The rete mirabile. Concerning this great laboratory of the animal spirits see Galen. It is formed from a network of the branches of the carotid arteries and completely surrounds the hypophysis on all sides. It extends from the sides of the sphenoid bone ... Bauhin contradicts Vesalius and maintains that it does exist in the human head ...[41]

Perhaps Harvey's disinclination to give a personal opinion is a sign of caution and the requirements of lecture presentation; but certainly there is little doubt or questioning to be found in his writing. That doubt over an anatomical structure could put traditional theory into question is clear from the example of Vesalius' and then Realdo Colombo's conclusions on the pores in the intraventricular septum and from the case of Argenterius and the *rete mirabile* in section five of this paper. However, the principle of doubting a theory which flowed from a controverted anatomical structure was, as we have seen, not acted upon consistently. In renaissance anatomy the falsificationist philosophy of Sir Karl Popper and his acolytes may have been recognised but tradition would have held back its implementation. The choices open to the anatomists were few. The Aristotelian alternative was not really viable: Galen had amply demonstrated the anatomical impossibility of the heart's being the origin of sensation and hence the producer of the spirits of sensation. There was no other established theory to which the anatomists could turn; they had either to create a new theory or to cover up the unfortunate discovery that the *rete mirabile* was not to be found in man. In this case, the underlying teaching of Galen was preserved and even the denial of a detail - the *rete mirabile* - was by no means clear-cut; there was compromise, prevarication and a general 'fudging' of the picture.

As there had not been a general challenge to Galenic medicine apart from the Paracelsian alternative, this perhaps was inevitable. The university based physicians generally rejected Paracelsus and remained in the Galenic camp; their only alternative was to move towards Aristotle. The fact that anatomists taught at universities is important. In the latter part of the sixteenth century what has been called 'academic anatomy' developed.[42] Anatomical books were essentially text-books and the teaching element was prominent throughout anatomy in this period. The anatomists argued and taught by extensive citation of ancient and modern authorities on a particular topic. This was essentially a traditional form of writing and was applied by writers like Andreas Laurentius and Caspar Bauhin to questions of theory and function. Observational matters might be decided by the sight of the writer but the solution of theoretical issues had to be the outcome of an argument produced out of various authorities as well as personal opinion. Given this framework it is perhaps not surprising that originality in observation was not carried over into theory which might then have produced a complete rejection of the Galenic system of the body. There were changes in the theory of the body's functioning but these were usually Aristotelian in origin and therefore hardly radical - after all Galen was influenced by Aristotle.

I now turn to a subject where the physicians tried to extricate themselves from the influence of the philosophers.

I

III

Medical Method

Any paper on Galen in the Renaissance should at least allude to the debates on method centred on the opening lines of Galen's *Ars Parva*. The complexity of the subject is great and a separate and lengthy article would be needed to do it justice. I limit myself, therefore, to some comments on the state of historical work on the topic and to some suggestions concerning interpretation.

Various historians have noted that Leoniceno separated Galen's three orders of teaching mentioned at the beginning of the *Ars Parva* from their identification with the methods of dialectic being developed by the Aristotelian Paduan philosophers.[43] Thus, the philological and philosophical research of Leoniceno led to the claim that the physicians could have their own methodology. Leoniceno's newly defined order of resolution began not from effects to causes as in Paduan resolution but from the end or purpose of the art. Edwards has emphasised this point and written that Leoniceno's order of resolution began from "the end of a whole science or art".[44] As such, the physician's order of resolution was, according to Edwards, either a teaching device or, more importantly:

> it offered a plan for the reconstruction of any science, or even the construction of a new one. It does not seem surprising, therefore, that before much time had elapsed, the manner of the presentation of a science ceased to be the *commentary* on an appropriate work of Galen, of Aristotle, etc., and became instead the independent treatise. These independent works were at first unoriginal, and amounted to little more than a recasting of the materials contained in works that had been university texts for centuries. But the opportunity to reconceive and reconstruct a science (such as natural philosophy) *de novo* was there, and began to be exploited towards the end of the sixteenth century.[45]

Edwards has produced an interesting speculation on the influence of method. He has also raised here the question of continuity and innovation which I now want to consider before looking at the content of the writings on medical method. Not all writings in the mediaeval period were commentaries. For example, Bradwardine's *De Proportionibus*, his *Geometria Speculativa* and his *De Causa Dei* are all independent works. In medicine, the *Isagoge* of Johannitius, Avicenna's *Canon* and Mondino's *Anathomia* come readily in mind as works which, if not original, are not commentaries but similar to the "recasting" of older materials which Edwards suggests occurs in the sixteenth century. It is true that noncommentative works dealing with large sections of medicine increased in the sixteenth century, and they often had an introductory section on medical method. But the influence of the latter upon the former is debatable.

Leoniceno did spark off a general interest in medical method and this is reflected in the inclusion of introductory discussions on medical method in medical text-books. An examination of the context of these discussions shows that they were placed into a traditional format. Medical methodology did not stand alone in the introductions of treatises on medicine; nor was its inclusion new. In fact, an introductory discussion of method was traditional; it forms, after all the beginning of the *Ars Parva*, which then goes on to teach the whole of medicine by definition. In addition to methodology it was also traditional to give an introductory discussion of the history of medicine, of the philosophical status of medicine as an art or science, and of the subject matter of medicine. Both of the latter can be found in the opening of Johannitius' *Isagoge* and of Avicenna's *Canon*. In Book IV of Isidore of Seville's *Etymologies* there is an account of the history of medicine and this formed the preface to his description of medicine. Additionally, Isidore included a description of the three sects, the methodists, empiricists and logicians described by Galen. As well as relating to the history of medicine it also served as the methodological part of Isidore's introduction.

In Champier's *Practica Nova* we find in the introduction the elements of the history of medicine, a discussion of the status of medicine, and descriptions of the methodology and subject matter of medicine. In addition to descriptions of the medical sects the opening parts of the *Ars Parva* are included.[46] There is little discussion and it is not clear what function this material serves except to fulfil traditional requirements; for Champier's book is largely a description of pathological states of the body and the resolution from the end of the art mentioned by Champier in the opening of the book in no way informs the ordering of the rest of the book.

In the work of Leonhard Fuchs there was still a debt to tradition. The introduction to his text-book on medicine, the *Methodus seu Ratio Compendaria Cognoscendi Veram Solidamque Medicinam* (1550), followed the traditional format, though with some sections expanded. Then, without in this work having discussed Galen's 'orders of teaching', Fuchs divided the whole of medicine into three orders ('universae medicinae in tres ordines distributio').[47] The orders with which the book is structured consist of the traditional categories found in Johannitius – the naturals, non naturals and the things against nature.[48] In Fuchs' very similar *Institutionum Medicinae Libri Quinque* there is a discussion of the *Ars Parva* and its three orders, and this discussion is enriched by citation

I

of other methodological works of Galen.[49] Although there is much that is traditional in Fuchs' text-books, there is no doubt that he was affected by the new debates on medical method begun by Leoniceno, Manardi and Montanus. One can reasonably conclude that although the practice of structuring medicine and the way in which Fuchs did it was traditional, yet his justification, or even legitimisation, of his practice was based on the new discussions on method.

Although I have stressed the traditional element in Fuchs it cannot be denied that there was a new interest in the Renaissance as to how a text-book on medicine should be taught and structured. In the work of Montanus the problem of how an art should be taught and arranged becomes almost an end in itself. This is clearly seen in the *Medicina Universa*[50] put together after Montanus' death. Here there is a long opening section on method and order in an art, and then the student is explicitly taught the substance of medicine 'methodically' in the rest of the book. Montanus was, however, exceptional in including so much discussion of medical method, in what was after all a compendium.

As Edwards hinted in the quotation above, there was an increase in text-books in the Renaissance. The general growth of compendia and methodical treatises[51] was mirrored in medicine – though again there had been similar mediaeval developments. Arnold of Villanova (d.1311) had rebuked those who "study not in the writings which convey the art of Galen and Hippocrates but in booklets and summas".[52] As Bates[53] has pointed out, the use of tables as teaching devices, and the schematising of medical information, can also be associated with the 'methodical' mind of the Renaissance – but here again the 'Tree of Porphyry' reminds one that nothing is new.

To sum up: I have tried to stress the traditional elements in the text-books, and to point out that the compressing of many authorities and especially the works of Galen into one book was not new – though the practice increased. The discussions on medical method may have helped to justify the practice of ordering or structuring medicine, but it is doubtful if they actually caused it. I suspect the growth in compendia and in discussions on method have common origins, but that would lead us far away from Galen in the Renaissance.

I want to turn now to the content of the discussions on medical method. Galen's *Ars Parva* and his other methodological works were the starting point for the medical writers but they also referred extensively to Plato, Aristotle and to the commentatory tradition. What is at issue is the status of medical method and its relation to the methods of the philosophers.

Close analysis of the work of Leoniceno and others would be out of place here. Instead I want to discuss how the recognition by the renaissance writers – in opposition to Avicenna[54] – that medicine was an art as Aristotle and Galen had taught them, led to the development of a methodology appropriate to an art as opposed to 'scientia'. This new approach began when Leoniceno emphasised that the order of resolution begins with the end of an art as opposed to the Paduan method of resolution from effects to causes. In doing so he followed the Aristotelian ends – means description of an art found in the *Ethics*. Leoniceno wrote in explaining the order of resolution:

> Now the fact that the orders under which each science can be taught are only three is proved as follows: either the science which is taught is taught in the same order in *which it is found and first established in the mind*, and this order of teaching is called the resolutory; or it is taught in the opposite order, and this order is called the compository (Leoniceno here ignores the order of definition).
>
> It is as if someone wishing to teach the art of building a house should first teach the form and material of which the roof should be constructed, second, how the walls are to be erected, third that foundations should be made and last how the earth should be dug out. He would be observing the resolutory order of teaching which begins from the conception of the end. For covering and defence from cold and rain is the end which a man who wants to build a house establishes for himself. [My italics].[55]

Leoniceno added in elucidation of resolution, "the first resolutory order is the same as the order in which the rationale of building a house is discovered". On the other hand, the compository order is that in which a house is actually built.[56] As the renaissance medical writers emphasised, medicine was an art and Leoniceno was giving here a description of the ordering of an art of which Aristotle would have approved. Certain knowledge for Aristotle was *episteme*, and in order to be certain, it had to be unencumbered by the limited and specific ends of the artisan.[57] As such *episteme* involved demonstrable (certain) knowledge a point which the Paduan philosophers attempted to develop.[58] On the other hand an art like medicine was concerned not with demonstrating knowledge but with achieving or producing a specific good-health. This was not a subject for analysis, which was reserved for the means whereby the good or end would be achieved. In Book III of the *Nicomachean Ethics* Aristotle wrote:

> We deliberate not about ends but about means. For a doctor does not deliberate whether he shall heal, nor an orator whether he shall persuade ... They assume the end and consider how and by what means it is to be attained.

Aristotle continues:

> ... It seems, then, as has been said, that man is a moving principle of actions; now deliberation is about the things to be done by the agent himself, and actions are for the sake of things other than themselves. For the end cannot be a subject

of deliberation, but only the means.. If we are to be always deliberating, we shall have to go on to infinity.[59]

Leoniceno echoed this part of Aristotle's teaching when he wrote that "the idea of an end does not come from resolution but precedes resolution".[60] He wrote that he would repeat again and again that the notion of the end precedes resolution ("ut etiam magis ac magis postea declarabimus notio finis antecedit resolutionem").[61] For Leoniceno, therefore, the discovery or setting out of the means to achieve an end is the task of the order of resolution. The starting point, the end of the art, is a given. For as Leoniceno wrote, citing Galen's De Constitutione Artis Medicinalis, the conceived purpose of an art was from the mind and was not derived from any method.[62] Therefore the conception by the mind of the end of an art was for Leoniceno a basic datum from which the order of resolution proceded to make sense of the activities and products of artists.

One can see in Leoniceno's discussion of order a conservative tendency. Here is no method for discovering a priori new knowledge in the manner of Descartes; for a priori conceptions of the mind are not subject to method. The other way of arriving at new knowledge is also barred as Leoniceno does not discuss the use of the resolutive method (as opposed to order) as a means of arriving at knowledge a posteriori from effects to causes.

One of the most enthusiastic followers in the methodological discussion begun by Leoniceno was Montanus. He went beyond Galen and Leoniceno in his ideas on medical method. In his commentary on the Ars Parva he tried to define the difference between resolutive method and order. He wrote:

> They [resolutive method and order] differ in this, that the resolutive way is not multiple but simple and directs itself towards a particular goal in knowledge; but order is multiple and directs itself to no particular goal in knowledge but rather to a universal end. So that when anyone declares the purpose in the medical art, which end is health – and it is a universal end – then he divides it into its principles by dividing into matter and form. And many resolutions [i.e. methods of resolution] and also many divisions and many definitions and many demonstrations are made in the parts and in all the divisions.[63]

For Montanus, therefore, it seems that the order of resolution analyses a multiple end – health – which is then separated out into its constituent principles. Then the four ways or methods of dialectic – division definition, demonstration and resolution – take over from the orders and analyse the principles. Method thus defined therefore comes after, and is in a sense subordinate to order.

It is important to realise that Montanus was developing a philosophical analysis of an art and not a science. Wightman[64] and Bates[65] have pointed to the obscurity and pedantry of this sort of discussion. Yet it is understandable that Montanus is difficult; after all the philosophers triumphed. We do not talk of an 'ordology' (!) but a 'methodology'. The attempt to develop a specifically medical methodology failed, for the whole philosophical tradition from Aristotle (but not from Plato)[66] was against the possibility of an art (techne) having its own methodology and being the equal of a science (episteme).[67] Polanyi's term 'tacit knowledge'[68] which describes the artistic or craft component in modern science is a sign that philosophy has still not developed an analytical language to describe the knowledge of an art. The problems of translating and understanding Montanus' still-born attempt to do this are therefore formidable. The difficulties of interpretation have been made worse by the tendency of writers like Gilbert[69] and Lisa Jardine[70] to judge the work of the medical writers on method in the dichotomous terms of discovery or teaching. This is further discussed below. For the moment I simply want to make the point that using these categories may lead to misunderstanding Montanus.

That Montanus was really concerned with developing a methodology for an art is clear when he describes how the doctor needs to apply particulars to universals. He wrote that particulars are known by the senses, causes by the mind. The two are separate:

> But since we are concerned with particulars and on that account we are called sensitive artificers, we ought to discover the causes of diseases; but we cannot do this (discover them) in particulars because we are made aware of particulars by the senses, which do not make causes known to us; for causes are universals and are to be perceived only by the mind: consequently causes are hidden from the senses.[71]

The discovery of causes from the phenomena à la Randall's Paduans was not of interest for Montanus. What was involved was the recognition that a cause explains a particular sign of illness. Montanus wrote that a sensory impression could be conceptualised by the mind and, by some means which he does not clearly describe, the hidden causes or universals which are appropriate to the sign are then evoked from the depths of the mind. Some form of analogy between sign and cause seems to be involved. The cryptic lecture notes of Montanus state:

> We ought to proceed to the recognition of causes by way of a sign evident and apparent to the senses. And when that effect is perceived, since it is a particular sign and perceptible to the sense it arouses the sense then is carried back to the intellect and forms a concept in it. Then (the intellect) refers (the sign) to the hidden causes (i.e. universals), and draws an analogy which is a certain relation (of the nature) of the particular to (that of) the universal.[72]

Montanus developed this description and wrote that when a particular

I

sense impression is placed before the intellect "it joins itself to the causes recognised already by the intellect" and from recognition that a particular depends upon a specific cause, knowledge emerges.[73] The whole emphasis of the argument was against induction or the methodical derivation of knowledge from particulars. The causes were already in the intellect, and as Sanctorius was to write, not a thousand thousand particulars could produce a universal. The only function of the perception of particulars was for it to act as a trigger whereby the mind is excited into producing the correct cause of the perception. This, therefore, was no dialectical method of discovery in which the discovery is publicly proved. Here a private process was involved. As such it could be interpreted as a teaching method, for a type of learning seems to be involved whereby general knowledge is related to particular phenomena or indications. Lisa Jardine, in fact, has argued that the medical writers on method fooled themselves into thinking that they were discussing the discovery of knowledge, whereas they were in fact dealing only with teaching.[74] This would be true only if we were to deny the possibility of *a priori*, innate, knowledge. If we do not do this, and do not require knowledge to be derived from the phenomena in the first place, then Montanus need not be reduced to a writer on the teaching of medicine. However, I do not think that either discovery or teaching are satisfactory explanatory terms in this case. Perhaps for the Renaissance an art was constituted from eternity or from its mythical moment of invention and was not "discovered" and then taught but rather uncovered. The problem is that we do not possess the terminology to express what Montanus meant.

The stress by historians upon the concept of discovery is the product of Randall's influential study of Paduan Aristotelianism.[75] Randall saw the Paduan discussions concerning a method of discovering new knowledge from the phenomena as one of the roots of modern science. The medical writers tend therefore to be contrasted with Paduan Aristotelians. This is historically sound, as Leoniceno self-consciously divorced medical method from that of the philosophers, whilst Zabarella on behalf of the philosophers denied the claims of Montanus.[76] However, it is too easy to dismiss the medical writers as *only* concerned with teaching. It is true that Montanus, Manardi and Fuchs were concerned with teaching but the ordering of an art went beyond teaching. The problem is that the medical writers themselves had to use the categories of teaching and discovery. Note how Fuchs used not one or the other but, both:

> Thus far therefore we have learned from Galen that there are three ways or modes by which any art can be certainly taught or written down with order. For indeed the resolutory (order) is most apt for the invention (uncovering) of an art (ad artis inventionem) ...[77]

Coming back to Montanus the question to ask is where does the knowledge of an art come from in the first place? An art could be taught using the three orders but the multiple end of medicine which was laid out by the order of resolution consists of principles already inhering in the mind of the artist-physician, if they did not do so the conceptions of the end of the art could not have been in the physicians's mind in the first place. The essentials of the art of medicine like its end are therefore already given – and it is the same thing if we talk of discovery or teaching when we lay them out in an ordered fashion and thus recognise that we have achieved knowledge.

Whether my view of Montanus or that of Gilbert and Jardine is correct the end result is the same in either case. Discovery of new knowledge is not an issue. I have indicated that to understand a writer like Montanus we should try to perceive the problems that he faced and not borrow the standards of the Paduan philosophers. However, in terms of Galen in the Renaissance it is clear from either interpretation that discussions of medical methodology did nothing to lossen Galen's authority or to replace his writings. Indeed, Galen's authority gained, as it was in his name that the debate originated. In practice in the lectures of a teacher like Montanus we find that when he goes on to discuss the principles of medicine such as the elements, qualities, temperaments and disease categories, his mind recognises only those 'hidden causes' that tradition and Galen have taught it.

A last point to mention is the development of a therapeutic method from Galen's *Methodus Medendi*. This has been discussed by Bates in a recent article[78] and I will not enlarge upon it.

In the end, the physicians' attempt to philosophise did not lead far. In the next section I consider a topic – astrology – where the need to create a new philosophy was notably absent.

IV

Medicine and Astrology

Some modern historians have written that astrology and medicine were inextricably linked in the Renaissance. This is rather surprising. It is true that the third book of Galen's *De Diebus Decretoriis* is astrological in content, being concerned with the influence of the moon on critical days. Also one spurious work on astrology, the *Prognostica De Decubitu*, was sometimes attributed to Galen. These works are, however, entirely swamped by the massive number of writings produced by Galen which

I

make no allusion to astrology. Bouché-Leclercq in his chapter on ancient medical astrology makes no mention of Galen,[79] whilst Thorndike writes that, "In the ordinary run of Galen's pharmacy and therapeutics there is very little mention or observance of astrological medicine".[80] If sixteenth-century medicine was so influenced by Galen, we would expect, *prima facie*, that there would be opposition to astrological medicine from Galenic physicians. Yet Frances Yates and Keith Thomas[81] claim that astrological medicine was practised by all physicians and was to be found in all medical treatises.

Of course, as many writers have pointed out there *was* a great deal of medical astrology in the Renaissance.[82] This is not surprising if one considers the popularity of medical astrology in the mediaeval period with the introduction of the Arabic system of elections to complement judicial astrology,[83] and that the teaching of astrology to physicians in the universities occurred at this time.[84] However, in the Renaissance there were many medical treatises in which there is no mention of medical astrology; in some, in fact, medical astrology was explicitly condemned. In this section therefore I want to point out that there were some medical writers who did not use medical astrology and who were true to the overall tenor of Galen's teachings. As we shall see the problem for some of these writers was that when they condemned astrology they also had to repudiate Galen's own *De Diebus Decretoriis*.

From at least the time of Augustine,[85] astrology, especially judicial astrology, had come under attack, but at the end of the fifteenth century there appears to have been a renewed antipathy to astrology, paradoxically Ficino was at the same time giving respectability to magic and making it remarkably popular.[86] Indications of this new feeling of hostility to astrology can be found in the publication in 1496 of Pico della Mirandola's *Disputationes Adversus Astrologiam* and the condemnation of Simon de Phares at Lyons and then in Paris in 1494 for practising astrology.[87] Richard Lemay in a recent paper states that the moment when astrology and medicine in Paris were divorced came in 1537–1538, when the medical faculty proceeded in Parlement against an astrologer named Villanovus.[88] The action against Phares was taken by the theologians, but in the case of Villanovus it was the medical faculty which explicitly condemned astrology, and one could point to similar action taken by the medical faculty around this time against Jean Thibault.[89]

I want to turn now to some of the renaissance writers in order to make the case that astrology was not always linked to medicine, and also to consider how some of them dealt with Galen's *De Diebus Decretoriis*. I shall examine in some detail the writings of Manardi and Fuchs, and then look more generally at the topic.

Manardi helped in the editing of Pico's attack on astrology, and in his letters he showed a clear antipathy to the use of astrology in medicine. In his leter to Martinus Melerstadius he wrote against astrological explanations of illness. He attacked an author called 'Simon' who "betakes himself to the common refuge of doctors as if it were to a harbour or a protecting god, when he claims that this disease (syphilis) comes about by an occult property which emanates from celestrial bodies".[90] Manardi then went on to say that diseases:

> ... do not have their origin in the sky apart from, as it were, a universal cause as Io. Pico, the splendour and glory of our age has proved by many arguments in that superhuman work against astrologers, which we have recalled from the darkness to the light by great efforts.[91]

Given this dislike of astrology, Manardi was concerned to minimise the effect of those passages in the standard medical literature which could be taken as supporting astrology. For instance, he wrote in the same letter that many references to the influence of the sky should be read as the influence of the air. He quoted Vergil and Galen's commentary on the first book of the *Epidemics*, as authorities for the view that 'sky' should be taken to mean 'air'.[92] Manardi continued and again used the authority of Galen to say, "For as I have pointed out above, that exposition of Galen wholly convinces me in thinking that we do not read a word about judicial astrology in Hippocrates".[93]

When, however, Manardi came to the awkward fact that Galen himself in *De Diebus Decretoriis* favoured astrology he could not argue about the interpretation of words. His tactic was to state that Galen wrote not as a physician but as an astrologer.[94] Furthermore, Galen had written in *De Diebus Decretoriis* about the length of the moon's phases in a way which went counter to established opinion. Manardi was, therefore, able to write concerning the truth of Galen's teaching that the stars and especially the sun and moon controlled the critical days:

> Otherwise if (those things) are true which he wrote in his book about critical days they rather detract from any belief in to-day's astrology than promote it, since he believed that the motion of the moon is different from what it is to-day. Therefore if he recognised the true motion of the moon the astrology which is practised to-day which follows another theory of the motion of the moon is false: but if not, it necessarily follows that his system of critical days falls to the ground, because it rests on no foundation and base.[95]

In his well known letter to Castellano,[96] Manardi wrote at greater length against the use of astrology in medicine. His arguments were essentially similar to those mentioned above. He tried to show that neither

GALEN: PROBLEMS AND PROSPECTS

Hippocrates, Plato nor Aristotle approved of astrology. It was especially important to Manardi that Hippocrates was shown not to be in favour of astrology, because then Manardi could oppose Galen as astrologer with Hippocrates. Manardi wrote that the Hippocratic *Airs, Waters and Places* "is seen to favour astrology most", but he explained:

> He (Hippocrates) says that the risings and settings of the dog star, Arcturus, the Pleiades, and the solstices and the equinoxes should be taken into consideration by a doctor for no other purpose than to discover through them the changes of seasons in harmony with which he says that mens stomachs are changed.[97]

Having defused Hippocrates and discussed Aristotle and Plato Manardi turned to Galen. He was faced with the difficult position of supporting Galen and yet also being against astrology. So he devoted much space to his discussion of *De Diebus Decretoriis*, for as he wrote, "the authority of Galen himself counts far more with me who in his book about critical days, a book which is certainly his, is known openly to have supported the delirium of astrologers".[98]

Much of Manardi's discussion is taken up with a technical attack upon Galen's enumeration of critical days. Setting Hippocrates against Galen, he wrote that Galen's system of critical days was abhorrent to the teaching of Hippocrates[99] and he also stated that "The more therefore we turn to astrology the more we diverge from Hippocrates".[100] To condemn Galen, Manardi thus turned to the older (and purer?) authority of Hippocrates, having first made sure that the latter could not be accused of astrological leanings. Manardi concluded his discussion with an outright rejection of Galen as an astrologer:

> These and many other factors bring me to depart from Galen in this respect and not only form him, but from all men who seek to foul and to contaminate the glorious and most pure art of medicine.[101]

Leonhard Fuchs in his *Methodus Seu Ratio Compendaria Cognoscendi Veram Solidamque Medicinam* also came out against medical astrology. However, unlike Manardi, Fuchs seemed to agree with Galen's description of the length of the periods between critical days. He wrote that experience and Hippocrates concur with Galen's account.[102] He minimised the astrological component in Galen by claiming that Galen's discovery of critical days was based far more upon experience than upon his theory of the course of the moon. Fuchs stated that "therefore (*sic*) Hippocrates by his observation and experience deserves to be given credibility and we should not lend our ears to the vain fabrications of astrologers". Fuchs went on to denounce the astrologers and wrote that students of medicine should guard themselves from those who strive with the superstitution of astrology to contaminate and foul our most distinguished and pure art".[103]

Unlike Manardi, Fuchs did not explicitly condemn Galen for his astrology, but, by writing that Galen gave less weight to his theory of the moon's course than to observation, Fuchs mitigated the case against Galen. The prominence of Hippocrates, experience and the condemnation of astrology in Fuchs' discussion make it clear that Fuchs disagreed with Galen. Perhaps his regard for Galen prevented his coming out in open opposition.

Writers who wrote on the general question of astrology sometimes discussed Galen's *De Diebus Decretoriis*. Thomas Erastus in his anti-astrological work *De Astrologia* (1580) wrote that Galen was not an astrologer though in his *De Diebus Decretoriis* he could be seen as writing in the role of astrologer or philosopher.[104] The reason for Erastus' interest in Galen was that he felt that Galen's authority could be used by astrologers to support astrology.[105] This in fact, was what the astrologer Thomas Bodier did in his *De Ratione et Usu Dierum Criticorum* (1555) where he cited the spurious Galenic *De decubitu* and Galen's *De Diebus Decretoriis* as well as the *Methodus Medendi* in support of the need for astrology in medicine.[106]

I want now to move away from discussing the way in which renaissance writers dealt with Galen the astrologer, and to look very briefly at the general issue of astrology and medicine. A good example of a university teach of medicine is Montanus. Montanus, unlike Manardi and Fuchs, did not condemn astrology, but the practice of astrology in the form of judicial astrology and in the making of elections is markedly absent from his work. In neither the *Opuscula* nor the *Medicina Universa* editions of his writings have I found any specific teaching of medical astrology. However, Montanus did recognise the influence of the heavens. In his chapter on the causes of mixture Montanus cited Aristotle's *De Generatione et Corruptione* on the influence of the heavens, and also Galen's *De Diebus Decretoriis* where the Sun is entitled King and the Moon is called Queen. Montanus wrote that the sun is the fountain of heat and efficient cause (and male) whilst the Moon is Queen of the humours and thus the material cause (and female). He also described the effects of the planets – Mars dominating and making men angry and so forth.[107] Montanus, therefore, was not against astrology and in his *Consultationes* he referred to the "most skilled astrologers".[108] However, he did not practise or teach medical astrology. A similar attitude of general acceptance but not of practise can be found in the writings of many others, such as those of the late renaissance Galenist Andreas Laurentius.[109]

I

Perhaps Montanus did not write about medical astrology because he felt it was a discipline different from his own, though the medical astrologers would have denied they were merely a complement to medicine. However, I believe that in the Renaissance medicine and astrology did move away from each other. If this is the case it represents a move towards the general tenor of Galen's writings and constitutes a great change in the formal teaching of medicine. That medical astrology continued is clear from the many works on the subject, but it certainly was not an inseparable part of medicine in the Renaissance.

V

Sanctorius Sanctorius

In the work of Sanctorius Sanctorius (1561–1636), sometime professor of the theory of medicine at Padua, can be found some of the themes that have been discussed so far. He stands at the end of our period and though favourable to Galen he was by no means uncritical of him. He also had some originality of mind and he unconsciously prefigures some of the new trends in seventeenth century science. Although neither he nor his fellow Paduan physicians knew it, Sanctorius stood at the moment before the Aristotelian-Galenic picture of the world and body disappeared;[110] and, in what we can see as an end point of time, we can note how some of the debates of the Renaissance concluded for a Galenist.

Sanctorius gave the customary lectures on Galen's *Ars Parva*, on Avicenna's *Canon* and on the *Aphorisms* of Hippocrates. He published these lectures as the *Commentaria in Artem Medicinalem Galeni* (1612), the *Commentaria in Primam Fen Primi Libri Canonis Avicennae* (1625) and the *Commentaria in Primam Sectionem Aphorismorum Hypocratis* (1629) respectively. He also wrote the *Methodi Vitandorum Errorum Omnium Qui in Arte Medica Contingunt* (1603) a work concerned with applying universals to particulars by means of signs. The most famous work of Sanctorius was his *Ars de Statica Medicina* published in Venice in 1614 which has been viewed as an early example of the introduction of quantification into medicine. However, the pre-eminence of the *Statica* becomes less when it is realised that, as various writers have pointed out,[111] Sanctorius' quantitative experiments in the *Statica* and his measuring instruments such as his thermometer and his pulsilogium were developed by him in order to have greater certainty in the practice of Galenic medicine rather than to challenge Galen.

Sanctorius' attitude to the authority of Galen was ambiguous. He agreed that the renaissance anatomists had successfully contradicted Galen. On the question of whether the cerebellum or the cerebrum is harder he wrote in his Commentary on the *Ars Parva*:

> Galen teaches in book 9 of *De Usu Partium* that the cerebellum is harder than the cerebrum and, moreover, that the nerves originating from the cerebellum are harder, which appears false since proper inspection teaches the contrary. Furthermore, the anatomists Vesalius, Columbus and many others bear witness that the cerebellum is not harder than the cerebrum; we have more than once confirmed from Galen and Aristotle that experience and the senses should always be believed more than authorities.[112]

Sanctorius is here being true to the teachings of Aristotle and Galen concerning the value of the senses and at the same time he is taking some of the sting away from the anatomists' challenge to Galen. Again, when together "with our anatomists" he contradicts Galen on the position of the stomach he lessens the force of the criticism by writing that Galen has a proper excuse since he wrote in chapter two of *Anatomical Procedures* that he had seen only two imperfect cadavers.[113]

In the *Methodi Vitandorum Errorum* Sanctorius pointed out some of Galen's anatomical errors, praised Vesalius, and wrote that the attack by Sylvius on Vesalius had been completely unjustified.[114] There is no doubt that Sanctorius accepted the achievement of the anatomists and it was they who give him confidence in trusting to reason and the senses more than the authorities – though he did also argue from 'experience, reason and Galen'.[115] However, Sanctorius was at pains to point out that the anatomists were following the teaching of Galen in trusting to observation,[116] and that Galen was handicapped in his supply of anatomical material.

On matters of physiology Sanctorius defended Galen more strongly. He was against the Aristotelian opinion that the veins originated in the heart and not in the liver. Vesalius had given weight to the Aristotelian teaching and Argenterius had used it, together with the anatomical doubts concerning the existence of the *rete mirabile*, to argue against the natural and animal spirits and to posit instead a single spirit coming from the heart. Sanctorius stated his belief that the heart is the source of some heat but not of all heat.[117] However he was faced with Aristotle's claim that the heart was the principle of the arteries and of the veins and therefore the heat of the blood came from the heart and not the liver. Sanctorius continued:

> Averroes and all the Peripatetics keep the same opinion. Moreover Peter of Abano and Plusquamcommentator (Torrigiano dei Torrigiani) and now Vesalius the most expert of the anatomists of our present time constantly state

that the veins originate from the heart. And therefore the heat of the blood will proceed from the heart and consequently the liver in no way heats the whole (body).

Sanctorius responded:

> The reply of all physicians is that the vena cava and all the rest lead the source (of heat) from the liver, the physicians and all anatomists apart from Vesalius think likewise.[118]

Having thus expressed the issue in the traditional form as a dispute between the philosophers and physicians, Sanctorius then supported his own view with the testimony of Hippocrates and Galen. However, although both of these helped his argument, Sanctorius clearly felt that experience was the deciding factor. In the *Methodi Vitandorum Errorum* he wrote that in the present day the insanity grows stronger in many universities of Europe of trusting more in Aristotle, Galen and Hippocrates than in one's own senses. As an example of this tendency Sanctorius cited the Aristotelian head of a university (Gymnasiarcha) who believed what Aristotle said concerning the origin of the veins rather than in autopsy and his own senses.[119] Clearly Sanctorius here wanted to defend a Galenic anatomical statement upon which the 'Galenic' doctrine of the three spirits depended. In order to do this, Sanctorius appealed not to authority but to eye-sight observation, the newly emphasised criterion of the anatomists.

From Sanctorius' references to the Peripatetics it is clear that he felt he belonged to the rival camp of the physicians or Galenists. Although he had read Zabarella and was sympathetic to some of his teaching, when he came to another Aristotelian, Argenterius, his judgement was clear: Argenterius could not understand the secrets of Galen, and he had fallen into six hundred errors in his commentary on the *Ars Parva*.[120]

Sanctorius' attack on Argenterius for positing a single spirit flowing from the heart shows how he tried to defend Galen. Again anatomy entered the argument. Argenterius had used the non-existence of the *rete mirabile* to deny the animal spirits.[121] In reply, Sanctorius wrote that Argenterius could not have seen for himself the anatomy of the human brain, for in it the retiform plexus is conspicuous.[122] Argenterius had asked why, if net-like structures are necessary for the generation of spirits, there are no such nets in the heart where the vital spirits are generated.[123] Sanctorius in response gave the various opinions concerning the place where the vital spirits were, in fact, generated. When he reached Ulmus he noted that Ulmus had postulated a plexus for the generation of vital spirits (the splenic arteries) and felt able to conclude:

Behold that at least from the teachings of Ulmus a plexus is given for the generation of the vital spirits, and therefore the argument of Argenterius is forsaken by all men.[124]

Despite Sanctorius' loudly proclaimed belief in the evidence of his senses it is clear that authority still counted a lot for him especially on matters of theory and function. The irony is that he used a theory of Ulmus' which had been developed against Galen's idea of the function of the spleen.[125] However, Sanctorius' desire to defend Galen was unambiguous, and so was his recourse to authority in matters of theory.

I would like now to turn to Sanctorius' attitude to medical method. In his Commentary on the *Ars Parva* he again placed himself amongst the physicians when he wrote in defence of Galen that definition was a distinct and separate order, and that Zabarella was wrong to dismiss the order of definition.[126] However, Sanctorius appears to have agreed with Zabarella that the order of resolution could not be anything more than a way of teaching an art. Sanctorius wrote in support of Zabarella that the end from which the order of resolution begins is not a principle of a thing but is our end and is a mental or ideal concept.[127] The implication here is that the order of resolution is concerned only with teaching, and not with finding the principles of health as Montanus would have wanted. Therefore, on this substantial issue Sanctorius was in agreement with the Peripatetics, and his agreement reflects their victory.

In more general terms, for a man who was to be famed for his quantitative experiments and for his instruments, and who praised the value of observation, Sanctorius was surprisingly suspicious of the logical worth of experience.

Here he was influenced by Galen's dislike of the empirical school. In the *Methodi Vitandorum Errorum* Sanctorius attacked present-day empiricists who, if a remedy worked two or three times, then gave it to everyone with injurious results.[128]

In the following chapter, Sanctorius argued that one could not logically reach any conclusion from experience:

Further, when experience shall be collected from particulars, it is not conclusive because out of pure particulars nothing follows. And do not object that experience is not collected from two particulars but from many; because we reply that if you gather it from a thousand, you are not able to infer a universal conclusion or rather if you induce through a thousand thousand, still you cannot derive a universal conclusion, since each species of the universal contains in itself infinite particulars.[129]

He considered the objection to his view. He wrote that there was a great doubt concerning his conclusions about induction, for by the authority of

I

Aristotle when a particular remains in the memory, then it begins first to be a universal in the mind, but as particulars are conserved in the memory by virtue of induction or experience, therefore induction or experience may produce universality. Further, experiences are seen to produce recognition of causes and demonstration 'quia', and this is because recognition of causes is a universal, therefore experiences lead to a universal, and this is confirmed by many examples. The two examples given by Sanctorius are that guaiacum is the cause of the cure of syphilis, and rhubarb of bile.[130] Sanctorius replied that when the particular in the memory begins to be a universal in the mind this is because in every particular there is included its total universal nature, and the intellect separates a universal from singulars by its own proper light[131] and not by induction and experience. Sanctorius maintained, furthermore, that the propositions concerning the cure of syphilis and of bile were indefinite and not universal propositions: only some guaiacum cured syphilis, and only some with syphilis were cured by guaiacum.[132] Sanctorius took the consequences of his view of the limitation of experience to their logical conclusion. He wrote:

> Secondly, while they say that experience, since it proceeds from effects to causes, is demonstration, *a posteriori* concerning the reason for the way things are, so it produces a universal. We reply that experience does not proceed from effects to causes, but from effects to particular and indefinite subjects.[133]

Sanctorius clearly was not going to be the man to produce a method for the new science of the seventeenth century with its ideology of deriving causes from effects (neglecting Descartes for the moment).

In Sanctorius' Commentary on the *Ars Parva* the influence of Galen on his views concerning method is obvious. Sanctorius wrote:

> Doubt arises as to why Galen has written that medicine is not about particulars, for it is seen that the physician is concerned with particulars ...
>
> It is replied that the doctor in no way treats or cures particulars as such...[134]

Sanctorius cited various passages in Galen which held that: "the expulsion of disease is indicated by a specific condition; therefore what is cured is specific and not singular".[135] Sanctorius went on to write that a study of a particular case does not of itself enable the doctor to cure it; reference must also be made to universals. If in fact a cure was effected, and this was solely derived from the particulars, then medicine would be laughable. Sanctorius was probably thinking of the empiricists in this context. He wrote:

> Moreover, if medicine cures singular cases (only) as they are singular cases, then

vain is the art ... because art and all intellectual dispositions are universal and not particular as Aristotle teaches ... because nothing is contained in particulars ... if particulars are cured, their indications do not show us the remedies because the progress from particular to particular is not allowable; therefore the medical art is altogether vain and ridiculous (because the cure would be by chance)[136]

Sanctorius argued that neither by induction or particulars nor from a single particular can we make the connection between the indications given to the doctor in a particular case and the cure itself.[137] Sanctorius concluded from Galen:

Therefore they (particulars) are most vain indications and conclude nothing. Hence Galen 9. *Methodi* cap 6, says, in universals is the method of healing, in particulars, in fact, only the method of practice. We gather therefore that medicine is centred around universals and not particulars.[138]

There was a connection for Sanctorius between effects and universals but this could not be reduced to a method. In the *Methodi Vitandorum Errorum* in a passage reminiscent of Montanus, Sanctorius did find experience useful:

We do not deny, however, that induction or experiments (experimenta) can contribute towards knowing a universal; because as Boethius said in (his commentary on Aristotle's) *Categories*, experience is the collection of examples, and after the collection, the intellect is urged on by its own light to separate the natural universals from the individual, for the whole universal nature is in any individual.[139]

Sanctorius also repeated the opinion of Averroes that induction infers the recognition of universals from accidents because the collection of many examples frequently places before the intellect a universal which is included in every particular.[140] Sanctorius is arguing about the suggestive power of experience. There is however no infallible way or method from experience to universals. The mind itself must grasp the reality out of the appearances.

Galen's attacks on the empirical school and the obvious dangers of empiricism in the practice of medicine lay behind Sanctorius' paradoxical distrust of experience. Although elsewhere he praises the use of the senses, it is clear that for a Galenic physician like Sanctorius there was no method of proceeding from effects to causes, and this may help to explain the attitude of some of the medical writers on method.

As for astrology, Sanctorius was against it. At least he was against judicial astrology. Like Montanus he did allow that the heavens influenced happenings down on earth but unlike Montanus he was explicitly hostile to astrology. Sanctorius wrote that those who deny judicial astrology do not deny that 'the heaven acts down here'. The voice of wisdom is unanimous that the heaven through innumerable motions introduces into this lower world various impressions and various degrees of termperaments. However, he added that these influences are indescribable, inexplicable and altogether imperceptible by the human intellect.[141] Sanctorius' position is similar to that of Augustine, accepting the principle of the influence of the heavens, but not the practice of judicial astrology. In fact, he damned judicial astrology, calling it ridiculous and vain.[142]

When Sanctorius came to Galen's *De Diebus Decretoriis* he claimed that Galen was not being serious. He stated that Galen always praised astronomy and not astrology and that the third book of *De Diebus Decretroiis* was written at the behest of inquisitive men. Sanctorius felt able to say that Galen did not follow such vanities by quoting Galen's apparent deprecation of the worth of the third book and his statement that it was written unwillingly at the request of certain friends.[143] Here, certainly, Sanctorius felt the need to excuse Galen and to lessen the impact of the book three of *De Diebus Decretoriis*. One work of Galen's, however, was not sufficient, as we have seen, to prevent some medical writers from condemning the practice of astrology. Even for the followers of Galen, Galen's authority was not sacrosanct.

Finally, in this review of where Galenism had got in the early seventeenth century we can note Sanctorius' attempt to reduce occult qualities to three-dimensionality.[144] As Pagel[145] has noted, the Galenists were far more materialistic and reductionist than Aristotelians like Harvey who could write that there was an inherent spirit in semen and blood "acting superiorly to the powers of the elements".[146] In his reduction of occult forces and properties to three-dimensionality Sanctorius again prefigured, unconsciously, the mood of the new science of the seventeenth century. Even in its old age Galenism could still be innovative.

I would like to thank Dr Nick Fisher, Dr George Molland, Mr Tom Pearce and Dr Charles Schmitt for their help in preparing this paper and in particular I thank Dr Walter Pagel and Dr Andrew Cunningham who as always freely gave their advice and knowledge.

Footnotes

1. Owsei Temkin, *Galenism*.
2. R. J. Durling, *Census*; R. J. Durling, 'Linacre and Medical Humanism' in F. Maddison, M. Pelling, C. Webster, eds, *Essays*, p.76–106.
3. See, for instance, M. Boas, *The Scientific Renaissance 1450–1630*, London 1962.
4. R. J. Durling, *Census*, p.243.
5. Io. Manardus, *Epistolarum Medicinalium lib. duodeviginti* ..., Basle 1535, p.13.
6. The quotation is taken from L. R. Lind's translation of N. Massa, *Anatomiae Liber Introductorius*, Venice 1536 in L. R. Lind, *Pre-Vesalian Anatomy*, Philadelphia 1975, p.175.
7. On the conservatism of university medical curricula see V. Nutton, *John Caius*, p.373–391.
8. See Temkin, *Galenism*, p.69.
9. For a medieval attack by an Aristotelian on Galen's theory of generation see M. A. Hewson, *Giles of Rome and the Medieval Theory of Conception*, London 1975. Linda Deer is currently working on the renaissance version of the Aristotelian-Galenic debate on generation.
10. Manardus, *Epist.Med.*, p.294.
11. See A. Vesalius, *De Humani Corporis Fabrica*, Basle 1543, Preface, p*2r. "Galenus post Hippocratem medicinae princeps".
12. L. Fuchs, *Methodus*, p.4.
13. Ibid., p.3.
14. Ibid., p.3.
15. Ibid., p.4.
16. See W. F. Edwards, *Leoniceno*, p.291.
17. R. Antonioli, *Rabelais et la Médecine*, Geneva 1976, p.215.
18. Temkin, *Galenism*, p.126–7, n.82. See also B. P. Copenhaver, *Symphorien Champier and the Reception of the Occultist Tradition in Renaissance France*, The Hague 1978.
19. S. Champier, *Practica Nova in Medicina*, Lyons 1517.
20. Walter Pagel, 'Medical Humanism – A Historical Necessity in the Era of the Renaissance' in Maddison, Pelling and Webster, *Essays*, p.381.
21. W. Pagel and P. Rattansi, 'Vesalius and Paracelsus', *Med.Hist.* 8, 1964, p.323–326. Pagel and Rattansi make it clear that 'prisca' in this context does not have the connotations of 'prisca' in the Hermetic tradition.
22. Pagel, *Medical Humanism*, p.380.
23. This historical truism has been challenged by Neal W. Gilbert, 'A letter of Giovanni Dondi Dal'Orologio To Fra' Guglielmo Centueri: A Fourteenth Century Episode in the Quarrel of the Ancients and Moderns', *Viator* 8, 1977, p.299–346. Gilbert writes, 'The Quarrel of the Ancients and Moderns had its beginnings, for modern Europe at least, in the rich soil of fourteenth century Italy: it did not wait for the achievements of seventeenth-century science to break out.' (p.299).
24. W. Pagel, *William Harvey's Biological Ideas*, Basle and New York 1967.
25. Temkin, *Galenism*, ch.4.
26. Jacques Roger, *Les Sciences De La Vie Dans La Pensée Française Du XVIIIe Siècle*, ed.2, Paris 1971, ch.2.
27. Jerome Bylebyl, 'Nutrition, Quantification and Circulation', *BHM* 51, 1977, p.369–385.
28. Temkin, *Galenism*, p.150.
29. See, for example, Charles Singer, *A Short History of Anatomy and Physiology from the Greeks to Harvey*, New York 1957, p.97 and p.132.

I

[30] Galen, *Galen on the Usefulness of the Parts of the Body*, tr. M. T. May, Ithaca, New York 1968, p.61 and p.430-433.
[31] Vesalius, *Fabrica*, p.642. I have used the translation of C. Singer, *Vesalius On the Human Brain*, London 1952, p.58.
[32] Ibid., p.622-623 (Singer p.3).
[33] Realdo Colombo, *De Re Anatomica*, Venice 1559, p.191.
[34] Ibid., p.191.
[35] Archangelo Piccolomini, *Anatomicae Praelectiones ...*, Rome 1586, p.253.
[36] Ibid., p.253.
[37] Andreas Laurentius, *Historia Anatomica Humani Corporis*, Frankfurt 1599, p.390.
[38] Ibid., p.391.
[39] Helkiah Crooke, Μικροκοσμογραφια, *A Description of the Body of Man. Together with the Controversies Thereto Belonging Collected and Translated out of All the Best Authors of Anatomy, Especially out of Caspar Bauhinus and Andreas Laurentius*, London 1615, p.516.
[40] Caspar Bauhin, *Theatrum Anatomicum*, Frankfurt 1605, p.609. Translation from Crooke, ibid., p.470.
[41] W. Harvey, *The Anatomical Lectures of William Harvey*, ed. G. Whitteridge, Edinburgh and London, p.335-337.
[42] The term 'academic anatomy' is taken from R. K. French, *Anatomical Education in a Scottish University, 1620*, Edinburgh 1974. I have used the Aberdeen, Equipress, 1975 edition p.XVI-XIX. See also A. Wear, *The Spleen*, p.56. Of course there was academic anatomy before the sixteenth century but the author's viewpoint was usually less defined and obtrusive than in the sixteenth century.
[43] N. W. Gilbert, *Renaissance Concepts of Method*, New York 1960, p.102-103; this is an essential work for any study of renaissance discussions of method. W. P. D. Wightman, 'Quid Sit Methodus? Method in Sixteenth Century Teaching and Discovery', *JHM*, 19, 1964, p.367-369. A. Wear, *Contingency and Logic in Renaissance Anatomy and Physiology*, Unpublished London Ph.D. thesis, 1973, ch.6, and Edwards, *Leoniceno*.
[44] Edwards, *Leoniceno*, p.298.
[45] Ibid., p.300.
[46] Champier, *Practica*, fol.IIIv-VIv.
[47] Fuchs, *Methodus*, p.17, title to ch.VII.
[48] The Galenic origin of these categories is very problematic. See L. J. Rather, 'The six things non-natural'. A note on the origins and fate of a doctrine and a phrase', *Clio Medica* 3, 1968, p.333-347. S. Jarcho, 'Galen's six non-naturals: A bibliographic note and translation', *BHM* 44, 1970, p.372-377: J. Bylebyl, 'Galen on the non-natural causes of variation in the pulse', *BHM* 44, 1970, p.482-485.
[49] L. Fuchs, *Institutionum Medicinae*, I have used the Basle 1594 edition, p.25-33. Nutton, *John Caius*, has drawn attention to the general growth of renaissance interest in medical method. D. G. Bates, 'Sydenham and the Medical Meaning of Method', *BHM* 51, 1977, p.324-338; discusses the multiplicity of meaning of the term 'method', which reached beyond the philosophical to the therapeutic.
[50] J. B. Montanus, *Medicina Universa*, Frankfurt 1587.
[51] On Compendia see: Gilbert, *Renaissance Concepts*, p.112-115. W. S. Howell, *Logic and Rhetoric in England, 1500-1700*, New York 1956. On Ramus and the structuring and methodising of knowledge see: W. J. Ong, *Ramus' Method and the Decay of Dialogue*, Cambridge, Mass. 1958.
[52] Quoted by Luke Demaitre, 'Scholasticism in Compendia of Practical Medicine,

GALEN IN THE RENAISSANCE

1250-1450', *Manuscripta* 20, 1976, p.84 from Arnold of Villanova, *De Consideratione Operis Medicinae* in *Opera*, Lyons 1509, fol.90v.

[53] Bates, *Sydenham*, p.326. See also K. J. Höltgen, 'Synoptische Tabellen in der Medizinischen Literatur und die Logik Agricolas und Ramus', *AGM* 49, 1965, p.371-390, cited by Bates.

[54] Avicenna held in the opening chapter of the *Canon* that medicine consisted of practical and theoretical knowledge, he did not use the term 'art'. In the translation of Gerard of Cremona (standard for the Renaissance) the terms used are *scientia* for knowledge and *theorica* and *practica* for theory and practice. See Avicenna, *Canon Medicinae*, Venice 1595, Liber Primus, Fen Prima, Doctri. Prima, p.6.

[55] N. Leoniceno, *Nicolai Leoniceni Vicentini De Tribus Doctrinis Ordinatis ...*, in *Opuscula*, p.73r-73v.

[56] Ibid., p.73v.

[57] See for instance Aristotle, *Met.* 981^b-982^a, 982^{a}20-25, 982^{b}15-25.

[58] See J. H. Randall, Jr., *Padua*, Padua 1961.

[59] Aristotle, *Nic.Eth.* Book III, tr. J. L. Ackrill, *Aristotle's Ethics*, London 1973, p.81-82 (1112^{b}13-16, 1112^{b}31-1113^{a}2).

[60] Leoniceno, *Opuscula*, p.81v.

[61] Ibid., p.69v.

[62] Ibid., p.82v.

[63] J. B. Montanus, *In Artem Parvam Galeni Explanationes*, Venice 1554, p.42r-42v.

[64] Wightman, *Method*, p.373.

"After reading Da Monte's eight folio pages addressed to a mature audience ... I feel more than a little sympathy for these erring professors (who confused the 'instruments' of teaching with the 'orders'), as I think did John Caius".

[65] Bates, *Sydenham*, p.327.

"It does seem, though, that Renaissance debates over method were often a mere wrangling over logical procedure, with an inescapable stamp of the scholasticism against which the seventeenth century approach to scientific method was a reaction".

[66] See especially the passages in the *Phaedrus* which describe the principles of definition and division necessary in rhetoric, the description of what it is to have real understanding in the art of medicine, and the necessity of knowing the whole (nature of the body) by means of method. (*Phaedrus* 265d-271b). Note that the examples used by Plato relating to method concern the 'arts' of rhetoric and medicine rather than certain knowledge (in fact the distinction is not made in this way by Plato).

[67] The problems are made worse for the renaissance writers as *techne-episteme* are not equivalent to *ars-scientia*. And of course an art did have its own procedure.

[68] M. Polanyi, *Personal Knowledge*, London 1958, and *The Tacit Dimension*, New York 1966.

[69] Gilbert, *Renaissance concepts*, p.102.

[70] See below, note 74.

[71] Montanus, *Methodus Universalis Signorum* in *Opuscula*, Basle 1558, p.112.

[72] Ibid., p.112.

[73] Ibid., p.112.

[74] L. Jardine, *Francis Bacon, Discovery and the Art of Discourse*, Cambridge 1974, p.40.

[75] Randall, *Padua*, note 58.

[76] Zabarella, *De Methodis* in *Opera Logica*, Lyons 1587, p.56. Here Zabarella stated that method proceeded from the known to the unknown whilst order merely disposed or set out knowledge which was already known. On Zabarella see A. Poppi, *La Dottrina Della Scienze In Giacomo Zabarella*, Padua 1962.

[77] Fuchs, *Institutions*, p.30.

I

[78] Bates, *Sydenham.*

[79] A. Bouché - Leclercq, *L'Astrologie Grecque,* Paris 1899, ch.15.

[80] L. Thorndike, *History,* p.178.

[81] F. Yates, *Giordano Bruno and the Hermetic Tradition,* London 1964, p.62: "It was absolutely inevitable that a medical treatise of the Middle Ages or Renaissance should make use of astrological presuppositions universally taken for granted". K. Thomas, *Religion and the Decline of Magic,* London 1973, p.339. "Different signs of the zodiac were thought to rule ever different parts of the body, and a proper election of times had to be made for administering medicine, letting blood or carrying out surgical procedures. This was generally recognised by all sixteenth century physicians".

[82] See for example: D. C. Allen, *The Star-Crossed Renaissance,* Durham, North Carolina 1941, Appendix. C. Camden, 'Elizabethan Astrological Medicine', *Annals of Medical History* 2, 1930, p.217-227. K. Sudhoff, *Iatromathematiker vornehmlich im 15 und 16. Jahrhundert* (Abhandlungen zur Geschichte der Medizin) Breslau 1902. A. Chapman 'Astrological Medicine' in C. Webster (ed.), *Health, medicine and mortality in the sixteenth century,* Cambridge 1979, p.275-300.

[83] T. O. Wedel, *The Medieval Attitude Toward Astrology,* Archon Books 1968, p.53-55.

[84] Richard Lemay, *Astronomy,* p.206-209.

[85] Augustine, *City of God* Book 5, chps. 1-10. Also note other patristic attacks upon astrology - Wedel, *Astrology,* p.15-20.

[86] On the popularity of magic and on Ficino see E. Garin, *Medioevo e Rinascimento,* Florence 1954. D. P. Walker, *Spiritual and Demonic Magic from Ficino to Campanella,* London 1958.

[87] For Phares, see Thorndike, *History,* ch.62.

[88] Lemay, *Astronomy,* p.215-217, unaware that this is Michael Servetus.

[89] C. D. O'Malley, *Michael Servetus. A Translation of his Geographical, Medical and Astrological Writing with Introduction and Notes,* Philadelphia 1953, p.169-171.

[90] Manardi, *Epist.Med.,* p.16.

[91] Ibid., p.16.

[92] Ibid., p.18.

[93] Ibid., p.19.

[94] Ibid., p.19.

[95] Ibid., p.19.

[96] See the arguments put forward against the opinions contained in Manardi's letter by G. A. Magini, *De Astrologica Ratione, ac usu dierum criticorum,* Venice 1607.

[97] Manardi, *Epist.Med.,* p.341.

[98] Ibid., p.343.

[99] Ibid., p.345.

[100] Ibid., p.348.

[101] Ibid., p.348.

[102] Fuchs, *Methodus,* p.200v.

[103] Ibid., p.200v-201r.

[104] T. Erastus, *De Astrologia Divinatrice Epistolae D. Thomae Erasti,* Basle 1580, p.41 and p.85.

[105] Ibid., p.17.

[106] T. Bodier, *De Ratione et Usu Dierum Criticorum,* Paris 1555, p.5r-5v.

[107] Montanus, *Medicina,* p.108-110.

[108] J. B. Montanus, *Consultationes Medicae,* Basle 1572, p.1018.

[109] Laurentius, *Historia* Book I, ch.2.

[110] Although there were definite differences between Aristotelians and Galenists, their

GALEN IN THE RENAISSANCE

differences become minor when seen against the backcloth of the new seventeenth century approach to nature.

111 On Sanctorius see M. D. Grmek, *Istatski liječnik Santorio Santorio i njegovi aparati i instrumenti*, Zagreb 1952 (with an English summary): M. D. Grmek 'Reflections Sur Des Interpretations Mécanistes De La Vie Dans La Physiologie Du XVIIe Siècle', *Episteme* 1, 1967, p.17-30. Also Grmek's article on 'Santorio' in the *Dictionary of Scientific Biography*. H. Miessen, *Die Verdienste Sanctorii Sanctorii um die Einführung physikalischer Methoden in die Heilkunde*, Düsseldorf 1940. See also chapter 5 of my thesis and Temkin, *Galenism*, p.159-160.

112 S. Sanctorius, *Commentaria*, p.195.

113 Ibid., p.472.

114 S. Sanctorius, *Methodi*, p.80v.

115 Sanctorius, *Commentaria*, p.422.

116 Sanctorius, *Methodi* p.74v.

"Nec mihi obiijciant, quod omnino temerarium sit Galenum reijcere, quia respondemus ex propria Galeni sententia 6 de morb, vulg. comm. 2. citata: illos potius, qui magis credunt auctoribus, quam experientiae, et rationibus esse temerarios . . . "

117 Sanctorius, *Commentaria*, p.300.

118 Ibid., p.330-331.

119 Sanctorius, *Methodi*, p.74v.

120 Sanctorius, *Commentaria*, p.333.

121 J. Argenterius, *In Artem Medicinalem Galeni Commentarii Tres*, Mondovi 1566, p.64.

122 Sanctorius, *Commentaria*, p.182.

123 Argenterius, *In Artem medicinalem*, p.188.

124 Sanctorius, *Commentaria*, p.182.

125 See Wear, *The Spleen*, p.53-55.

126 Sanctorius, *Commentaria*, p.26 and p.28. On Zabarella and the order of definition see Edwards, *Leoniceno*, p.295.

127 Sanctorius, *Commentaria* p.25.

128 Sanctorius, *Methodi*, p.187r.

129 Ibid., p.188v.

130 Ibid., p.189r.

131 Ibid., p.189r.

132 Ibid., p.189v.

133 Ibid., p.189v.

134 Sanctorius, *Commentaria*, p.61-62.

135 Ibid., p.62.

". . . ex Galeno enim lib. de optima secta et primo ad Glauconem habetur, morborum expulsionem a specifico affectu indicare: ergo quod curatur est specificum, et non singulare".

136 Ibid., p.62.

137 Ibid., p.62.

138 Ibid., p.62.

139 Sanctorius, *Methodi*, p.189v-180r.

140 Ibid., p.190r.

141 S. Sanctorius, *Commentaria in Prima Fen primi libri Canonis Avicennae*, Venice 1626, p.73.

142 Ibid., p.75.

143 Ibid., p.79.

The passage reads: "Quo ad Galenum arbitramur semper laudasse astronomiam, et

I

non astrologiam. Dum vero tertio de diebus decretorijs agit de astrologia, Respondemus illum librum esse factum propter curiosos. Quod vero Galenus non sequatur illas vanitates, ipsemet eodem libro affirmat cap. 10. ubi habet hanc sententiam, 'laudo librum primum et secundum; ab hoc tertio vero tanquam de rebus a ratione alienis, omnes debent abstinere', additque, 'illum tertium librum invito scripsisse, idest, precibus quorundam amicorum', scilicet curiosum, non ut fidem aliquam his nugis, sed ut aliquid auribus stultorum daret, quorum numerus erat, sicuti modo, infinitus". For the passage in Galen see *De dieb. decret.* III.10:IX,934.

[144] See for example Sanctorius, *Methodi*, p.151v-162v. I hope that a paper I have written in which these matters are more extensively discussed will be published.

[145] W. Pagel, 'William Harvey Revisited', *History of Science* 8, 1969, p.21-22. Also Pagel, *Harvey's ... ideas*, p.251-255. That Galen was not a complete materialist is noted by D. Sennert, in his *Hypomnemata Physica* Frankfurt 1636, p.50, where he states that Galen believed poison acted by its 'whole substance' rather than by its constitutent elements.

[146] W. Harvey, *On Generation*, tr. R. Willis, London 1848, p.506.

NOTE

For expansion of footnotes see below:

D.G. Bates, 'Sydenham and the medical meaning of Method', *BHM* 51, 1977, p. 324–338.

R.J. Durling, 'A chronological census of Renaissance editions and translations of Galen', *JWCI* 24, 1961, p. 230–305.

W.F. Edwards, 'Leoniceno and humanist discussion of method', in *Philosophy and Humanism*, ed. E.P. Mahoney, Leiden 1976.

L. Fuchs, *Institutiones medicinae*, Basle 1594.

L. Fuchs, *Methodus seu ratio compendiaria cognoscendi veram solidamque medicinam*, Paris 1550.

N. Leoniceno, *De tribus doctrinis ordinatis*, in *Opuscula*, Basle 1532.

V. Nutton, 'John Caius and the Linacre tradition', *Med. hist.* 23, 1979, p. 373–391.

J.H. Randall, Jr., *The school of Padua and the emergence of modern science*, Padua 1961.

S. Sanctorius, *Commentaria in Artem medicinalem Galeni*, Lyons 1632.

S. Sanctorius, *Methodi vitandorum errorum qui in arte medica contingunt*, Venice 1603.

O. Temkin, *Galenism*, Ithaca, London 1973.

A. Wear, 'The spleen in the Renaissance anatomy', *Med. hist.* 21, 1977, p. 43–60.

II

Explorations in renaissance writings on the practice of medicine

Summary

In this chapter I discuss the general characteristics of a genre of renaissance medical writings which dealt with the practice of medicine (the *practica*). To begin with I trace how the *practica* changed over time and consider how humanistic values with their emphasis on classical purity of language and of source material altered the *practica* as did the needs of educationalists. At the same time I point out the continuation of a medieval tradition alongside the new renaissance products. I shall set out a case example drawn from the *practica*, that of vertigo. Most historians when discussing the nature of a particular type of medical literature concentrate on the general structure of the books in question and on their author's intentions as seen in prefaces and introductions and rarely look at the subject matter in any detail. I also begin with this approach but then, by looking at the topic of vertigo in detail, I show how the general conclusions regarding changes in the *practica* can be illustrated by a specific example. At the same time, the material on vertigo can be briefly analysed to discover how internal pathological processes taking place within the body were described by writers on practical medicine, and I hope to bring out the extent to which such causal accounts of illness based themselves on localized events taking place within the body rather than on a generalized imbalance of the humours. Finally, I touch upon some of the problems associated with fitting new explanations of disease into the methodical framework of Galenic medicine; and I point out how, although the application of method in medicine was suited to teaching Galenic medicine, it posed difficulties when innovation was envisaged. The chapter is exploratory and more concerned with sketching out and reporting findings in a largely unresearched area than producing an argument around a single issue.

119   *Explorations in renaissance writings*

Introduction to the renaissance practica

If a student or practitioner wanted to have information on the practical side of medicine – (diagnosis and treatment) he could use the writings of Hippocrates, Galen, Avicenna and other writers. However, in addition to these disparate sources, there was also available to him the frequently published (and presumably frequently used) *practica*. Yet with one notable exception[1] hardly anything has been written on the sixteenth century *practica*.

The *practica* were books used as primers for medical students and handbooks or 'vade mecums' for the practising physician. They followed the format of the medieval *practica* and taught 'particular' diseases in a head to toe order *a capite ad calcem* and they also dealt with the 'universal' diseases of fevers; in addition there might be separate sections on plague, arthritis, dislocations etc. The *practica* were related to university teaching in that the professors of the practice of medicine followed the same format in their lectures.[2]

The medieval *practica* continued to be available in the sixteenth century at the same time as renaissance writers were attempting to 'humanize' and reform them. They had dealt with the affections of the body in a reasonably brief manner, giving the causes (though not always) and the signs which would identify the disease and then detailing its treatment. The new renaissance *practica*, on the other hand, became increasingly verbose and concerned to define, divide and discuss their subject matter. It is not surprising therefore, that medieval *practica* continued to be printed in the renaissance (and also that a partial reaction set in later in the century deploring the concern with words and rhetoric). The *Praxis Medicinalis* of Arnald of Villanova (1240?–1311) was printed in 1585 and included his *Compendium Medicinae Practicae* which was also published separately in 1586[3]and in German in 1619. The *Practica* of Johannes Savonarola (1382–1462) was reprinted in 1559 and that of Marcus Gatinaria (d. 1496) in 1560.

The *De Medendis Humani Corporis Malis Enchiridion* or 'Vade Mecum' of Petrus Bayrus the personal physician to Charles III Duke of Savoy gives us a sense of how a renaissance editor might view his medieval material for it was edited and brought to publication in 1561 by the Swiss humanist physician Theodor Zwinger. It was frequently reissued in the following fifty years. Zwinger viewed Bayrus as a medieval writer though he had died in 1558, and he wrote, in typical humanist vein, that his language and mode of argument was not in keeping with the times. Yet, Zwinger found something of value in his author and wrote in his dedicatory letter:

He is barbarian I admit, but speaking in this barbarous manner he will be better understood than if he were forced to stammer in Latin, especially by those who can read without distaste Savonarola, Montagna, Gatinaria and the other writers of the same ilk. I am sending you this Medicina of Bayrus put together in twenty-four books, never before printed, with the odious repetitions of distinctions and tractates excised.[4]

For Zwinger the positive virtues of Bayrus lay in his attempt to join the dogmatic and empirical approaches together (a desideratum of any humanist and Galenist), though he did not know 'if the attempt was greater than its success'.[5] He also praised his method which consisted in setting forth 'shortly and succinctly as necessity seemed to demand the nature and essence of all diseases, the causes, signs, differences, prognostics'.[6] Method here was not the complex hydra of Montanus drawn from Galen's *Ars Parva* and the *Methodus Medendi* but was, in effect, the medieval way of writing a *practica*. Such a view of method was always possible in the renaissance since the word could be equated with brevity and a 'methodus' was often a synonym for a compendium. However, as we shall see Bayrus in practice was often so brief that Zwinger's hopeful advertisement that the nature, causes, signs of disease would be considered was misleading.

Another medieval *practica*, the *Rosa Anglica* of John of Gaddesden (c. 1280–1361) was first printed in 1492 and 1502 and reissued in 1595 by Phillip Schopfius. The *Rosa Anglica* was the exception to the rule of *a capite ad calcem* and Schopfius remedied this by putting the contents of the book into the traditional order. Schopfius felt that there was a market for the book and he wrote that a new printing was necessary as copies of the original printing were no longer available and people could not understand its abbreviated print.[7] His comments on the text itself show how he produced a compromise between humanistic values and the intrinsic usefulness of the original text. He wrote that he corrected the Latin 'lest men of more polished literary tastes should be detracted from reading it'. However, he emphasized that 'we have left unchanged some technical words and formulae although they are rather rough, lest we should lose truth in our zeal for elegance of language or lest we should interpret the author's intention less correctly'.[8] The ultimate justification of the *Rosa Anglica* for Schopfius was based on the claim that the medieval writers were better than the modern ones:

Now to come to the age immediately preceding our own I believe that there is no-one so unjust or bold as to prefer the writings of the moderns of our time to the memorials of those most excellent physicians I mean Valescus, Arnaldus de Villanovus and John the Englishman seeing that these men in treating diseases methodically, in prescribing remedies and setting out and solving questions applied such care, labour and diligence as no other applied or will apply.[9]

This inversion of the normal renaissance view of things•might be explained by the date of the publication – 1595. The first flourish of the renaissance was coming to an end, even for science and medicine which had been late starters. Elegance of language was becoming less important (see also the attack on humanistic rhetoric by the later editors of Avicenna's *Canon* which is discussed by Nancy Siraisi) whilst that of content, of attention to the 'things themselves' was increasing. Schopfius wrote:

> There are many who are unable to read the writings of the medical barbarians who lived in an earlier age because these writings are very far from the purity and elegance of the Latin tongue and because they produce disgust and nausea to students of that tongue. This is true but it is not everyone who feels this way but the majority, and especially of those that are best in judgment, think that one should place more of one's energy in the discovery and examination of things rather than in mere elegance, splendour and charm of language.[10]

In the renaissance an attempt was made to transform the manuscript *practica* which had evolved during the middle ages within the Arabo–Latin tradition into a humanistic production. By looking at one or two writers it is possible to find out how this change was envisaged. In 1539 the German humanist physician Leonhard Fuchs produced a *practica* whose title expressed its purpose *De Medendis Singularum Humani Corporis Partium. A summo capite ad imos usque pedes Passionibus ac Febribus*. In the dedicatory letter Fuchs set out his aims. He not only wanted to revert to a pure and uncorrupted medical terminology (that is, classical), but he also wished to produce a method or *ratio* for treatment which would reflect Galen's views, especially as they related to the indications for cure.[11] Jerome Bylebyl has written at length on this topic: how some renaissance writers tried to replace medieval indications of the cause of an illness with those of Galen and how others sought to introduce Galen's idea of indications arising from the individual patient as an input into treatment. (As Bylebyl has covered the ground so well I will leave the subject of the indications rising from the patients to one side.)

Fuch's love of all things classical and his dislike of the Arabs and of the 'barbarians' (the medieval writers) further emerged when he wrote that his book was written for those who were frightened away by the great length and difficulty of the works of Galen and of the Greeks, and who consequently forsook Galen's reputation for the Arabs and for 'the most inept mob of barbarian doctors'.[12] Here Fuchs must have recognized that neither Hippocrates nor Galen – with the questionable exception of *De Locis Affectis* – had produced a compendium which could provide a doctor with a handbook for easily recognizing and treating an illness. The medieval *practica* did fulfil precisely such a need, but for a humanist doctor such *practica* were, because of their origin, corrupt. Fortunately, classical alternatives were at hand and the works of Aëtius and Paul of Aegina provided the materials from which a compendium based upon classical sources could be produced. Both Aëtius (fl. *c.* 500) and Paul (625–90) had extracted and summarized previous Greek writers, and both in a sense had produced a *practica*. The third book of Paul's *Libri Septem*,[13] in fact, had the same head to toe order as the *practica*, whilst the second dealt with 'universal fevers' which were also to be included in the *practica*. Moreover, Paul had the further advantage of being very close to Galen, Conrad Gesner reports that Manardi called him Galen's ape ('Galeni simiam'). Guenther von Andernacht, who was to become a translator of Galen and a prominent humanist and anatomist in Paris, had seen Paul's merit and translated him into Latin in 1532.[14] His reasons for doing so were to help the *practici* whom he recognized as a specific group:

Among others I first tackled turning the whole of Paul of Aegina into Latin, an excellent writer of medicine and one who was missing for a thousand years, for this cause and reason: that next to those full doctrines of Galen our schools should have some compendious author from whom they could reliably learn that way of healing which they call practical. Since Paul indisputably excels all recent writers from Galen in compendiousness, order, skill, perspicacity and doctrine. Add to this the fact that he treats of many things with erudition which are either left untouched by others, or even unknown to them.[15]

Fuchs wrote that his own *practica* or method of healing was 'conflated from the works of Aëtius and Paul who follow Galen for the most part', and that it had been composed so that men who had forsaken trustworthy judgement and rashly followed anyone could return to virtuous goodness and hence reform.[16] Fuchs' new *practica*, by going back to the Greeks, would revert to a new *prisca medicina* even if not using the original and 'prolix' words of Galen. Here the humanistic ideal of reverting to the classical world for one's knowledge and the pragmatic necessity for brevity went hand in hand.

Fuchs gave two foundations for his method of treatment:

. . . the method of the treatment of the ancients is composed especially from two things, from precepts of course, which show whence the indications for treatment are to be sought, and in medicines which repel illnesses.[17]

With regard to indications Fuchs stated that he followed the ancient Greek writers, who had set them down 'most correctly', rather than the Arabs and barbarians.[18] In contrast to indications, knowledge of medicines could not be recalled to its pristine state:

For there are many medicines both simple and compound which they used in overcoming diseases which escape the knowledge of all who live to–day and therefore cannot be recalled to use. So we are, as it were, compelled by necessity to make use in their place our own habitual remedies, especially those of which the forms and faculties are known to us.[19]

Moreover, Fuchs wrote, in order to be understood by the apothecaries he had sometimes to use words which were not in Latin but which were familiar to them.[20] The humanistic programme of retrieving ancient knowledge could not always be carried out, and the restoration of linguistic purity sometimes had to bow to the needs of business. The medical humanist could be very aware of the claims of the here and now. An example of this was Fuchs' use of well-tried local remedies in his *practica* rather than ones drawn from exotic far away places. He wrote:

I have been on my guard against exotic and expensive medicaments and those which are difficult to prepare only because there is a danger of many of these being adulterated, since they are insufficiently known either by those that sell them or by those who buy them. And the merchants in extracting them (such is their insatiable avarice) are principally concerned to sell inferior ones, and while they do this those which are good being kept too long or eaten by mould and maggots become worse. Now the apothecaries, almost all of them being no less eager for profit than the merchants and paying out money, buy only the worst ones. And although even amongst this kind there are good men to be found nevertheless, because, for the most part they are unlearned and ignorant of better things, they purchase only the familiar materials which are for the most part adulterated for making up their medicines. Wherefore, I am not able to give my approval to the practice of foolish and unlearned physicians who in practising use no medicines except those which they compose from the four parts of the world.[21]

Although I do not consider treatment in detail in this paper a cursory reading of the *practica* shows that there might be broad agreement on what was necessary in treatment but its detailed implemention could vary very much. So that if purgatives were prescribed the ingredients making up the purgative varied from author to author. The element in the *practica*, therefore, which escaped the hold of the ancients lay in the prescriptions given in the sections of the *practica* on treatment ('curatio').

After Fuchs many renaissance *practica* became more methodical and philosophical, partly in response to educational needs and practices. Fuchs himself in his *Institutionum Medicinae* (1555) produced a book which began with the theory of medicine and ended with its practice. The contents included the definition of medicine, the division of medicine, the elements, qualities, humours, the parts of the body, its actions, a description of the non-naturals, the causes and definition of illness, brief accounts of fevers and a short exposition *a capite ad calcem* of the affections of the body and then a discussion of signs and diagnostic matters such as uroscopy and the taking of the pulse. The format of the book reminds one a little of Avicenna's *Canon* which contains both the theoretical and practical parts of medicine. However, Fuchs in his *Institutiones* concentrated more on theory and on explaining the theoretical underpinning of concepts such as symptoms used in the practice of medicine, which the traditional *practica* took for granted and had seen no need to explain at length. On the other hand, the central element of the practice of medicine, that concerned with the nature, recognition and treatment of diseases was reduced by Fuchs to a mere enumeration of the names of illnesses and of their definitions.

Writers like Montanus, Altomari, Capivaccio and Massaria wrote at much greater length and with more concern for theory when producing their *practica* than had their medieval predecessors, and were more concerned with educating medical students than providing handbooks for practitioners. (Montanus did not write a *practica* but lectured on the *practica* of Rhasis.) Bates and Bylebyl[22] have also pointed out that such men attempted to transform the *practica* into treatises of methodical therapeutics following the example of Galen's *Methodus Medendi*. Apart from the wish to restore Galenic teachings and to educate students, one motive for this may have been to bolster the claims of university-trained doctors over the providers of medical expertise in the renaissance, namely: priests, wise-women, magicians, herbalists, travelling empirics and so forth. In an age when licensing and regulation of doctors was lax, a claim to have a proper 'method' of healing which only the properly educated could practise could be a means of excluding outside competition. The renaissance physician could use as a model Galen's attack on the empirical sect and his praise of the dogmatic[23] physician who knew the causes of diseases as well as its signs. When Montanus lectured on Rhasis' ninth book *ad Almansorem*, which listed diseases *a capite ad calcem* and formed one of the models of the medieval *practica*, he castigated Rhasis for writing empirically and contrasted this with his own approach which was 'dogmatice et methodum' and a few lines later 'dogmatice et ex methodo'.[24] The reform of the practice of medicine was not to be undertaken only by method but also by the allied but much wider concept of dogmatism or rationalism (the latter being concerned to cure by discovering the causes of disease, the former curing by rational indications derived from the patient). That knowledge of the causes of disease and knowledge of disease from the patient himself came to be linked together as representing expert knowledge and opposed to the ignorance of the empiric can be seen in one of Johann Lange's letters where he attacked the ignorance of empirics and uroscopists. He wrote that the method of healing consisted in the knowledge of the causes of diseases, whilst:

. . . the ignorant and inexperienced crowd of philosophers, seduced by old women's superstition and by the impostures and false appearance of knowledge of the Jews and pseudodoctors whose effrontery knows no bounds, thinks falsely not that the causes and the natures of illnesses can be discerned by pathognomic symptoms or by dyscrasia of the affected part or organ . . . but that the natures of the illnesses can be discerned by a mere inspection of urine.[25]

Lange went on to say that the uroscopist also ignored the way of life of the ill patient. Uroscopy, where the practitioner could be sent the urine without seeing and examining the patient, set at nought the lengthy education of the university physician and the Galenic mores of knowing the causes of a disease and taking into account the patient's specific nature.

As such it was an obvious target for opposition by the rational physicians of the renaissance.

Sentiments such as Lange's, attacking the competition and defending the virtues of the Galenic doctor, can also be found in the introductions to some of the renaissance *practica*. The Frankfurt physician Johann Hartmann Beyer, in his dedicatory letter to the *Practica Medica* (1594) of his former teacher at Padua Girolamo Capivaccio, quoted Galen to the effect that the physician defeats disease by being instructed by reason and that 'the best doctor is a philosopher'. At the same time Galen was cited as commending experience by means of which the precepts of the theoretical part of medicine were confirmed.[26] Beyer considered *ratio* and *experientia* and wrote that though he liked both he would have to give the palm to reason.[27] Then, from this rather abstract discussion of reason and experience he moved to the empirics and the quacks, and he clearly saw his support of reason as a defence against them. For, he wrote 'what is more cheap than empirical physicians' and every place was full of well tried (medicinal) recipes:

You can see that mad, deaf, toothless witches, priests, barbers, porters, Jews, murderers and criminals who are deserving the cross and further people who are bereft of reason, are all rich with remedies so that the waters could more easily fail the Rhine than empirical remedies fail this class of people.[28]

How far this fear of empiricism was real and how far it was an ancient literary device should become clearer from other chapters in this book. However, it is possible that the opposition to empirics made for a conservatism in which reason (that is, Galenic doctrine) was defended to the exclusion of new knowledge gained by experience.

Beyer contrasted Capivaccio with the empirics and praised him as being most studious about method and order and 'he leans everywhere on the solid foundations of philosophy'.[29] As we shall see later on Capivaccio certainly applied a philosophical approach to his *practica*, so much so that it is doubtful if it was much use as a *vade-mecum*; brevity, which is one sense of 'methodus', being sacrificed for the prolixity of philosophical distinctions.

Peter van Foreest (1522–97) the town physician of Delft wrote at the end of this period a series of medical observations arranged in the head to toe order of the *practica* (medical observations, *consilia*, *consultationes* were the practice of medicine brought to the level of the individual case and formed a counterpart to the general approach of the *practica*). Foreest, the 'Hippocrates of Holland' was a practical physician par excellence and in the prefaces to his books of medical observations we get the views of someone looking back, rather dispassionately, at a panorama of medical views. He made it clear that his intention was to make doctors rather than orators[30] and that he preferred knowledge of treatment to eloquence, the thing itself rather than the decoration of words.[31] He was not therefore a humanist who would exclude the Arabs and the medieval writers. He admitted that he did 'not fear to bring forward now the Greeks, now the Latins, now the Arabs or even the Barbarians and on occasion to follow these same people'.[31] Although Foreest wrote a violent diatribe against uroscopists and empirics[33] he was willing to acknowledge that within 'proper' medicine there had been criticisms and disagreements. He listed some of the comments made against particular philosophers and physicians, when he came to Galen he wrote that he had been attacked for excessive prolixity and for the fact that he had written in 'a certain order which is not suitable for practise'. He continued:

Furthermore, quite a number of people embrace Avicenna and neglect Galen. On the other hand, others reject Avicenna because of the barbarous medical terms. They receive Galen with both arms. Or rather the ears of some people are so fastidious that they admit no other doctor unless one who has written in pure language, Greek or Latin, and that briefly. But they turn away from all practici (practicos) as though they were barbarians and loath them. So, that they do not deign even to read the Arabs however much they might have produced remedies for us. All the same the Arabs and the barbarians have each their reputation, they have been more fertile in remedies than the Greeks themselves and there are certain people who just as they blame the prolixity of Galen so they blame the brevity in Paulus of Aegina and not a few consider him an ape of Galen.[34]

From this passage it is clear that the humanists had not been able to have it all their own way. There still remained an undercurrent within medicine which, paying less attention to ornament and more to the things themselves, valued the Arabs and the traditional practici. The attraction of the new, reforming, movement within medicine and the articulateness of humanist physicians has meant that more attention has been paid to them than to the old-fashioned practitioner and his needs. Nevertheless, Foreest made it clear that such people did exist, and that he himself was not so besotted by classical eloquence that he would reject what could be of use.

Francis Bacon felt that the middle ages and the renaissance could be characterized as having too much empty argumentation to the detriment of the study of 'substance'[35] and too much elegance of style so that 'men began to hunt more after words than matter . . . Then grew learning of the schoolmen to be utterly despised as barbarian'.[36] We have also found these generalizations in the medical writers cited above. However, like all generalizations they were too exclusive. The Arabic and medieval writers were valued by some physicians despite the attempt by renaissance writers to reform the teaching of the practice of medicine by 'humanizing' its language and by producing a philosophically based (that is, concerned with causes) and methodically ordered form of practica.

Continuity is equally strong in the structure of the practica. Firstly, the traditional order of classical origin, a capite ad calcem, is found not only in

Galen[37] and Paul of Aegina but also in Rhasis, Albucassis and Avicenna amongst the Arabs and in Constantine the African, Gariopontus and Petrocellus in the Salernitan period and in writers such as Gilbertus Anglicus, Arnald of Villanova, through to Sylvius, Fuchs and then to Capivaccio and Massaria at the end of the sixteenth century. It was not until Theophile Bonet in 1682 wrote his *Mercurius Compilatitius* that an alphabetical listing of diseases was produced as a substitute to the head to toe order. The latter had distinct advantages. It ordered the body into regions such as the head, the upper chest, belly, sexual organs and so forth. Within these sections one could list the illnesses or affections that could befall those areas of the body. (Affection or illness is a better word to use than disease, as some affections could be symptoms of an underlying disease.) Secondly, the list of affections remained reasonably constant over time and kept recurring in nearly all writers up to the end of the sixteenth century. So, for instance, headache, migraine, vertigo, phrenitis, epilepsy and melancholy would almost certainly be found in any medieval or renaissance account of affections of the head. The existence of a new disease such as syphilis might be admitted in the renaissance but in general the list of possible disorders remained remarkably constant from Greek times to the renaissance.[38] As I explain below, in my study of vertigo, the question of whether an affection was a disease (*morbus*) or not could arise, but apart from such issues which were meat and drink to the men applying method to medicine in the renaissance, there was no attempt to discover new illnesses unless they were thrust into the consciousness of physicians.

Vertigo and the description of illness

There was nothing novel about vertigo for the medieval and renaissance writers. It was a condition known from Greek times and was one of the affections regularly discussed in the *practica*. In other words, it was ordinary and well established, and although lacking the interest of a new disease like syphilis for contemporaries and historians, it can be used as a representative example of what was contained in a *practica*.

A difficulty faced by anyone undertaking a case study of this sort is how much space to devote to questions of provenance and how much to an analysis of the material in its own right. Such was the derivative nature of medieval and renaissance medicine that if a particular slice of medical knowledge is studied it will inevitably involve a consideration of its provenance. This is a proper way of proceeding since both medieval and renaissance writers were concerned to draw their knowledge from past authorities, and the latter often took great care in detailing the sources that they used, so that by tracing the provenance of a piece of medical knowledge the historian is engaged in the same sort of activity as the writers that he or she studies. Yet, such an approach can have its dangers.

For instance, we may find that the description of say, migraine goes back in all its essentials to an account by Galen and consequently we may ignore its content or meaning leaving that to people who write on Galen – although such an account would not have lost meaning for the middle ages and renaissance merely because it was derivative. It is notorious that analysis of the content of ideas is undertaken by philosophers and historians at their point of origin, and only some innovatory ripple within the calm sea of tradition – for instance, developments in anatomy – stimulates an investigation of content. In my discussion of vertigo I will consider provenance but I will run counter to the normal trend and also look briefly at content. I want to bring out three things. First to demonstrate the change-over from medieval to renaissance *practica* and the developments that occur within the latter. My specific example will mirror the general points made in my introduction to the *practica*. Secondly, by briefly analysing Arnald of Villanova's explanation of vertigo I give an exposition of humoural medicine which contradicts some commonly held assumptions. Lastly, I hope to give the reader some taste of what was in the *practica* and this means that I have included more material than is strictly necessary.

The Arabic and medieval writers

Rhasis' ninth book *Ad Almansorem* was frequently used in the middle ages and commented upon in the renaissance. The *Articella*, which formed a basis for medieval medical teaching was often printed together with it. Rhasis' account of vertigo did not discuss the provenance of the information given – though some was ultimately derived from Galen – and it had little if any discussion of causes, but instead it was concerned with identifying the affection in its various forms and giving instructions as to treatment. The chapter on vertigo began:

When someone sees what is before him move in a circle and his eyes are darkened and he wants to fall down and his face and eyes grow red at the same time and the veins also which are behind the ears swell prominently you must perform venesection, and cupping glasses must be placed on his neck and shin-bones. But if the aforementioned veins do not appear and the face is ruddy the blood is to be lessened by drawing it from the basilic vein and the cupping glasses must be applied to the shins.[39]

As Montanus and Massaria[40] realized Rhasis proceeded empirically; there was no discussion of the causes that produced the symptoms. What we are given are the visible signs to be found in the patient and instructions on how anyone with those signs is to be treated. However, other Arabic and medieval writers did discuss the causes of vertigo and should not be stuck with the label of empiricists.

Avicenna wrote at length, in a vein of natural philosophical enquiry, on how external impressions could impress themselves within the subject's brain so that when one saw a rotating wheel its impression would remain within a susceptible individual (such as a sick person) even when it was no longer being sensed. Another explanation concerned vertigo produced by someone going round in a circle; in this case Avicenna thought that the vapours in the brain were given a sort of momentum so that they continued moving in the brain even after the motion had stopped. These explanations drawn from reasoning in natural philosophy were not taken up by later writers. Avicenna also wrote, in more of a medical manner, of vertigo which occurred from causes within the body. Vapours, either from bile or phlegm originating in the stomach or in the womb, could rise up and affect the animal spirits within the brain. Avicenna differentiated vertigo from epilepsy by its greater duration and lack of spasm, but he wrote that when vertigo came from phlegm it was close to epilepsy (epilepsy being thought to be produced by phlegm). He went on to write about the signs which preceded vertigo such as pains in the head, tinnitus and heaviness of the head, he also gave the differentiating signs which would distinguish whether the humour involved was phlegm or bile. Finally, Avicenna detailed the treatment for vertigo.[41]

Avicenna's account of vertigo was very unlike that of Rhasis and certainly combined reason and experience in a manner that the renaissance should have approved of. Avicenna's ability to look at the phenomena from more than one point of view is not untypical of medieval authors, though their renaissance successors tended to oversimplify the tradition by seeing all medieval medical writing as an undifferentiated whole.

Constantine the African gave an account of vertigo which combined a discussion of its causes with an account of the signs of the condition in its different forms.[42] The shadowy Salernitan writer, Gariopontus, on the other hand, seemed to favour the approach of Rhasis. His discussion of 'scotomia' (darkening of the eyes, black-out) or vertigo began in an empirical fashion with no discussion of causes: 'Those people who suffer from scotoma have these signs . . .'[43] However, in the next chapter he again discussed vertigo, but this time did write something on its causes. He wrote that scotomia arose in bibulous men and in those who frequently cleansed (*purgant*) their heads in the sun. According to Gariopontus when the head was heated its veins opened up and haemorrhoids in it would be inflated. In a more general sense, he saw vertigo as resulting from bile coming from the top part of the stomach to the head and in that case the stomach had to be cured.[44] Elsewhere in the book the empirical approach based on signs and treatment, and the dogmatic founded on causes, signs and treatment alternated.

Other medieval writers discussed the cause of vertigo as well as its signs and treatment. Arnald of Villanova tried to grapple with the causes of vertigo, and his attempt is worth analysing. First of all Arnald used his imagination to describe the inner happenings of the body. The distinction between a sign and an internal cause in all the writers that I discuss is that a sign was visible whilst a cause was invisible. Therefore, in the case of the latter one had to produce a description of something that could not be observed but which, nevertheless, was believed to be taking place in the body and producing visible signs. However, the story was not totally imaginary. It was given shape by reference to well known, if invisible entities, such as the animal spirits, vapours in the body, and hidden but known structures such as the optic nerve, and by the use of concrete analogies drawn from the visible world to explain the hidden world inside the body. For Arnald, vertigo was a revolution of the spirit in front of the eyes (in the anterior ventricles of the brain?) or an enveloping of the brain whereby the spirit of vision was impeded. First the definition, then came the cause. This was from some material existing in the brain itself or coming from the stomach. Smoke was formed from material in the stomach and coming up to the optic nerve it closed it up. This blockage in the optic nerve produced a change in the essence of the animal spirits and the interactions of smoky vapour and the animal spirits produced a circular motion in the optic nerve just as when two winds of equal force create a whirlwind.[45] This was essentially a story, a narrative of generally unverifiable events and it was given verisimilitude by the references to generally-agreed-upon structures within the body; the imaginative part had been to produce a narrative of happenings within the body that would account rationally for the visible manifestations of the condition; hence the trick was to show how the animal spirits themselves could be put into a motion analogous to the spinning motion that people feel while they have vertigo.

This analysis, I would argue, holds for most accounts of illness in the medieval and renaissance period. A point that emerges, and which I will develop later is that even if the ultimate cause of an affection was humoural there was, nevertheless, a very specific and localized element to causal explanations of illness (one effect of this would be to allow identifiable conditions to be defined, not only from signs, but from causes). One can also note that many writers referred to external causes of vertigo. These were specific rather than general and also, by the very fact that they had an external origin, they run counter to the internal causality that is usually thought to have been required by humoural medicine.

Some accounts may have been more persuasive or rational than others (though how contemporaries could judge the matter is usually impossible to tell). In the *Rosa Anglica* of John of Gaddesden the explanation of vertigo is less convincing (to me) because there was no clear connection between what was said to be going on inside the body and the outward signs of vertigo. John wrote that in vertigo the cause was a more subtle material than in scotoma (he was one of the few to separate the two). This material was trapped with flatulence inside a humid viscous matter that had no exit, and so went round and round just as children are used to do when they spin themselves round like wheels.[46] John's analogy between the motion of children who, of course, produce vertigo by their action, and the motion of the subtle material is blurred because we are not given enough details as to what happens to the subtle material in the body: where is it situated? how did it arise? what is its nature? how is it set in circular motion? and so on. From the analogy of children spinning themselves dizzy John came to his conclusion:

So vertiginous man, when he sees a wheel revolving or water rushing in a torrent or in a revolution as occurs in whirlpools in water or moving clouds swiftly driven by the wind, thinks that he is being swung round with them and therefore he grasps onto things near at hand because he absolutely must sit down or fall down. Hence in scotoma and vertigo there is a corruption of the vision and an injury to the procreation of images . . . as if the optic nerves have been shaken and consequently injury is produced in the common sense and as a consequence judgement is corrupted in the imaginative (faculty).[47]

Neither the 'So' at the beginning of the passage nor the 'Hence' towards the end is justified, for the two conclusions have little connection with the antecedent material. In a sense John of Gaddesden was not, at least in this case, a convincing or rational story-teller and perhaps this partly explains why some medieval writers thought poorly of him.[48]

In the renaissance there was a similar method of giving an explanation of what was going on inside the body. However, the story becomes more uniform and this is because the three sources of Galen, Aëtius and Paul of Aegina, although not always agreeing with each other, provided the materials from which a causal account of the affections of the body could be produced. The Arabic and medieval writers, of course, also ultimately drew upon Greek writers[49] but the derivation was not so clear cut and, as the differences in their accounts of vertigo show, there was no agreed explanation of the condition, though the description of the outward signs of the condition was reasonably uniform.

The Greek sources for renaissance writers

At this point it is necessary to give a brief exposition of the opinion of Greek writers on vertigo as this will help to put the renaissance writers into context.

In *De Locis Affectis* Galen wrote[50] that scotoma and vertigo occurs on trifling occasions. This was often repeated, as was his next comment that people subject to vertigo fall down after one rotation whilst it takes many spins to make other people fall down.[51] Galen wrote that vertiginous persons also get dizzy watching someone else spinning round, or when they see a wheel turning or something else in a circular motion or when they look at whirlpools. The vertigo occurs more readily if they have been exposed to the sun or if their heads have been overheated for some other reason.[52] Galen went on to argue that in normal people the effect of dizziness or spinning round many times is produced by an irregular, turbulent and disordered motion of the humours and the spirit.[53] Therefore, logically, the same should occur in the disease condition. The affection, Galen argued, could be primary and situated in the head or it occurred by sympathy with the opening in the stomach[54] (a view found later in Avicenna and some medieval writers), and he cited Archigenes to this effect. Galen also repeated Archigenes' differential signs: vertigo which was a primary affection of the brain produced tinnitus, pain and heaviness in the head, whilst vertigo originating at the stomach was preceded by *cardiogmon* (pain in the heart area) and by nausea.[55]

The two compilers, Aëtius and Paul of Aegina, differed in one or two instances from each other. Aëtius, who drew his material from Archigenes and Posidonius, argued that hot and acrid vapours carried to the brain disturbed the animal spirit,[56] whilst Paul stated that:

The affection of vertigo arises when a cold glutinous humour occupies the brain whence men even fall down straight away on the slightest occasion as when they see certain things outside them going round such as wheels, whirlpools or when they spin themseves round.[57]

Aëtius described similar precipitating causes:

If the ill persists they are affected with vertigo from a slight cause so that they sometimes fall down, especially when they spin round in a circle, for what befalls others as a result of many revolutions befalls them from one revolution. But also if they see someone else spin round they are affected with vertigo, or if they see a wheel or something of that kind going round they suffer the same thing.[58]

The similarity in the descriptions by Galen, Aëtius and Paul of what external causes brought on the condition is striking. In the Latin editions of Galen and Aëtius the same adjectives were used to describe what happened to the humours and the spirit when they were excited by an outside cause – 'inaequalem et turbulentem et inordinatum'[59] – and the renaissance writers often repeated them.

The renaissance

In the renaissance as in the middle ages there was no uniformity in discussions of the affections of the body. Some writers, especially in the second half of the sixteenth century, might write at length on causes whilst others could be very brief. The intention of the writers also differed and some concentrated more on treatment and giving prescriptions than on detailing the causes of the conditions, which others, more concerned with education than practicalities, emphasized.

Sylvius, the Paris humanist and Galenist, in his *practica*, rather surprisingly only alluded to the causes of vertigo and was more concerned with treatment. He divided the causes of vertigo into external and internal, the former consisting of spinning round and of getting drunk, the treatment being to stop the activity in question, and additionally in the case of drunkenness the applications of clysters.[60] An internal cause could be produced by the immoderate and disordered movement of spirits and for that Sylvius advised staying in a dark room and gave a detailed prescription consisting of cold ingredients for quietening and settling the turbulent motions of the spirits.[61] Sylvius' real interest lay in treatment and he went on to advise that the patient should be given external applications to repel the material flowing into the head; he also prescribed remedies for vertigo caused by the different humours.[62] In effect, what Sylvius did was to assume that his reader already knew the causes of vertigo and would understand his allusions to them. In other words, he was not concerned with educating his reader in the theoretical part of medical practice.

In the *practica* of Bayrus, as edited by Zwinger, the explanation of the cause of vertigo was minimal. The chapter was organized on the lines of: 'if vertigo arises from bloody matter there should be cut first the vena basilica' and so on through each of the four humours with a final section devoted to the treatment of vertigo arising from 'foetid vapours'.[63] What was important was the treatment; how to recognize which humour was involved was left to the reader who might need to have recourse to some other *practica* to find this out. Yet, despite Zwinger's complaint, this is no barbarian *practica*; for the author was aware of Galenic teaching since he quoted the one piece of advice concerning treatment to be found in the chapter on vertigo in *De Locis Affectis.*[64]

Rather than taking the renaissance *practica* to be an undifferentiated whole we should see them as having a range of interests and approaches. Bayrus (via Zwinger) had the clear intention of producing a *practica* in which treatment ('curatio'), the essence of practical medicine, was more important than 'causa', even though the lack of the latter might condemn an author with the label of empiricism. (Zwinger's doubt as to whether Bayrus succeeded in his attempt to unite dogmatism and empiricism was more than well founded, as Bayrus had hardly anything on the causes of disease.)

Leonhard Fuchs, on the other hand, being a good Galenist and a student of method in medicine and a humanist to boot, produced in his *practica* a totally different account of vertigo from that of Bayrus. His chapter was structured in the following manner. There was a discussion of the name σκότωμα which he held to be Greek for the Latin 'vertigo', and he pointed out that the 'barbarians' had corrupted the word to 'scotomia'.[65] This was a typical opening to a renaissance-humanistic *practica*, reflecting the concern to produce a correct and pure terminology. The chapter then dealt with causes, signs, regimen, treatment, venesection, purgation, local remedies and cautery. It would be tedious to go into much detail, but Fuchs followed Galen's account in *De Locis Affectis* and also used Aëtius and Paul. Fuchs mentioned how a trivial occasion could bring the condition on, and how one spin rather than many would make a person prone to vertigo fall down.[66] Also present was the idea that vertigo is either a primary affection of the brain or came by sympathy from the mouth of the stomach with the excretions in the stomach producing vaporous exhalations which drove the animal spirits round.[67] Fuchs used the same adjectives – 'turbulentus, inequalis, inordinatus'[68] – as had Galen and Aëtius to describe the motion of the spirit and the humours. The account was not totally derivative for some creative work was involved in producing agreement where one's sources clashed with each other. The contradiction between Paul and Aëtius on what were the humours which caused vertigo was resolved by Fuchs when he described the humour as 'thick and slow' from which a vaporous spirit was released by the heat of the ill person.[69] In this way the cold glutinous and the hot acrid humours of Paul and Aëtius respectively were reconciled. There was, however, no explicit discussion of the issue and Fuchs' *practica* like many others did not involve lengthy argument, with the juxtaposition of conflicting authorities and the solution of contradictions so beloved of medieval and renaissance writers. Although, as we shall see, the *practica* did not always retain their claim to brevity, there yet runs throughout the genre the style of assertion rather than of dialectical argument.

The regimen that Fuchs advised was explicitly rational, for there was a connection between the cause of the condition and its avoidance and treatment. Food should lack 'flatus' and everything steamed should be avoided (so that vapours causing vertigo could not be generated – though Fuchs did not spell this out) and things going round in a circle should also be avoided.[70] As for venesection, Fuchs repeated the advice of Aëtius and recommended that only a small amount of blood be let since people with vertigo fell on the slightest occasion.[71]

Fuchs had produced a brief and rational account of illness. From the time of Montanus onwards there was an effort to apply the idea of method to therapeutics. As I mentioned before, Jerome Bylebyl[72] has discussed how the indications arising from the individual patient came to be included in the discussion of what should be the correct treatment. In what follows I will concentrate on the question of the cause of the affection and its signs rather than on indications from the patient. I do this in order to illustrate the general point that the philosophical/logical approach applied to therapeutics was also co-existent with discussions of method. Leoniceno and Manardi had explored the instruments of method – definition, division, demonstration and resolution and the three orders of resolution, composition and definition, but they did not apply it to the practice of medicine. Montanus, however, also produced interesting ideas on the question of method and order in medicine, and he did go on to apply method to the practice of medicine.

The contrast between Fuchs and Montanus is quite striking. This is partly because when Montanus wrote on vertigo it was in a lecture course commentating on Rhasis' ninth book and not in a *practica*. He, therefore, explicitly pointed out the contradictions between Aëtius and Paul, gave the opinion of modern writers – that all the humours could cause vertigo – and from various passages in Galen concluded that Galen's opinion was that it was caused by a cold humour.[73] Montanus' solution to the conflict of opinion was that vertigo fixed in the head was caused by a cold humour, his reason being the Galenic one that because of a lack of heat the excrements could not be properly concocted and consequently vapours would be produced which agitated the animal spirits. On the other hand, vertigo which was not fixed in the head could be caused by any humour, as in cases of drunkenness, or of too much blood or bile in the stomach.[74] This discussion and conciliance of previous views shows how the past served as a repository of knowledge out of which one could arrive at one of the objects of method in medicine, that of definition. Montanus wrote:

From this the correct definition of vertigo is obvious: vertigo is a disordered motion of the spirits in the anterior ventricles of the brain which motion arises because of the thick and confused vapours in them.[75]

What is significant here is that Montanus, the great teacher of clinical medicine at Padua, drew his knowledge of the causes of vertigo not from his experience but from the ancient authorities. This perhaps was inevitable, because to have knowledge of causes was to be rational, and reason as we have seen was sometimes contrasted and opposed to experience (and by extension to the empirics). The reliance on authority meant also that whatever might have been the potential flexibility of the humoural system for a writer producing an explanation of illness, in well recognized affections at least, physicians like Montanus did not have a great deal of freedom, for in practice they did not go beyond previous authorities.

The application of method to practical medicine involved both logic *and* experience – despite my comments above. In the case of logic, Montanus pointed out that vertigo was a symptom or accident and not a disease. It resulted from the action of the humours, and as the animal spirits were injured so the many actions which depends upon them were also injured.[76] This concern to have a proper classification was a characteristic outcome of the renaissance concern with method. At the same time the method of division brought the physician close to experience (that is, in his examination of the patient). Montanus produced a 'syndrome of signs' to be found in the patient from which the physician could deduce which particular humour was causing vertigo. The signs common to all types of vertigo were the feeling of everything going round, blacking out, hearing ringing in the ears and a corruption of the motive faculty so that the sufferer thinks he is falling.[77] But the signs which allow one to distinguish between the different causes producing vertigo were according to Montanus of three kinds: those arising from the injured function, those seen in the excrements and those found in the common accidents (or qualities).[78] The signs from the injured function originated from the animal faculties and could be divided into sensitive and motive signs, and the sensitive was further divided into interior and exterior.[79] Montanus continued in this vein and argued that if blood was the cause of vertigo the natural functions of the patient will make him imagine cheerful things, he will be inclined to sleep, he will feel heavy in the head and have happy dreams as did those of a sanguine temperament 'and in this way you will know from the internal operations of the brain what it is that has dominion'.[80] Montanus went on through the different division of signs:

So far as the vital functions are concerned you have the pulse which is felt to be great, vehement, resisting the touch, soft to the touch, full rapid, infrequent so that it would demonstrate to those that were blind the predominance of the blood . . . As far as the excrements are concerned they must clearly indicate the predominance of the blood, the urine is thick, red, which is the perpetual property of blood, the stools are concocted and the excrements which descend from the head are somewhat moist and if there are tears in the eyes they will be hot but not stinging and trickling down. And besides this, coming down to the mouth, the mouth will be somewhat sweet, and if it is the blood that predominates he will have ringing in the ears and heaviness in the head.[81]

Montanus then enumerated the signs taken from accidents which consisted of the first qualities, namely the habit and disposition of the patient, and of the secondary and tangible qualities such as the gentle heat felt on the patient's head.[82] Montanus concluded 'From all these things you will have so clear a syndrome of signs that you cannot be in error. You will say absolutely the same about bile . . .'[83]

One can see how the methodical approach of Montanus, by using the method of division, allowed him to fulfil Galen's requirement of applying universals to particulars. Moreover, it also helped the student (for Montanus had him in mind) and the physician to infer systematically rather than in a haphazard way what particular form of illness affected the patient. It also gave further verisimilitude to the explanation of the cause of the affection; for by means of the syndrome of signs one moved from the visible to the hidden, and inferred what was going on inside the body. Of course, the inference is not a real one, for what is happening is that the syndrome of signs reflects the causal account and without the latter's pre-existence would make no sense. In reality, the signs are not a research tool, independent of theory whereby new causes are discovered. For, as we saw, the causes are to be first established by an examination of ancient opinions and were not discovered *de novo* from signs in the patient. The signs merely indicated which amongst a set number of predetermined causes is the operative one. Montanus' general discussion of signs confirms this interpretation.[84]

Whether the signs were drawn at all from contemporary clinical experience is difficult to say. Some of them were clearly traditional such as the feeling of heaviness in the head, others such as ringing in the ears could be read in Galen and found in clinical practice. From Montanus' *Consilia* it is pretty clear that the signs were not only run through in a set order, but that their interpretation was uniform. In the case of the Venetian senator Bernardo Naugerio, Montanus went through the three types of signs and he was guided by authority not only in his choice of what signs to look for (for example, the colour of the face) but also in his interpretation of them (as in the case of the senator's urine).[85] This should not be too surprising, for not only was the modern idea of progress alien to the renaissance physician but we are here faced with the practice of medicine, a practice, moreover, to be undertaken methodically. Now, even the modern practice of medicine tends to be conservative in approach and revolves around well-tried methods and this was certainly the case in the renaissance where the distinction between teaching and discovery was unclear, and discovery often consisted in uncovering and teaching the proper views of the ancients.[86] Classification, as seen in Montanus' methodical approach to a problem, where he defined it and divided it up, was also essentially conservative, as the categories used were normally well established ones.

To end my case study of vertigo I will look briefly at the *practica* of Capivaccio and Massaria. Montanus exemplified a thoughtful application of philosophy and method to practical medicine; Capivaccio and Massaria who followed in Montanus' footsteps as professors at Padua show how the methodical approach could be taken to extremes, and how the *practica* were being changed from handbooks for practitioners to teaching texts for students.

Capivaccio's account of what happened inside the body is less graphic in detail and more ponderously abstract, being almost baroque in style:

> . . . the animal spirit which resides in the ventricles of the brain is affected with a morbid motion so that when this morbific motion tends towards the circular the brain is affected in repect of the heat of the imaginative faculty, so that the substance of the brain is affected by an affection which does not produce darkness as in melancholy, which is not fiery as in mania, but is circular. Hence the imagination is corrupted so that the patient imagines that objects are going round . . .[87]

Perhaps Molière had this sort of writing in mind when he considered the medicine of his time. Capivaccio went on to give the definition of vertigo and then took each term of the definition and differentiated it:

Vertigo therefore is a corruption of a principal function of the anterior brain along with injury of the vision and of the motion of the whole body dependent upon a circular affection of the brain. The function is said to be corrupt as differentiated from being destroyed and removed. The function is said to be principal as differentiated from non principal. It is said to be a function of the brain as differentiated from any other of the viscera . . .[88]

There is a certain sense of Aristotelianism about this which is confirmed by Capivaccio defining the 'form' of the vertigo.[89] This application of logic to medicine was the sort of thing that Ramus might have objected to; certainly it lacked the sense of enquiry and concern with substance that one finds in Montanus' application of method to medicine (in fact one might argue that the injection of Aristotelianism into medicine in the second half of the sixteenth century tended to produce a frame of mind which was at home with forms, specific qualities and occult qualities and would make something which appears abstract to us seem concrete – perhaps this is how we should see Capivaccio's 'morbific motion' and 'circular affection'.)

Massaria also applied logic in his discussion of what vertigo was. Whereas Montanus asserted that vertigo was a symptom, Massaria wanted to prove it (in fact his 'proof' was also close to an assertion):

Now since vertigo is a thing contrary to nature and the things contrary to nature are threefold, namely disease, cause of disease and symptom the question is under which heading it is to be placed. First of all it is not a disease because it is not a dyscrasia and not a lesion in the continuity of the body nor an abnormality in the composition of the body. Secondly, neither is it the cause of a disease since there is no disease produced by it and so it remains, as it should be, a symptom. Now since symptoms are of three kinds, injuries of the functions, change in the excrements, change in the qualities, it is obvious that the excrement is not changed nor the quality, therefore it will be an injury to the action. But once again since functions are threefold, the natural, the vital and the animal and since in the present case neither the vital nor the natural function are injured it does follow of necessity that it is an animal function which is injured. But since functions of this kind are threefold . . .[90]

This type of argument explains why the renaissance writers found it convenient to use tables to encapsulate the information they wanted to communicate (that is, moving from the general to the specific by the use of inclusive brackets as in a family tree but horizontally left to right across the page). However, clear as such *practica* might have been to the reader they tended to put great emphasis on theory and its sytematic presentation and less on treatment. Capivaccio had little on treatment in relation to the space that he devoted to discussion of the affection itself. It is a moot question if practising physicians found such *practica* useful, as they were designed more for teaching students (Massari's *practica* was produced from his lecture notes) to acquire a philosophical and methodically ordered

II

knowledge of medicine (note how the ordering of the information in the passage above into three becomes a mnemonic device for students). Furthermore, the question could be raised: what happened to new ideas or findings which could not be fitted into the categories that the application of method to medicine had produced? The *practica* at the end of the sixteenth century, therefore, seemed not only to have restored Galen's teaching but to have codified it in such a way that the original purpose of the *practica* was being lost sight of, and at the same time a potentially inflexible system was being raised inimicable to innovation. Before discussing the last point I turn first to the question of how the causes of illness were described.

The description of disease

So far, with the exception of my discussion of Arnald of Villanova, I have discussed the approach rather than the content of the writers of *practica*. A look at content may prove worthwhile, for it will show that whatever might be the ideal explanation of illness, in practice it contained a specific and localized element which is at variance with the commonly accepted view that medicine until the nineteenth century was holistic and concerned with general disorders within the body.

Certainly the latter might at first sight seem to be the case. In the passage above from Massaria a disease was defined as either a dyscrasia (humoural imbalance) or, a lesion in the body or an abnormality in its composition (this was a standard definition).[91] Most internal illnesses appear to be produced from a general cause since they would fall under the heading of dyscrasia or ill temperament (the varieties of ill temperament were eight plus a ninth, the neutral state). The treatment of dyscrasia could involve other general considerations such as the habits and disposition of a patient. Furthermore, although symptoms were specific they were clearly differentiated by renaissance writers from diseases for, as Manardi wrote in his letter on the principles of medicine, we recognize diseases from symptoms.[92] At first sight, therefore, the specificity of symptoms should not be seen as extending to diseases. Yet in a sense it does, for there was a continuity from the symptoms to the diseases. As Manardi put it symptoms were more readily apparent and it was this that allowed us to infer what disease was involved,[93] but it is clear that for this to happen the symptom must be connected with the disease. The bridge between the two was the story of the hidden events in the body that were producing the symptoms. These events could ultimately be caused by a qualitative or humoural dyscrasia such as too much heat or blood in the body. This pattern, from symptom to hidden event to dyscrasia can be seen in the 'curatio' of the renaissance *practica* in which many of the remedies were not only concerned to treat the dyscrasia but also to treat the symptoms and to rectify the internal course of events (for example, Fuchs' advice to avoid the sort of food which could produce vapours that might affect the brain, and Lange's prescriptions).[94] In fact, a great deal of treatment was concerned with altering what was occurring in the body, and this is a sign that importance was attached to local pathological events and not only to the underlying humoural balance. Moreover, the dyscrasia itself could be localized rather than general, Montanus stated:

The vapours can ascend from any humour existing in the stomach or the spleen or the liver or the bladder and the whole body as well . . . But that this symptom (falling) arises from a quality, this you have from Galen book 3 chapter 7 of De Locis Affectis where he gives two cases, one of a child of thirteen years of age from whose shin a certain quality begun to rise which he did not know how to name which arose from part to part as far as the brain and at length he fell down. In the other case, a youth, from whose large toe a cold quality ascended to the brain . . . and which produced and caused epileptic fits.[95]

Here the origin of the dyscrasia itself was a local one though its ultimate cause might be of a general nature; and although Montanus did not go into detail, its journey to the head was localized for it 'arose from part to part'.[96]

It is understandable, given the nature of the practica, that renaissance writers should have held not only a general concept of illness but also a specific view in which localized events within the body produced symptoms. The practica were concerned with particular affections. These were given specific names such as 'lienteria', 'dysentery', renal stone, phthisis, dropsy and others, and they were often explained in semi-mechanical, concrete terms. As we have seen in the case of vertigo, these explanations tended to be uniform, especially after the retrieval of Greek medical texts. Jerome Bylebyl has pointed out that writers like Montanus tried to make treatment less standardized (that is, they were against the view of one treatment for one condition). However, the dogmatic tradition within medicine (which held, against the empiricists, that hidden causes produced disease) ensured that there was always a tendency to emphasize the causes of the illness rather than the indications originating in the patient and thus to conceive of illness in universal rather than individualistic terms (Montanus' phrase 'dogmatically and methodically' thus expressed a hidden tension as well as agreement).

New diseases and new explanations

Vertigo was a well-known affection, but how did the renaissance deal with a new illness? Here I will turn away from the practica per se and I will briefly look at Montanus' influential explanation of syphilis. I then consider how new explanations could be seen to fall outside of the ambit of methodical medicine and this will illustrate the difficulty that Galenic medicine as codified by the methodical *practica* faced in accepting innovation. My comments are very limited and exploratory.

A new disease like syphilis could be easily assimilated into the *practica* tradition. Montanus employed the same techniques to explain the newly arrived disease as he and others had used to describe well-known conditions. Story-telling, a localized and detailed account of what took place in the body to produce syphilis, was the key to Montanus' explanation.

Montanus first stated the dogmatic proposition that in order to teach the treatment of syphilis its nature and essence had to be discovered,[97] he continued 'I say that it is a bad hot and dry dyscrasia impressed in the liver by means of contagion.'[98] From this assertion or definition Montanus went on to unfold his story. The disease begun with intercourse with an infected person from whom emanates a certain poison 'in which exists that evil and poisonous quality'.[99] This attaches itself into the foreskin or to the mouth since these parts are loose (permeable) and more suitable for receiving the poisonous quality. We now proceed on a journey to the liver. Montanus wrote that gradually the quality creeps to the small veins then to the larger ones until it arrives at the liver. Once there it takes over and changes the liver's natural temperament. Because the liver is so changed it burns all the humours which are in it, which are transmitted to all parts of the body for nourishment. However the parts of the body do not accept these humours, the body then becomes full of sharp excrements which produce ulcers, blisters, joint pains and infinite other symptoms.[100] Montanus went on to give other graphic details of the action of this bad quality upon the body.

Montanus was telling a story with a beginning (intercourse, and the permeability of the foreskin), a middle (the liver) and an end product (the symptoms). Verisimilitude is given to the journey of the bad quality by referring to the bodily structures passed along the way, the permeable skin, the small and large veins, and the liver. The enormity of the disease is stressed by the damage it does to one of the primary organs of the body. In Galenic theory the liver was the source of nutriment to the body, changing chyle to blood, with the different parts of the body attracting blood as food for themselves as needed. The arrival of the 'mala qualitas' at the liver, and its destruction of the liver's natural temperament made the consequences fully understandable to Montanus' readers, given their knowledge of the liver's function.[101] In other words, not only did Montanus use anatomical points of reference but also ones drawn from theory. In fact, his whole account is within the ambit of Galenic qualitative theory.

However, the qualities involved could be either manifest (that is, those we can feel such as hot, cold, dry and wet) or occult. Occult, hidden qualities were often associated with the concept of *tota substantia*[102] that is discussed in Linda Deer Richardson's chapter. Both concepts were used to explain the inexplicable. The action of poisons, drugs, the magnet, the electric discharge of the torpedo fish were unexplainable in terms of manifest qualities so recourse was had to hidden qualities or to the action of the total substance (that is, the action of a poison might appear far greater than might be expected from its manifest quality, hence either a hidden quality was at work or the poison acted by its whole substance). Here was an addition to traditional theory (albeit having its origins in Galen). However, Montanus did not accept occult qualities as an explanation of disease. Those who teach nothing, he told his audience when lecturing on plague, flee to two things: to occult qualities and to unknown and obscure names.[103] Montanus did, rather grudgingly, consider the possibility of occult qualities in pestilential fevers stating that Galen 'your teacher and mine' advised that occult qualities should not be neglected if the manifest qualities could not be discovered.[104] As, however, Montanus believed that he had found out a manifest quality for plague the discussion was academic. Similarly, for syphilis Montanus gave a manifest 'hot and dry' quality as the cause, rather than an occult one. Yet, he stated that remedies for syphilis could operate either by manifest or by occult qualities. He excused this inconsistency over occult qualities by recourse to Galen.[105]

Why was someone like Montanus so hesitant to use occult qualities and *tota substantia* as explanatory concepts? After all a 'mala qualitas' transmitted by contagion has a similarity to the action of the magnet. Apart from the obvious point that in using occult qualities one was employing the unexplainable to explain the inexplicable, which is what Montanus implied in his castigation of those who teach nothing, there were more concrete objections.

Montanus raised a problem related to the practice of medicine. He stated that those who taught that pestilent fevers were caused by an occult quality derived knowledge of the different types of fevers from unknown differences in the qualities. Furthermore, if the differences in the qualities were unknown how could one discover the proper treatment?[106] As we have seen, in the methodical practice of medicine the different qualities could produce different forms of an illness, and unless the particular quality was known (and by definition an occult quality was unknown) no rational treatment could be given.

Apart from Montanus' very practical objection there was a more general problem. For some physicians occult qualities and the concept of *tota substantia* did not fit into the general scheme of methodical medicine. Moreover, for the rational physician the two concepts were tainted, for they seemed only to be known by experience. (Cesalpino, in his chapter on poison in the *Artis Medicae*, in fact tried to show that such a charge was unfounded.)

Argentarius, one of the *bêtes-noir* of the Galenic establishment, was by

II

no means hostile to the idea of *tota substantia* but he was also very much in favour of the methodical approach of Montanus (he joined Montanus with Vesalius as a man who had to suffer much opposition at first before his views prevailed).[107] When, therefore in *De Morbis* Argentarius discussed how many different kinds of diseases were to be put into the category of *tota substantia* he was perplexed. He stated that although the different types of diseases arising from the four qualities were eight (that is, the eight types of dyscrasia) the diseases produced by the pestilential air and by poison were diverse and as yet unknown. A definite number of diseases could not be assigned to *tota substantia*.[108] Argentarius continued and developed a line of thought from Galen:

To this is certainly relevant the fact that Galen is accustomed everywhere to write that the remedies which are beneficial through the *tota substantia* are discovered through experience alone, but are not established by any reasoning. But of things for which there is no reason there can be no definite species.[109]

Occult qualities and *tota substantia* did not fit into the rational, classificatory scheme of methodical medicine and this in a sense reflects the latter's conservatism. Of course, as with any scheme accommodations could be made. Thomas Erastus in a letter to Capivaccio wrote that he agreed with him that when we consider the genus or the differences of diseases, that a disease of *tota substantia* could not immediately fall into the realm of methodical doctrine. But Erastus went on to say that this was not because of any inherent difficulty in fitting an anomaly into a classificatory system as his correspondent thought, but because a disease of *tota substantia* did not exist anywhere and never had.[110]

Erastus then embarked on an interesting line of thought. Some people, he wrote, believed that diseases of *tota substantia* are known by experience and did not fit into methodical teaching. He denied this, and argued that everything found by experience had been placed within the method of medicine.[111] This claim contradicted the dichotomy and tension between experience and reason in renaissance medicine that I have been pointing to in this paper. Galen, of course, had written at length on the need to unite experience and reason, and renaissance authors were aware of his teaching (though the fear of empiricism could make a writer prefer reason). It was natural, therefore, for Erastus to feel that methodical medicine, as one might call the systematic practice of Galenic medicine, should always be able to include any findings from experience. However, as with all systems, methodical medicine was not open-ended but structured around the mainstream of Galen's theories. Therefore, a bad mixture of the qualities rather than an occult quality *had* to be the beginning of the disease process. Anything that did not fit into the standard eight combinations of the qualities did not fit methodical doctrine.

Erastus' solution in his letter was to integrate and assimilate the new ideas of disease causation embodied by *tota substantia* and seeds of disease into the old system. His example was the older disease of plague. He wrote that a method for treating the plague could be produced even though it was believed to be a disease of *tota substantia*. He argued that a 'morbus seminarius' (he seems to equate it epistemologically with *tota substantia*) did not act directly by pouring itself across from an infected person to someone else and then extinguishing his spirit and innate heat. Instead, the seeds of disease first affected the temperament or balance of the humours.[112] Erastus' solution thus brought one back to familiar territory for once the temperament was involved, therapy proceeded normally and rationally with the physician trying to discover the variety of ill temperament and initiating treatment accordingly.

Erastus' union of experience and method was a one-way process, with the latter altering the former into its own image. Perhaps the problem was that *tota substantia*, occult qualities and seeds of disease were not purely matters of experience but had a theoretical element alien to standard Galenic medicine. They could either transform Galenic medicine, they might themselves be transformed back into orthodoxy or the two could exist side by side.

By the end of the sixteenth century university teachers had bound the *practica* together with method. The benefits of this for them were that the practice of medicine could be systematically taught, and also differentiated from empiricism; at the same time, the localized element in explanations of illness which had been present from early on gave them detailed and specific material to classify and methodically digest. If there had been only a generalized notion of a humoural dyscrasia to account for illness it would have been difficult to produce the detailed differentiae of diseases and their treatments which gave such confidence to renaissance physicians. (Method was frequently associated with the avoidance of error.) Another benefit of localism was that a new illness could be placed within Galenic medicine. This was not so much because of the vagueness and flexibility of the humoural system, but because the techniques of telling quite a complex story could be applied to a new disease. The corollary of this was that, despite new ideas within establishment medicine such as occult qualities, the practice of methodical medicine might for some writers act as a barrier to change.

Conclusion

The keystone of Galenic practical medicine in the renaissance remained the list of fevers and affections contained in the renaissance *practica*. I have traced some of the changes that occurred in the *practica*. These were concerned with the restoration of Galenic medicine, and with the development of a methodical approach to the practice of medicine which was

II

designed to codify Galenic knowledge and to show how, in a logical manner, it could be put into practice. The brief excursion into new illnesses and new explanations illustrated how the need to have a rational methodical medicine might exert a strong conservative force dampening innovation. As I have shown, the writers on the practice of medicine could be creative and were far more specific and detailed in their explanations of illness than is sometimes thought, but ultimately they were constrained by the overall qualitative theories of Galen. Innovation did exist but its only systematic development lay amongst Paracelsus and his followers.

I thank Marie and Rupert Hall and Vivian Nutton for their helpful comments when I was preparing the chapter, the participants of the Cambridge Conference for their very constructive discussion, and especially Iain Lonie for giving a great deal of help in a short time.

Notes

1 Jerome Bylebyl has written an important article, 'Teaching *Methodus Medendi* in the Renaissance' which was delivered to the second Galen Conference, Kiel, 1982. The paper gives a good introduction to the *practica* and is concerned with how Galen's *Methodus Medendi* affected the genre. I am grateful to Professor Bylebyl for allowing me to refer to the paper in its preliminary draft stage. The papers of the Kiel conference will be published. On the medieval *practica* there is Luke Demaitre, 'Theory and Practice in Medical Education at the University of Montpellier in the Thirteenth and Fourteenth Centuries', *J. Hist. Med.*, 30 (1975), 103–23 and 'Scholasticism in Compendia of Practical Medicine 1250–1450', *Manuscripta*, 20 (1976), 81–95. Demaitre's, *Doctor Bernard De Gordon: Professor and Practitioner* (Toronto, 1980) also contains rather similar material on the *practica*. C. H. Talbot, *Medicine in Medieval England* (London, 1967) has good accounts of the writers of medieval *practica*. See also N. Siraisi 'Reflections on Italian Medical Writings of the Fourteenth and Fifteenth Centuries' in J. Dauben, V. Dexton (eds.) *History and Philosophy of Science: Selected Papers*, Annals of the N. York Acad. of Sciences Vol. 412 (NY, 1983), pp. 155–68.

2 Often there would be lectures on Rhasis' ninth book *Ad Almansorem* or on the third Book of Avicenna's *Canon*. Both listed affections in a head to toe order.

3 There is confusion as to the exact bibliographical details.

4 P. Bayrus, *De Medendis Humani Corporis Malis ENCHIRIDION. Quod vulgo VENI MECUM vocant* (Basel, 1578), sig. 7r–7v.

5 *Ibid.*, sig. 5v.

6 *Ibid.*, sig. 5v.

7 John of Gaddesden, *Ioannes Angli Praxis Medica 'Rosa Anglica' dicta . . . recens edita opera ac studio . . . Phillip Schoppfii* (Augsburg, 1595), sig. 3v.

8 *Ibid.*, sig. 3v.–4r.

9 *Ibid.*, sig. 3v.

10   *Ibid.*, sig. 3r.
11   L. Fuchs, *De Medendis Singularum Humani Corporis Partium A Summo Capite ad Imos Usque Pedes Passionibus ac Febribus* (Basle, 1539), sig. 2r.
12   *Ibid.*, sig. 2r.
13   C. Gesner, *Bibliotheca Universalis* (Zurich, 1545), p. 536v., entry on Paul of Aegina.
14   Paul of Aegina had previously been translated by Albanus Torinus.
15   Paulus Aegineta, *Opera a Ioanne Guinterio . . . conversa et illustrata commentariis* (Lyons, 1551), sig. a 4v.
16   Fuchs, *De Medendis*, sig. 2r.
17   *Ibid.*, sig. 2v.
18   *Ibid.*, sig. 2r.
19   *Ibid.*, sig. 2v.
20   *Ibid.*, sig. 3r.
21   *Ibid.*, sig. 3r. The argument for local remedies can also be found in Timothy Bright's *A Treatise wherein is Declared the Sufficiencie of English Medicines, for cure of all diseases* (London, 1581).
22   D. G. Bates, 'Sydenham and the Medical Meaning of Method', *Bull. Hist. Med.*, 51 (1977), 324–38. For Bylebyl see note 1.
23   I use the terms dogmatic and rationalist interchangeably.
24   J. B. Montanus, *In Nonum Librum Rhasis ad Almansorem Regem Arabum Expositio* (Venice, 1554), p. 6. Jerome Bylebyl in his paper (note 1) has noted Montanus' condemnation of Rhasis for writing empirically.
25   J. Langius, *Epistolarum Medicinalium* (Frankfurt, 1589), p. 999.
26   H. Capivaccius, *Practica Medicina* (Frankfurt, 1594), sig. 2v.
27   *Ibid.*, sig. 2v.
28   *Ibid.*, sig. 2v.
29   *Ibid.*, sig. 4r.
30   P. Forestus, *Observationum et Curationum Medicinalium ac Chirurgicorum Opera Omnia* (Frankfurt, 1634), sig. 1v (to the reader, books 1 and 2, Leyden, 1589).
31   *Ibid.*, sig. 2r (to the reader, books 3; 5, Leyden, 1589).
32   *Ibid.*, sig. 2v (books 1–2).
33   P. Forestus, *De Incerto, Fallaci Urinarum Judicio . . .* (Leyden, 1589).
34   Forestus, *Observationum*, sig. 2r (books 3–5).
35   F. Bacon, *The Advancement of Learning* 1, IV, 5.
36   *Ibid.*, 1, IV, 2.
37   The first use of the head to toe order is given by Demaitre in his *Doctor Bernard De Gordon*, p. 55, n 103 citing C. Talbot *Medicine in Medieval England*, p. 15 who gives Pliny's *Natural History* as an early example (Talbot, despite Demaitre, does not write that the order originates with Pliny) and L. Mackinney, 'Medieval Medical Dictionaries and Glossaries, in J. L. Cate and E. N. Anderson (eds.) *Medieval and Historiographical Essays in Honour of J. W. Thompson* (Chicago, 1938), p. 243, who gives Scribonius Largus as the originator in the *Compositiones Medicamentorum*. Galen used the order in *De Locis Affectis*.
38   See how Manardi discussed whether lycanthropia existed; the fact that the Greeks did write about it was enough to justify its existence for him.

I. Manardus, *Epistolarum Medicinalium, Libri xx* (Venice, 1557), book 4, letter 5, p. 207.

39 *Articella* (Lyons, 1519), p. 363. See text at note 95 for the Galenic significance of the shin.

40 A. Massaria, *Practica Medica* (Venice, 1642), pp. 1–4. In his 'Preaefatio methodica' Massaria wrote that Rhasis 'agit . . . Empirice omnino'. I am grateful to Iain Lonie for drawing my attention to this edition and passage in Massaria's *Practica*.

41 Avicenna, *Liber Canonis* (Venice, 1544), book 3, fen 1, tract. 5, ch. 1, pp. 209v–210v.

42 Constantinus Africanus, *Operum Reliqua* (Basel, 1539), pp. 11–12.

43 Gariopontus, . . . *Ad Totius Corporis Aegritudines Remediorum* ΠΡΑΞΕΩΝ Libri V (Basel, 1531), p. 3r.

44 *Ibid.*, pp. 4r–4v.

45 Arnaldus De Villanova, *Praxis Medicinalis* (Lyons, 1586), p. 35 (second part of book).

46 John of Gaddesden, *Rosa Anglica*, p. 29.

47 *Ibid.*, p. 29.

48 Guy de Chauliac wrote of Gaddesden's work as 'Rosa Fatua'. C. Talbot, *Medicine in Medieval England* thinks better of it. Maybe I am too hard on Gaddesden – he did perceive the relativity of motion.

49 Galen's *De Locis Affectis* was known in the middle ages from a translation by Burgundio of Pisa and one possibly by Peter of Abano. See L. Thorndike and P. Kibre, *A Catalogue of Incipits of Medieval Scientific Writings in Latin* (London, 1963), col. 831.

50 Galen, *De Locis Affectis*, book 3, ch. 12 (Kühn, VIII, pp. 201–4). I have been guided in my rendering by R. Siegel's translation in his *Galen on the Affected Parts* (Basel, 1976), pp. 98–9.

51 *Ibid.*, (Kühn) p. 202.

52 *Ibid.*, p. 202.

53 *Ibid.*, p. 202.

54 *Ibid.*, p. 203.

55 *Ibid.*, pp. 203–4.

56 Aëtius, *Aetii Medici Graeci Contractae ex Veteribus Medicinae Tetrabiblos a I. Cornario . . . Conversa*, 4 vols. (Lyons, 1560), II, p. 204.

57 Paulus Aegineta, *Opera*, p. 127.

58 Aëtius, *Tetrabiblos*, pp. 204–5.

59 Galen, *De Locis Affectis*, (Kühn, VIII) p. 202, Aëtius *Tetrabiblos*, p. 205. The Greek adjectives were also the same: Galen, *De Locis Affectis*, p. 202 and Aëtius, *Librorum Medicinalium Tomus Primus* (Venice, 1534), p. 101.

60 I. Sylvius, *Opera Omnia* (Geneva, 1634), p. 405.

61 *Ibid.*, p. 405.

62 *Ibid.*, p. 405.

63 Bayrus, *Enchiridion*, pp. 45–6.

64 *Ibid.*, p. 45, referring to cutting the arteries behind the ears.

65 Fuchs, *De Medendis*, p. 23.

66 *Ibid.*, pp. 23–4.

67 *Ibid.*, p. 23.

68 *Ibid.*, p. 24; see also note 59.
69 *Ibid.*, p. 23.
70 *Ibid.*, p. 24.
71 *Ibid.*, p. 25.
72 See note 1.
73 Montanus, *Rhasis*, pp. 77r–77v.
74 *Ibid.*, p. 77v.
75 *Ibid.*, pp. 77r–78v.
76 *Ibid.*, pp. 76r–76v.
77 *Ibid.*, p. 89v. In my thesis pp. 219–24 (see note 84) I point out the importance of division for Montanus; J. Bylebyl also does this (note 1).
78 *Ibid.*, p. 89v.
79 *Ibid.*, pp. 89v–90r.
80 *Ibid.*, p. 90r.
81 *Ibid.*, p. 90r.
82 *Ibid.*, p. 90r.
83 *Ibid.*, p. 90v.
84 Montanus wrote that signs formed the bridge between universals and particulars: 'And at this point we begin to show, obscurely, how universals are applied to particulars. And around this order the medical art turns proceeding by means of signs, with which we deal at length afterwards.' The 'universals . . . are to be perceived only by the mind: consequently causes are hidden from the senses'. Causes, therefore, could not be derived from the senses but signs could indicate the cause appropriate to some particular. The causes are already present, the problem is to recognize which is the relevant one: '. . . we ought to proceed to the recognition of causes by way of a sign evident and apparent to the senses. And when that effect is perceived, since it is a particular sign and perceptible to the sense it arouses the sense then is carried back to the intellect and forms a concept in it. Then (the intellect) refers (the sign) to the hidden causes (that is, the universals) and draws an analogy, which is a certain relation (of the nature) of the particular to (that of) the universal'. The three passages come from the *Medicina Universa* (Frankfurt, 1587), p. 26, and *Opuscula Varia* (Basel, 1558), p. 112 and p. 112 respectively. I have cited these passages from my Ph.D. thesis 'Contingency and Logic in Renaissance Anatomy and Physiology' (London University, 1973).
85 Montanus, *Consultationes Medicae* (Basel, 1572), col. 77.
86 See my discussion of this issue in 'Galen in the Renaissance' in V. Nutton (ed.), *Galen: Problems and Prospects* (London, 1981), esp. pp. 239–44.
87 Capivaccio, *Practica*, p. 131.
88 *Ibid.*, p. 132.
89 *Ibid.*, p. 132 'Forma igitur vertiginis, est corrupta imaginatio, cum laesione visus et motus.'
90 A. Massaria, *Practica Medica* (Frankfurt, 1601), pp. 49–50.
91 See Manardus, *Epistolarum*, p. 76.
92 *Ibid.*, p. 77.
93 *Ibid.*, p. 77.
94 The remedies in Lange, *Epistolarum* are concerned to alleviate specific

conditions as well as underlying causes – p. 873, 'Decoctum cephalicum' to be used with appropriate pills for epilepsy, vertigo, dimness of the eyes and floaters; pp. 873–86 decoctions for pain in the teeth, cough and asthma, heat of the liver and choleric fevers, and diseases of black bile; p. 888, infusions for renal stones, for burnt humours and quartan illness; p. 890 'Syrupus Mercurialis' for headache by sympathy from the stomach and the womb; p. 899 syrup in continuous choleric fever. Here one runs through the whole range, from symptoms to internal causes/events to underlying humoural causes.

95 Montanus, *Rhasis*, pp. 89r–89v.
96 Galen went into a little more detail: the condition went from the shin to the thigh and to the ribs and then to the neck and head. Galen, *De Locis Affectis* (Kühn VIII), p. 194 (book 3, ch. 11).
97 Montanus *De Excrementis . . . Tractatus etiam de Morbo Gallico* (Paris, 1555), p. 227r.
98 *Ibid.*, p. 227r.
99 *Ibid.*, p. 227v.
100 *Ibid.*, pp. 227v–28r.
101 Montanus wrote, *ibid.*, p. 230v 'Pariter mirum non debet videri, quod ex parva pustula vel ulcusculo istius morbi venenosi inficiatur totum, si quidem inficiatur hepar, quod est principale membrum toti deserviens: quod cum fuerit ita infectum, necessarium est omnia in deterius labi.'
102 Montanus wrote, *Opuscula* (Basel, 1558), II, p. 34 '. . . quaedam vero tota substantia agere videntur, ut scammonium bilem trahens', and in *De Excrementis*, p. 235v where the reference is to occult qualities: 'Duplex est via, una per ea quae a qualitatibus manifestis operatur, alia quoque a proprietate occulta. Ac quis insurget dicens: tu ergo concedis illam qualitatem occultam sive proprietatem quam tantopere ubique vituperas? Ad hoc dico quod Galenus interdum ad illam confugit, ut exempli gratia quare Scamoneum trahat bilem.' See also a letter by Thomas Erastus: 'Quaeris post haec, an eadem sit putredo, quae ex occultis qualitatibus atque adeo a tota substantia oritur, cum illa, quae e manifesta qualitatibus', in C. Gesner, *Epistolarum Medicinalium* (Zurich, 1577), p. 21.
103 Montanus, *Opuscula*, II, p. 338.
104 *Ibid.*, p. 279.
105 See note 102 the second passage by Montanus.
106 Montanus, *Opuscula*, p. 387.
107 I. Argentarius, *De Morbis* (Florence, 1556), p. 8.
108 *Ibid.*, p. 15.
109 *Ibid.*, p. 15. See Galen, *Methodus Medendi* (Kühn X, p. 895).
110 In C. Gesner, *Epistolarum Medicinalium* (Zurich, 1577), p. 77r. Thomas Erastus wrote at length on *total substantia* in *De Occultis Pharmacorum Potestatis* (Basel, 1574).
111 C. Gesner, *ibid.*, p. 77r.
112 *Ibid.*, p. 77v. On seeds of disease see V. Nutton, 'The Seeds of Disease: An Explanation of Contagion and Infection from the Greeks to the Renaissance', *Medical History*, 27 (1983), 1–34. The wider context of the

II

issues raised by Erastus' letter are currently being studied by Dr Nutton, and he is also considering the letters of Crato von Krafftheim, Capivaccio and Erastus around these topics.

III

WILLIAM HARVEY AND THE 'WAY OF THE ANATOMISTS'

The enigma that is William Harvey has been puzzled over by successive historians,[1] and my purpose in this paper is to offer material and interpretation within a limited scope which may help to elucidate the riddle further.

Harvey's methodology, his method of knowledge, can give us a clue to what he was trying to do in *De motu cordis*. This can be gleaned from *De motu cordis* itself, from the *Second letter to Riolan* and from the opening of *De generatione*: what emerges is a consistent approach in which knowledge comes from observation, both for the original discoverer and for the reader (who has also to see with his own eyes in order to gain knowledge). Discovery and teaching thus follow the same process. The role of reason is often minor if not nugatory. It was this empiricism, in part derived from the anatomical tradition, that Harvey tried to unite with Aristotelian methodology[2] (the two were not incompatible as both agreed that knowledge came from observation). Although in this paper I am solely concerned with the anatomical influence on Harvey's methodology this does not mean that I intend challenging the Aristotelian influence on Harvey; rather, I am adding a new source for his methodology.

In the desire to see Harvey as either a devoted Aristotelian or a pure modern or, paradoxically, as both,[3] the Galenic and anatomical tradition which underlay his Paduan training and against which he at times reacted has not been properly assessed as an influence in his work. Although Gweneth Whitteridge has rightly emphasized the anatomical and observational side of Harvey, her understanding of Harvey the anatomist has been coloured by modern views of scientific method. Jerome Bylebyl, on the other hand, has given a good account of Harvey's debt to the anatomical tradition but has limited its influence only to the first part of *De motu cordis* and has placed the crucial later chapters dealing with the circulation of the blood in the context of the Aristotelian methodology of a demonstrative proof.[4] This, as I will show, is to misunderstand what demonstration meant for an anatomist like Harvey and I will argue against both Whitteridge and Bylebyl that chapters 9 to 14 of *De motu cordis* should be seen in terms of an anatomical demonstration rather than a demonstrative proof. This discussion will provide an entrée into Harvey's general methodology *qua* anatomist and at the same time help to rescue it from an anachronism. Reference to the anatomical tradition represented in the writing of Andreas Laurentius will enable us to see how it was that Harvey perceived the circulation as an observable fact and not as a theory. More generally, it should also help us to understand how Harvey came to view observation as a form of knowledge in its own right (perhaps *the* epistemological discovery of the seventeenth century) by contrast to the Aristotelian position that knowledge of causes was the only knowledge.

Finally, my analysis of Harvey's methodology will show how Harvey came to the view that observation was a type of knowledge, and how it was consonant with his role as an anatomist. More specifically, such an analysis should give credence to the idea that Harvey's demonstration of the circulation was an anatomical demonstration and not a demonstrative proof, and at the same time the analysis will develop the general point that Harvey was propounding a new view of knowledge.

THE DEMONSTRATION OF THE CIRCULATION

In her recent translation of *De motu cordis* Gweneth Whitteridge has presented the world with a picture of Harvey proceeding according to the form of the academic disputation, and using one of disputation's arguments, that of demonstration, in chapters 9 to 14 (where the evidence for the circulation is set out). She writes:

> A demonstrative proof is one that is based on observations of phenomena tested by experiment, and its validity as a method of scientific enquiry and formal argument had been recognized since Galen's time.

She has also equated this with the 'hypothetico-deductive' method.[5] According to Whitteridge in a later paper, the overall structure of *De motu cordis*

> is as follows: chs 2–7 contain the anatomical evidence on which the hypothesis will rest; each piece is described, tested experimentally and established; ch. 8 states the hypothesis which seems to account for all the evidence set out in the preceding chapters; chs 9–17 prove the hypothesis by different methods; chs 9–14 set forth the demonstrative proof of the circulation and end with a formal conclusion in ch. 14. . . .[6]

Now this is a rather surprising methodology to find in Harvey, for it would not have been acceptable either to Galen or to Aristotle. It is essentially that of an inductive process leading to a hypothesis or generalization which is then tested and proved deductively. Galen, in his writings on demonstration, considered that the ἀρχαί, the first principles or primary premises, were axiomatic and were drawn from logic, thought and observation. Where empirical ἀρχαί were to be used (sometimes drawn from dissection) they could only be ἀρχαί if they were universally agreed to at the moment of observation by properly trained observers. Empirical premises or first principles were not subject, therefore, to proof or testing.[7] The three suppositions of chapters 9–13, which, according to

Whitteridge, once proved lead to the conclusion of the circulation, would not have been recognized by Galen as being part of a demonstrative proof (because the authentication of such propositions precedes the process of proof). Furthermore, demonstration in both Aristotle (especially in the *Posterior analytics* which Harvey knew) and Galen took the form of an argument from premisses to conclusion rather than starting with a hypothesis, testing it and drawing a conclusion.[8] Whitteridge's view that the early chapters should be seen as providing an inductive account leading to an hypothesis rests on a crucial error of translation in chapter 8. Here she has Harvey say, as if looking back to the early chapters, that it was questions of the size of the arteries, ventricles and valves of the heart that led him to the circulation as well as the amount of blood leaving the heart.[9] This is not, in fact, what Harvey wrote. We can also note that in Aristotle induction did not lead to hypotheses but to definite conclusions and that Galen explicitly rejected induction.[10]

If neither Aristotle nor Galen would have recognized Whitteridge's account of Harvey's method, would Harvey himself? In what follows I want to argue that in *De motu cordis* Harvey, as in his *Anatomical lectures*, saw demonstration[11] as a pointing out, in the anatomist's sense of involving personal visual experience of what was being described, with each and everyone of Harvey's readers being expected to go personally through this process of seeing for himself.

First, some examples of differences in translation that turn upon the question of whether demonstration is a proof or whether it is an experiential confirmation. I give the Latin text, the 1653 English rendering (which Whitteridge generally follows and which I also use as it is literal and close to the Latin, albeit in seventeenth century English) and that of Whitteridge. In the Epistle Dedicatory to Dr Argent:

> Nisi prius vobis proposuissem et per autopsiam confirmassem, vestris dubiis et obiectionibus respondissem.
>
> *If I had not first propounded it to you, confirm'd it by ocular testimony, answer'd your doubts and objections. . . .*
>
> *Unless I had first laid it before you, proved it by ocular demonstration, answered your doubts and objections.*[12]

Another example of Whitteridge's showing Harvey proving things is in the heading of chapter 14 of *De motu cordis*.

> Conclusio demonstrationis de sanguinis circuitu
>
> *The conclusion of the demonstration of the circulation of the blood.*
>
> *Conclusion of the demonstrative proof of the circulation of the blood.*[13]

There is a subtle but important difference between 'demonstration' and 'demonstrative proof' and 'confirm'd' and 'proved'. From these passages and elsewhere the overall impression given by Whitteridge's translation is that Harvey wrote according to the demonstrative proof as defined by her in her Introduction.[14] That is that Harvey was engaging in an extended and connected line of reasoning involving the testing and confirmation of an hypothesis. However, the translation of 1653 renders the verb *confirmo* by 'confirm' rather than 'prove' and this supports the view that demonstration was not an extended proof but an instant and direct appeal to observation (as in the case of Galen's empirical ἀρχαί). Such a view of anatomical ἀρχαί was also held by Archangelus Piccolomini, professor of anatomy at Rome in the late sixteenth century.[15] Furthermore, each one of the suppositions of chapters 9–13 appears from the chapter headings to be intended to give the reader experiential knowledge by themselves of the circulation of the blood (i.e., chapter 12, "Esse sanguinis circuitum ex secundo supposito confirmato"),[16] rather than all three suppositions forming an extended argument for the proof of the circulation. This supports the contention that Harvey was not producing a logical proof but rather a series of observations. Chapter 9, however, seems to argue that all three suppositions have to be confirmed (Whitteridge 'proved') and then the truth of the circulation follows and the fact is apparent to everyone: "tria confirmanda veniunt, quibus positis, necessario hanc sequi veritatem et rem palam esse arbitror."[17] The *rem* that is apparent is, however, not a theory but the observation of a motion: "His [the three suppositions] positis sanguinem circumire, revolui, propelli et remeare, a corde in extremitates et inde in cor rursus et sic quasi circularem motum peragere, manifestum puto fore." By translating *positis* as "being proved" and *manifestum* as "abundantly clear", Whitteridge loses Harvey's sense of the experiential nature of what he was showing and replaces it with the idea of the *theory* of the circulation being proved.[18] Chapter 14, which describes what the suppositions had confirmed, has more of the sense of a proof but equally there is also present the descriptive ability of an anatomist demonstrating or describing what he sees in the body to his audience.[19] The suppositions of chapters 9–13, then, whether taken singly or together, show rather than prove the circulation for Harvey.

Where Harvey did talk of proof was in chapter 16 which is headed "Sanguinis circuitu ex consequentis probatur", translated in 1653 as "The circulation of the blood is prov'd [tested] by consequence".[20] Harvey's rather apologetic tone at the beginning of the chapter — "arguments *a posteriori* are not altogether useless"[21] — implies that his proof here was weaker than his confirmations in the preceding chapters (9–14). One reason may lie in the indirectness of the proof, involving as it does more reasoning in understanding how the rapid spread of snake poison through the body helps to support the circulation, in contrast with the directness of the other observations that confirm it.

In order to develop and support the contention that the demonstration of the circulation involved simply the experience of observation I will first discuss how

one of Harvey's immediate predecessors, Andreas Laurentius, viewed observation and theoretical reasoning, and then I will consider the role that Harvey
himself assigned to reason and its relation to observation. In the process of doing
this a wider understanding of the anatomists' and Harvey's views on knowledge
should emerge which goes beyond the specific question of how to interpret
Harvey's demonstration of the circulation.

ANDREAS LAURENTIUS AND THE ANATOMICAL TRADITION

Harvey wrote little about his debt to the anatomical tradition stretching back to
Vesalius and ultimately to Galen, but the anatomical books on the parts of the
human body written by men like Caspar Bauhin and Andreas Laurentius
certainly influenced him. He made extensive use of Bauhin and Laurentius in his
Anatomical lectures, and his exposure to the anatomical traditions of Padua must
have been lasting. A sign of this is that Harvey's *Anatomical lectures* begin by
detailing the nature of anatomy which, he wrote, consists of the descriptions of a
part of the body (*historia*) and then the study of its use and action; this, together
with the idea that the parts may be either "containing, contained or causing the
force for movement",[22] could be found in previous anatomical writers.[23]
Although in *De motu cordis* and *De generatione* references to the comparative
anatomy and the Aristotelianism of his immediate teacher Fabricius abound, yet
these references are generally on matters of detail and there is a paucity of
programmatic statements by Harvey concerning the general nature of anatomy
other than those to be found in his *Lectures* and in his comments on comparative
anatomy. The latter were naturally emphasized by Harvey as they were more
novel, but part of the bedrock upon which he worked, although not emphasized
by Harvey, still remained in *De motu cordis*, namely the traditional anatomist's
categories of action and use.[24]

A representative anatomist of the late sixteenth and early seventeenth
centuries is Andreas Laurentius,[25] whose *Historia anatomica* Harvey used in his
Lectures. Laurentius was no zealot in overthrowing traditional views; he favoured
Galen and opposed Aristotle's influence in medicine, and his extended discussions of the methods to be used in acquiring anatomical knowledge could be
termed main-stream conservative. An exposition of his views on anatomy can
help us to understand how Harvey could have conceived the circulation as
something to be pointed out by anatomy rather than being proved by argument,
and it can also serve as a backcloth and introduction for the discussion that
follows of Harvey's views on knowledge and his elevation of the status of
observation.

Laurentius wrote that the art of anatomy could be established in two ways: by
αὐτοψία or inspection and by instruction (*doctrina*) and that both ways were
necessary. But, Laurentius added, the first way of inspection was more certain

and was historical or descriptive (*historicus*). The way of doctrine, on the other hand, was more noble and concerned with knowledge ("ἐπιστημονικός, id est, scientificus"). Inspection, *autopsia*, was concerned with observing the internal motion of the parts of animals and men either from anatomical drawings or from the bodies themselves. The way of doctrine could be taught viva voce or by writings and it was concerned, wrote Laurentius, with the final cause or purpose of the parts of the body and this cannot be known by inspection alone ("multa enim sola inspectione sciri nequeunt, quae describenda, ut cur tot et tales sint masculi, cur talis figura, magnitudo, et similia").[26]

Laurentius was thus contrasting the greater certainty of observation with the more noble concern of doctrine to elucidate the final cause which Aristotle and Galen had stated was the ultimate goal of the philosopher. This distinction was apparent in Harvey when, as we shall see, he extolled the certainty of observation over theory both in *De motu cordis* (the "*rationibus verisimilibus*" on the purpose of the circulation in chapter 15) and in the Preface of *De generatione*.

Later in the *Historia anatomica*, in his definition of anatomy, Laurentius repeated his two-fold distinction. There was the anatomy done with the hand, πρακτική established by experience, attained by inspection and section alone, and most necessary to the art of anatomy, its object being the structure of the parts. Doctrine, taught viva voce or by writings, on the other hand, was theoretical and rational and rose above the practice of the art to enquire into the causes, actions and uses of the structures. Laurentius called the way of doctrine a 'science' ('scientiam') because it has "universal theorems and common notions out of which, as they are primary, true, immediate and more well known, demonstrations are produced".[27] The anatomists, as part of their attempt to raise the status of their subject, inevitably gave importance to inspection by stressing its certainty. Yet they could not totally escape from Aristotle's praise of those who knew the causes of things over those ignorant of causes.[28] Knowledge of causes remained nobler than knowledge of structure. Indeed, when the Aristotelian Cremonini in 1627 attacked the pretensions of the anatomists,[29] he argued that anatomy was merely a stage in the progress to knowledge of causes; an instrument of *scientia* rather than *scientia* in its own right.[30] Though knowledge came from the senses, the sense in dissection was not always certain and had to be corrected by reason.[31] Cremonini's strictures show that he was aware that the anatomists were moving to the position of seeing observational knowledge as an end in itself.

As we shall see, the structure of Harvey's thinking seems to have followed along the lines of the two-fold distinction of the anatomists. He certainly increased the emphasis on inspection but already Laurentius had claimed greater certainty for *autopsia* over doctrine. But a problem remains. Laurentius wrote that the object of anatomy was not the whole body but the parts of the body. The anatomists had divided structure into situation, figure, magnitude, number, connection and origin of the parts, and this was the subject for inspection.[32] Harvey was not setting out such information in *De motu cordis* and, moreover, although concerned with the heart as a part of the body, when he came to the circulation he was not dealing with a single part but with a complex whole, which he discussed by means of comparative anatomy and vivisection.[33] Hence it was not the *structure* of the heart *per se* that concerned him but its action, and the action and use of the circulation.

Laurentius, following Galen and the sixteenth century anatomists, divided the topics of anatomy into those of structure, action and use. In the passage cited above action, together with use, came under the sway of doctrine and theory. However, elsewhere Laurentius was ambivalent. When condemning the practice of human vivisection he argued that one could use animals rather than humans since the actions and motion of the internal parts were similar in both. He also wrote that vivisection was needed to discern action — which part is moved by what muscle — whilst the anatomy of dead bodies would discern the situation, magnitude, connection, origin of the parts. Here action is being put on a par with structure as something to be observed, the one by vivisection, the other by dissection, and he went so far as to classify some actions as '*sensificas actiones*'. In other words some actions were known by inspection just like structure.[34] Laurentius went on to distinguish action from use. Action, being a motion of the operational parts, was different from the purpose of such a motion.[35] Action was, in a sense, what a working structure accomplished, and as such it was both a subject for inspection and for doctrine.

What Harvey did in *De motu cordis* was to follow the way of the anatomists and to use *autopsia* — seeing for oneself. In his work there was no ambiguity, the action of the heart *and* of the circulation (despite Bylebyl's claims to the contrary) was solely a matter for anatomical demonstration.[36] It was only the *purpose* of the circulation that was a matter for 'theoria'. Such was Harvey's emphasis on inspection and its certainty that the 'scientia' of theory and purpose was only *verisimilis*, but that after all was what Laurentius had meant when he stated that inspection was more certain than doctrine and 'scientia'.

Historians can be a little misled by their own preconceptions. Whitteridge writes that in his *Anatomical lectures* Harvey "is far more concerned with the action and function of the parts. In modern terminology, he is not primarily an anatomist, but a physiologist".[37] True, Harvey was concerned with action, more so in *De motu cordis*, but everything that he wrote points to his inspecting action first as an anatomist rather than as a philosopher searching for causes. For Harvey theory (modern physiology) was concerned with purpose or the final cause. Of course, today, teleology has been officially consigned to the scrap-heap, and action or function is now part of theory, but for Harvey teleology, rather than action, comprised theory and was vitally important.

It should now be apparent why Harvey has been taken to have used a demonstrative proof to establish the circulation — that is what one does when establishing a theory. But Harvey saw the action as opposed to the purpose of the heart and circulation as an anatomist saw the structure of the body, that is, by *autopsia*, with one's own eyes.

HARVEY ON KNOWLEDGE

Scattered through Harvey's writing there are references to the need to observe, to the role of reason and to knowledge in general. *De motu cordis* and the *Second letter to Riolan* (1649) can broaden our understanding of Harvey's attitude to observational knowledge, and of how he saw the circulation; whilst the extended discussion of knowledge in the Preface to *De generatione*, which I discuss later on, gives us a more philosophical treatment of the issues.

In the *Second letter to Riolan*, in a passage concerned with the nature of knowledge, Harvey made the distinction between logical argument and confirmation by observation of the circulation clearer:

> Frivolous and unexperienced persons do scurvily strive to overthrow by logical and far fetch'd arguments, or to establish such things as are merely to be confirm'd by Anatomical dissection and ocular testimony. . . . So concerning the Circulation of the blood, which all have had confirm'd to them for so many years by so many ocular experiments [*Sic de sanguinis circuitu, quem tot sensibilibus ad autopsiam experimentis confirmatum*] . . . nay by ocular testimony none ever offer'd to build up a contrary opinion.[38]

Sense and not reason was the arbiter of truth. Now this was not new. The anatomists before Harvey had a similar, if not as clear cut, view and both Gweneth Whitteridge and Walter Pagel have noted the empirical and sensualist element in Harvey. What has not been noticed is that Harvey put such emphasis on personal sensory experience that he practically excluded reasoned argumentation from his criteria of how the circulation should be discovered and accepted. For, as he wrote, no-one by ocular testimony (as opposed to argument) had put forward an alternative to the circulation.

Harvey argued that all sensory knowledge had to be personally experienced and that it was not enough to be taught that something was the case by someone else:

> It behoves him, who ever is desirous to learn, to see anything which is in question, if it be obvious to sense, and sight, whether it be so or no or else be bound to believe those that have made trial, for by no other clearer or more evident certainty can he learn or be taught. Who will persuade a man that has not tasted them, that sweet or new wine is better than water? With what arguments shall one persuade a blind man that the Sun is clear, and out-shines all the Stars in the firmament? So concerning the Circulation. . . .[39]

Where arguments failed, only direct sensory experience could prevail, according to Harvey.

Harvey went on to pose, in a difficult piece of Latin which I have rendered in a conservative fashion, the dilemma of what happens when sense, data and reason are opposed.[40] He wrote that there would be no problem for dispute if "nothing should be admitted by sense without the testimony of reason or sometimes against the dictate of an accepted reason".[41] Dispute occurs when the testimony of the senses stands by itself or even against reason. However, we can think best when sense and reason are in perfect harmony, where certain knowledge comes from the senses and is confirmed by reason as in geometry which draws its reasoning from *sensibilia*. Nevertheless, the dilemma remains of what happens when sense and reason are opposed. Harvey's answer (unlike that of Copernicus) was to choose sense over reason. He resolved his dilemma by stating that "Aristotle advises us much better" ("Melius multo Aristoteles admonet") when he wrote on the generation of bees to the effect that faith is to be given to reason if it agrees with what is perceived and when the matter is fully explored (by the senses) then the senses should be trusted more than reason. For Harvey, therefore, there are times when sense can contradict reason and stand alone without its support.

We have seen that Harvey felt that 'ocular demonstration' can teach the truth of something as well as discover it, and that reason of itself was not enough. Was Harvey excluding causes, which inevitably require rational argument? Of course Harvey considered, like contemporary anatomists, the final cause but there was a distinction to be made between the fact of the circulation and its purpose, the former was known by observation the latter by reason. In the *Second letter to Riolan*, Harvey wrote that one had at times to talk of the *causes* of fevers, of plague or drugs, yet he added, because we are ignorant of these causes it does not mean that we deny their existence.[42] So also with the circulation:

> . . . this is that I did endeavour to relate and lay open by my observations and experiments and not to demonstrate by causes and approvable principles, but to render it confirmed by sense and experience, as by the greater authority, according to the way of the Anatomists.[43]

This, again, indicates that the circulation for Harvey was an observable fact and not some theoretical construct like the faculty of 'coction'. The circulation is not a theory and therefore cannot be a hypothesis (*pace* Whitteridge). Nor can one ever *see* a hypothesis.

Harvey thus placed the circulation squarely within the ambit of anatomy (he wrote that only people experienced in anatomy could perceive anatomical observations),[44] and he defined the 'way of the anatomists' in such a way that demonstration 'by causes' was excluded; instead anatomy 'related', 'laid open', 'confirmed' by the senses, observations and experiments. Furthermore, there is an implication that the method of discovery (i.e. 'laying open') is the same as that of teaching (our modern method of justification) (i.e. 'related', 'confirmed'): in order to be taught one had to discover for oneself.

From the *Second letter to Riolan* it is clear that Harvey supported ocular rather than rational demonstration, and that he felt that in order to convince Riolan, the circulation had to be grasped as a sensory phenomenon and not proved by reasoned demonstration. Also, as we have seen, there is a conjunction between 'confirm' with ocular testimony and ocular experiments, just as there was in *De motu cordis* between "confirm" and the three suppositions of chapters 9–13. This has a particular significance for our understanding of *De motu cordis*. The confirmations of Harvey's suppositions in chapters 9–13 are not a demonstrative proof in Whitteridge's sense of belonging to an impersonal Popperian Third World, where the proof once published has an independent existence in the world of knowledge and books[45] (a world that Harvey explicitly rejected). Rather, the suppositions consist of descriptions by Harvey of observations and experiments which allow the reader to see what Harvey saw, and thus to recreate in himself Harvey's knowledge. As such, experiments are confirmatory instances but are also to be personally re-experienced. They serve both to teach and to act as agents of discovery in each reader — the distinction between private and public knowledge is not present in Harvey. How Harvey justified the need for personal experience will be discussed later when I consider Harvey's epistemology in *De generatione*.

For the moment I want to gather some further evidence from *De motu cordis*. In the Epistle to Dr Argent, Harvey wrote that his opinion on the motion and use of the heart and the circulation of the blood had been "confirmed by many ocular demonstrations for nine years or more in your sight, illuminated [*illustratam*] by reasons and arguments".[46] Harvey emphasized the eyes of the observer; the many demonstrations that were ocular and not verbal. The "reasons and arguments" are separate from the ocular demonstrations of the motion of the heart and blood and presumably refer to Harvey's second category, the *use* of the heart and circulation. Harvey went on to point out that he had many reliable witnesses from the Royal College of Physicians who had agreed with his ocular demonstrations.[47] Caspar Bauhin, Harvey's main source for his *Anatomical lectures*, had also stressed the fact that he had made many dissections faithfully demonstrated to the eye ("ad oculum fideliter demonstravimus") so that many spectators were able to act as witnesses.[48] Apart from emphasizing again the role of observation in demonstration, the stress on the need for witnesses points to the lack of mechanism whereby anatomists would introduce their findings into the realm of public knowledge and could then have them taught. This may partly explain why in the main body of *De motu cordis* the experiments and observations are designed so that the reader can repeat them and observe what Harvey had observed. For instance, in chapter 10, there is an appeal to the immediate perception of the reader's eye. Harvey discussed the return of the blood to the heart and wrote that by ligating the veins of serpents or of some fishes a little below the heart

> you shall quickly see the distance betwixt the heart and the ligature to be emptied so that you must needs affirm the recource of blood, unless you will deny your own eye-sight [*nisi autopsiam neges*]. The same shall clearly appear afterwards in the confirmation [Whitteridge — "proof"] of the second supposition [*in secundi suppositi confirmatione*].
> Let us conclude, confirming [Whitteridge — "by proving"] all these things with one example [*una exemplo confirmantes concludamus*], that every one may believe his own eyes. If any one cut up a live Adder. . . .[49]

In these two experiments Harvey is appealing to the reader to repeat them, see for himself and be convinced. Here Harvey is not only anatomist and demonstrator but is also giving instruction as to how the demonstration could be repeated so that the reader could follow Harvey's footsteps and see what he had seen. Another example of Harvey giving the reader instructions as to how he could see for himself occurs after the experiment with the live adder, when Harvey explained how death could occur from too little or too much blood in the heart. Of the former he wrote:

> The *vena cava* enters the lower part of the heart, the *artery* comes out at the upper part, now taking hold the *vena cava* with a pair of pincers or with your finger and thumb, and the course of the blood being stop'd a little way beneath the heart, you shall perceive at once that place which is between your fingers and the heart, through the pulse, to be almost emptied, the blood being exhausted by the pulse of the heart; and that the heart will be of a far whiter colour, and that it is lesser too in its dilation for want of blood, and at last beats more faintly insomuch that it seems in the end as it were to die.

Harvey then shows how the heart can stop beating from too much blood and concludes:

> So now there are two sorts of death, extinction, by reason of defect and suffocation, by too great quantity; here you may have the example of both before your eyes, and confirm the truth which hath been spoken concerning the heart, by your own view [*hic ad oculos utriusque exemplum habere licet, et dictam veritatem autopsia in corde confirmare*].[50]

It would not be an exaggeration to say that the early chapters, on the action of the heart, and the crucial observations and experiments that Harvey brought forward in chapters 9–13 of *De motu cordis* to convince the reader of the circulation are similar to the one above. Harvey is saying, "If you will do so and so, then you will see for yourself that such is the case". We should take Harvey's intentions seriously, especially as his epistemology in *De generatione* confirms his attitude — there we find that knowledge in order to be true knowledge, has to be personally experienced: it cannot be gained without that experience.

A reason for being blind to Harvey's intentions is that today we see teaching as taking place by the written word through articles and books; despite the rhetoric of the repeatable experiment few are actually repeated.[51] Harvey's 'rhetoric' in *De motu cordis* helps us understand in what sense he saw himself as a discoverer or teacher. He wrote that there was no point in being taught by books (the corollary of this is that Harvey did not want his reader to be taught by *his* book).[52] Moreover, Harvey saw himself as learning from dissections and from the fabric of Nature rather than from books and the axioms of Philosophers. ("Tum quod non ex libris, sed ex dissectionibus, non ex placitis Philosophorum, sed fabrica naturae discere et docere Anatomen profitear.")[53] The image of Nature replacing books and their authority is a powerful and important one in this period. Paracelsus referred to the "books of nature" and Galileo wrote, by implication, of the Book of Nature replacing the Bible in appropriate circumstances.[54] Caspar Bauhin wrote that his anatomical institutes were proved out of the Book of Nature and the authority of Hippocrates, Aristotle and Galen.[55] Harvey went beyond Bauhin and rejected authorities in general; to him Nature was much more trustworthy than writers, and so personal knowledge of Nature had to replace public knowledge embodied in books. This belief in Nature as *the* authority is what leads Harvey to write that he teaches (*docere*) as well as learns anatomy from Nature. In order to teach Harvey must take the reader to Nature herself, hence he must be given instructions as to how he can see what Harvey had seen. Thus demonstration was a pointing out of the parts of Nature rather than the establishment of some eternal truth to be taught by books.

DE GENERATIONE

Harvey did not discuss epistemology as such in *De motu cordis* and inferences as to his theory of knowledge drawn from that book may be considered strained. Fortunately, in his Preface to *De generatione* Harvey discussed how knowledge was to be acquired in the first place and this is consistent with the hints that he gives in *De motu cordis*. The first part of *De generatione* is now thought to have been written quite soon after the publication of *De motu cordis*;[56] its views on knowledge are certainly close to the latter but as the *Second letter to Riolan*, written in 1649[57] also shows similar ideas, one must conclude that Harvey held consistent views on the matter from 1628 onwards.

The opening of the Preface repeated and elaborated some of the themes in the Letter to Dr Argent in *De motu cordis*. Harvey wrote that the false assertions of the past will instantly vanish like phantoms of the night when the light of anatomical dissection dawns upon them; nor will they require any wordy refutation when the Reader himself, with his own eyes, shall discover the contrary by ocular inspection and find that contrary conformable to reason. Then will he at the same time understand how unsafe, nay base, a thing it is to be tutored by other men's commentaries without making trial of the things themselves especially since Nature's book is so open and legible.[58]

The need for personal visual experience, and the unproblematic evidence of the Book of Nature (clearly Harvey did not have our worries about the problems of interpreting observations) confirm what Harvey had written in *De motu cordis*. What is problematic is the idea that new knowledge gained from observation is 'conformable to reason'. One might object: the previous observations had been thought to agree with reason, but now reason supports the new ones. As we shall see, Harvey appears to solve the dilemma by making reason depend upon observation rather than being independent of it.

Harvey felt that he was expounding a new method; he wrote "by revealing the method I use in searching into things, I may set before studious men a new and if I mistake not, a surer path to the attainment of knowledge".[59] He went on to say that the method was to reject the "reading of books" and "the opinions of philosophers" and "to find out that nature of things by the things themselves". This Harvey concluded is "a much more open way to the hidden secrets of natural philosophy and one which leads less into error".[60]

Other anatomists had extolled the virtues of personal observation of Nature but none went so far as to reject in principle the value of paying attention to the opinions of previous writers. Vesalius rejected Galen's opinion on specific topics as did Bauhin later on but both men, when introducing anatomy to their readers, acknowledged the value of Aristotle and Galen, though emphasizing that they loved truth more.[61] This was a common attitude among the anatomical writers and Harvey's explicit rejection of all past writers is only paralleled by writers standing on the extremes of medicine such as Paracelsus and Argentarius.[62] In practice, however, Harvey often referred to Aristotle and Galen, and Fabricius and Colombo amongst the moderns (he called Aristotle his guide and Fabricius his general).[63] Nevertheless, the reiterated rejection in both *De motu cordis* and *De generatione*, in principle, of books and of previous authors helps to explain the lack of reference to authorities when Harvey demonstrated or pointed out the circulation in chapters 9–14 of *De motu cordis*. We should not dismiss Harvey's words as the rhetoric of introductions but take them seriously, as Harvey himself did.

Harvey closed the opening section of the Preface by emphasizing how other men's opinions lead to "uncertain problems and thorny and captious questions", whilst "Nature herself must be our adviser; the path she chalks must be our walk,

III

for thus while we confer with our own eyes and take our rise from meaner things to higher, we shall at length be received into her closet-secrets".[64]

THE PHILOSOPHY FOR THE NEW METHOD

What was the philosophical justification for the new method of looking into Nature's book for oneself? How was it to be applied? Harvey gave his answer in the next two sections of the Preface, which are entitled: "Of the manner and order of attaining knowledge" and "Of the same matters according to Aristotle's opinion". At first sight Harvey appears to base his own account of how we gain knowledge upon Aristotle whom he presents as an empiricist (in the modern sense of believing that knowledge comes from the senses). But Harvey's own views on the value of personal observation and the untrustworthiness of universals keep cropping up and are at variance with the teachings of Aristotle that he quotes — despite the fact that Harvey has carefully chosen those passages that presented the empirical Aristotle.

De generatione was more theoretical and more explicitly concerned with the final cause of things than *De motu cordis* and this accounts for Harvey's concern there to describe how we arrive at universal theories. Observation of singulars for Aristotle was merely a means to the end of arriving at universals.[65] However, such was Harvey's belief in the value of observation *per se* that he elevated singulars and conversely threw doubt on the trustworthiness of universals. Like Aristotle, Harvey would have agreed that the end of investigation was to have knowledge of causes but he would have added that observation itself gave a form of knowledge.[66] In Harvey's account of knowledge in *De generatione* there is, therefore, the Aristotelian strand of seeing observation as a stage on the way to knowledge of causes and there is the Harveian (anatomical) strand of accepting observation as of value in itself, giving more certain if less noble knowledge.[67]

Harvey began by describing the two-fold Aristotelian path to knowledge. He quoted one passage from the *Physics* where knowledge proceeded from universals to particulars, from things more known to us (i.e., concrete wholes-universals) to things more knowable by nature (i.e., elements and principles of the universals).[68] The other way of knowledge, which Harvey stated came from the *Analytics*, is, in fact a generalized epitome of an Aristotelian position. Harvey wrote:

> Singulars are more known to us and do first exist according to sense, for nothing is in the understanding which was not before in the sense. And although that ratiocination is naturally first and more known which is made by syllogism, yet that is more conspicuous to us which is made by induction; and therefore we define singulars with more ease than universals, for there lies more equivocation in universals. Wherefore we must pass from singulars to universals.[69]

III

The dual progress from universals to particulars and vice versa from singulars to universals is found in the *Posterior analytics* with the first method (syllogistic demonstration) being given more weight.[70] However, the phrase "nihil est in intellectu quod non antea fuerit in sensu" is a post-Aristotelian tag, though present in embryonic form in *De anima*.[71] Its place in the passage serves to underline the importance of the senses for Harvey and for his argument. Caspar Bauhin, in support of his view that in theoretical matters the senses are confirmed by reason, had cited Aristotle to the effect that "nothing is in the sense which was not first in the intellect".[72] Harvey, on the other hand, made the senses superior to reason where the issue was a matter of fact to be decided by observation. That there is more equivocation in universals ("aequivocatio")[73] is indicative of Harvey's preference for induction beginning with singulars over syllogistic demonstration beginning from universals, but it also anticipates Harvey's argument that universals can mean different things to different people and thus, by implication, throws doubt on any conclusion derived from induction.

Although Harvey plumped for the second Aristotelian way of knowledge, from singulars to universals, he appeared to accept the first when he wrote that although the two ways seem to clash, in fact they "hang very well together".[74] This concordance was produced by emphasizing that sensation itself is a universal in that what is perceived by sight is a singular, say a yellow colour, yet that which is abstracted from it by the internal organ of sense and judged and apprehended, is a universal.[75] (A similar view can be found in the Paduan philosopher Zabarella.)[76] However, different people may see the same thing yet have different notions of it. Harvey, using the example of painting, argued that different portraits of the same subject differ from each other and from the original sitter. This is because the painters have formed an idea or universal of the sitter but in so doing the corresponding representation between the mental picture and the actual face of the subject becomes blurred[77] (i.e., there is 'equivocation').

Although Harvey was arguing in the first instance that sensation is a universal or, rather, that it produces a universal and hence universals are perceived by the senses, his comments about the blurred correspondence between the universal and reality serve not only to illustrate the equivocation of starting with universals but also must question the validity of any inductive conclusion.[78] Harvey himself was silent on the validity of inductive conclusions, but his continued comments on the weakness of universals place doubt not only on universals as a starting point of inquiry but even as its end points, after they had been derived from singulars. Harvey wrote:

Now the reason for all this is that in vision or in the act of seeing, each particular by itself was clear and distinct; but the object being removed (as if, for example you shut your eyes), this same particular is abstracted in the imagination [*phantasia*] or laid up in the memory and appears obscure and confused, nor is it any longer apprehended as a particular but as some general universal thing.[79]

Harvey's approach was to denigrate universals and to praise sensation; as long as we are seeing then the object is clear and distinct (almost a Cartesian inversion), when we shut our eyes then the image of the object goes to the imagination or memory and is abstracted by the mind to produce an "obscure and confused" universal. What Harvey has done here is to use the well known Aristotelian description of how a universal is produced from singulars (singulars, to memory, to experience, to the universal)[80] to throw doubt on universals, but this process from singulars to universals was the second Aristotelian way to knowledge and the one that Harvey seemed to favour. The reason for this contradiction is that Harvey has his own epistemology which is at variance with the Aristotelian one that he was ostensibly supporting.

Reality, as Harvey went on to emphasize, consisted in singulars; that is, the object outside of ourselves. As long as we were perceiving them we would have a clearer representation of their nature than if we conceived them in the mind. He wrote:

> ... in both Art and knowledge that which we perceive in sensible objects differs from the thing perceived and is that which is retained in the imagination or the memory. The former, the thing perceived, is the exemplar, the idea, the form informing; the latter is the representation, the εἶδος, the abstracted notion. The former again is a natural object, a real entity; the latter a resemblance or likeness, an entity of the mind. The former is concerned with a particular object and is itself a particular and an individual; the latter is a universal and common thing. In every artist and man of learning, the former is a thing perceptible to the senses, clearer and more perfect; the latter belongs to the mind and is more obscure. For what we discover by the senses is more clear and more manifest to us than that which we discover by the mind, because the latter springs from these sensible perceptions and is illuminated by them. To conclude, sensible objects are of themselves and prior to the things in the mind; these things of the mind are after them and derive from them, nor could we attain to these intelligibles at all without the help of the sensibles.[81]

The purest form of knowledge is, therefore, for Harvey, that which we have as long as we perceive. The problems of how to interpret what we see come after we have stopped perceiving, when we form ideas of what we have seen. Nowadays, it is generally agreed that even *whilst* perceiving we interpret (*cf.* the well-known drawing that can be seen as either an old woman or a young girl).[82] Aristotle, unlike Harvey, felt that sensation cannot be understood or comprehended *per se* until a universal has been formed in the mind.[83] Moreover, Aristotle did not think that universals once derived from sense data were intrinsically questionable and thus had to be constantly corrected by reference to sensory experience.[84] Of course, as in the generation of bees, conclusions derived *from reason* could be corrected by the senses.

Harvey's epistemology is on all fours with his views on the need for personal observation and on the openness of the Book of Nature which, as long as it was being observed, would not bring forward the "thorny and captious questions" of other men's opinions. The purity of sense data and the doubtfulness of universals also help to explain Harvey's emphasis that each of his readers must see for himself.

Harvey, therefore, agreed with Aristotle that knowledge came from the senses but went beyond him, though still using Aristotelian terminology, and reflected the anatomists' view that observation was a form of knowledge in its own right. When Harvey related his epistemology to his anatomy he again put forward his own brand of empiricism:

Wherefore it is that without the right verdict of the senses controlled by frequent observations and valid experience, we make judgements entirely on phantoms and apparitions inhabiting our minds. . . . We must, I say, rely upon our own experiences and not those of other men. . . . Without experience and skill in anatomy, he will no better understand me than a man born blind can judge the nature and difference of colours or one born deaf of sounds. Therefore, gentle Reader, take on trust nothing that I say of the generation of animals.[85]

Since perfect knowledge came from the senses, Harvey added, we have to see that it is "safely grounded by using frequent dissections of animals". He rejected the value of anatomical drawings which predecessors such as Vesalius, Piccolomini, Laurentius and Bauhin[86] had pragmatically supported and wrote that it was not enough to see anatomical pictures which induce "a false representation of the reality".[87]

Harvey concluded this section of the Preface by reiterating two themes explicit and implicit in *De motu cordis*: that of the need to see for oneself (which is what Harvey's whole epistemology was based on) and the idea that his experiments were consciously designed to be actually repeated by his reader, since that was the only way that the reader could gain knowledge:

It has pleased me to set down these things as a foretaste so that you may understand by what helps I myself was assisted and upon what consideration *I was induced to communicate to the world these my observations and experiments; and that you yourself, treading the same path*, may be able not only to be an impartial umpire between Galen and Aristotle, but also, laying aside all cavillings and verisimilar conjecturings, that you may find out many things as yet unrevealed to others, and perchance more precious, by embracing the practice of viewing Nature with your own eyes [my italics].[88]

The third section of the Preface is entitled "Of the same matters according to Aristotle's opinion" and indicates Harvey's awareness that previously he had been putting forward his own views. Harvey stated that for Aristotle there was no innate knowledge, it all came from the senses. The disposition of the mind by which it acquired knowledge was for Aristotle, argued Harvey, quoting the *Posterior analytics*,[89] based upon the process whereby repeated sensory impressions were lodged in the memory producing experience and out of experience proceed "universal reason, definitions and maxims, or common axioms which are the most certain principles of cognition".[90] Reason itself is therefore based upon experience and hence upon the senses. The example that Harvey gave of reason or a common axiom was the seemingly *a priori* principle that "it is impossible that the same thing under the same conditions should both be and not be".[91] So, by basing reason upon the senses, Harvey denied that reason and sense were separate and distinct from each other, and hence reason will always be 'conformable' to the senses.

Harvey did not produce further philosophical analysis of this idea, and in general in his writings reason and the senses are treated as distinct entities which should agree with each other but with the senses being superior to reason in disputed questions.[92] In the remainder of the section Harvey emphasized that we must perceive things for ourselves and not accept other people's views. Books, he argued, are no substitute for personally experienced knowledge.

> For whosoever they be that read the words of Authors and do not by the aid of their own senses abstract therefrom true representations of the things themselves as they are described in the authors words, they do not conceive in their own minds aught but deceitful eidola and vain fancies and never true ideas. And so they frame for themselves certain shadows and chimaeras, and all their theory and contemplation [*theoria sive contemplatio*] which, none the less they count knowledge, represents nothing but waking men's dreams and sick men's fantasies.[93]

Harvey here associated books with theories and perhaps it is because he so distrusted the former that he did not consider how we can arrive at certainty in our theorizing except to say that it must be founded on the certainty of our observations;[94] indeed from his previous comments it seems that Harvey had no great trust in the sureness of theories. Certainly, Harvey was concerned with showing how we arrive at knowledge of causes but at the same time he emphasized not only the value of using proper and repeated observations at the starting point of the progress to universals but also he stressed the need to use observation to confirm the validity of universals; and in general Harvey concentrated on the purity of knowledge gained by personal perception, and so gave observation status as a form of knowledge whilst he explicitly played down the reliability of universals. Yet, for Aristotle, if a universal has been properly grasped by the mind it is irrefutable; that after all was Aristotle's purpose in setting out ways of arriving at universals.[95] Harvey's epistemology is one suitable for an anatomist concerned with pointing out, 'demonstrating', what he observed inside the body (Harvey's experiments are equated by him with observations and thus do not present him with the problem of distinguishing them from observations as was the case with Realdo Colombo).[96] Harvey's practical admonitions to his reader in *De motu cordis* and the *Second letter to Riolan* are reflected in the epistemology of *De generatione* and together they throw light on what Harvey was trying to do and remind us that Harvey was an anatomist who, by giving observation a certain epistemological status, was able to reject the authority of books and of previous theories and to advise his reader to see Nature for himself — a piece of advice that Harvey himself followed in *De motu cordis*. So the paradox of Harvey the physiologist who used both ancient and modern approaches disappears to be replaced by Harvey the anatomist pointing out the observable fact of the circulation and with a matching epistemology of observation. Moreover, Harvey the physiologist is now a more understandable creature — one using Aristotelian ideas to elucidate the purpose of the circulation, rather than being a mixture of modern and ancient.

ACKNOWLEDGEMENTS

I am grateful to the following for reading earlier drafts of this paper and for their helpful comments: Jonathan Barnes, Marie and Rupert Hall, Iain Lonie, David Mannings, Vivian Nutton, the late Walter Pagel, and Roy Porter.

REFERENCES

1. Gweneth Whitteridge and Walter Pagel have produced the present but conflicting inter-pretations of Harvey. For a good appreciation of the positions of Whitteridge and Pagel see Lloyd G. Stevenson, "William Harvey and the facts of the case", *Journal of the history of medicine*, xxxi (1976), 90–97. Whitteridge is characterized by Stevenson as being concerned to present a Harvey "who was simply and solely concerned with the phenomena — the Dale-type physiologist"; whilst Pagel presents an Aristotelian Harvey "who was all his life concerned with nature's purposes, nature's ends", as well as a man "concerned with the phenomena", p. 95. The major works of Pagel on Harvey are Walter Pagel, *William Harvey's biological ideas* (Basel and New York, 1967) and *New light on William Harvey* (Basel and New York, 1976). Gweneth Whitteridge has written, as well as her translations of Harvey's work which are noted below: *William Harvey and the circulation of the blood* (London and New York, 1971).

2. Harvey's Aristotelianism has been so very well set out by Walter Pagel that it needs little discussion in this paper. Dr C. Schmitt has written a paper, to be published soon, which gives

the Latin translations of Aristotle that Harvey used and examines the general context of his Aristotelianism.

3. See ref. 1.

4. Jerome J. Bylebyl, "*De motu cordis*: Written in two stages? Response", *Bulletin of the history of medicine*, li (1977), 130–50. My comments on Bylebyl's views are not in the main text of the paper (as they would interrupt its flow) but can be found in refs 33, 34, 36.

5. William Harvey, *An anatomical disputation concerning the movement of the heart and blood in living creatures*, trans. with introduction and notes by Gweneth Whitteridge (Oxford, 1976) (cited below as Harvey, *De motu cordis*, 1976), Introduction, xvii–xix.

6. Gweneth Whitteridge, "*De motu cordis*: Written in two stages?", *Bulletin of the history of medicine*, li (1977), 130–9, p. 138.

7. Jonathan Barnes, "Galen on logic and therapy", delivered to the Second International Conference on Galen, Kiel, Sept. 1982. The Proceedings are due to be published. References are to the edition of Galen's works by C. G. Kühn, *Claudii Galeni opera omnia* (Leipzig, 1821–33). Loci given by Barnes are, on the axiomatic nature of demonstration: Galen, *De optima doctrina*, i, 52; on logical axioms: *De Hippocratis et Platonis placitis*, v, 782; on axioms expressing the τί ἐστιν of something: *De methodo medendi*, x, 27; axioms expressing the φύσις of the object: *De methodo medendi*, x, 753; and its οὐσία or essence: *De Hippocratis et Platonis placitis*, v, 593. Empirical axioms: *De Hippocratis et Platonis placitis*, v, 226 — Barnes cites *De temperamentis*, i, 590, "the principles of every demonstration are things evident to perception and to thought". The axioms are non-demonstrable: *De methodo medendi*, x, 34, and *De naturalibus facultatibus*, ii, 184; 'evident': *De cuius libet animi peccatorum dignotione*, v, 94, and *De Hippocratis et Platonis placitis*, v, 782. Empirical axioms are, writes Barnes, immediately perceived and are not subject to assessment: *De optima doctrina*, i, 49. The axioms are agreed on by all men: *De methodo medendi*, x, 32; but they must be properly trained: *De methodo medendi*, x, 42. On Galen's dislike of induction Barnes cites *Ad Thrasybulum*, v, 812, *De semine*, iv, 581, and *De simplicium medicamentorum temperamentis ac facultatibus*, xi, 469–71. I am grateful to Jonathan Barnes for allowing me to cite his paper.

8. See Aristotle, *Posterior analytics*, 71b17–72b4; for Galen see ref. 7 above.

9. A separate paper would be needed to explicate the issue. Walter Pagel has pointed out (*New light on William Harvey* (ref. 1), 3–5) that Robert Willis in his translation of ch. 8 of *De motu cordis* (*The works of William Harvey*, trans. by R. Willis (London, 1847), 45) for "Sane cum copia quanta fuerat" had inserted the phrase "When I surveyed the mass of evidence". This made the circulation appear to be the result of the investigations of the previous chapters (i.e., a quasi-inductive process). However, "copia" must refer to the great abundance of *blood* because the chapter heading is "De copia sanguinis . . ." and in the same paragraph before "sane copia quanta . . ." we have "de copia . . . sanguinis" and after it we find "quanta scilicet esset copia transmissi sanguinis". It seems clear to me that with "sane copia quanta" we should understand "sanguinis", so that it was a meditation on the great abundance of blood that led Harvey to the circulation. Whitteridge translates the passage as "Now truly, when I had many times and seriously considered with myself the varied means of searching, and how varied they were! both . . .", *De motu* (1976, ref. 5), 74. She discusses the translation in her Introduction, xli–li, but she does not bring forward any convincing evidence that "copia" on its own means what she thinks. See also Jerome J. Bylebyl, "The medical side of Harvey's discovery", *William Harvey and his age*, ed. by J. J. Bylebyl (Baltimore, 1979), 99 n. 228. For the Latin text see William Harvey, *Exercitatio anatomica de motu cordis et sanguinis in animalibus* (Frankfurt, 1628), 41.

10. Aristotle, *Posterior analytics*, 71a1–71a27,81b7,92a37–92b3, on Galen see ref. 7.

11. Whitteridge in her translation and edition of *The anatomical lectures of William Harvey* (Edinburgh, 1964), 16, translates "Demonstrare propria illius cadaveris" as "Point out the peculiarities of the particular body". The anatomists also saw demonstration as a pointing out. Bauhin

III

wrote of his discovery of the ileo-caecal valve "anno 1579, inventam et demonstratam", Caspar Bauhin, *Institutiones anatomicae* (Basel, 1609), Ad Lectorem. See also ref. 48 below where Bauhin demonstrated his findings "faithfully to the eye".

12.   Harvey, *De motu cordis* (1628, ref. 9), 6; *The anatomical exercises of Dr William Harvey* (London, 1653), 3* recto (cited below as *De motu cordis* (1653) — I have used the 1653 translation extensively, though I have amended it in one or two places — and *De motu cordis* (1976, ref. 5), 6. Franklin's translation has "description" for demonstration: William Harvey, *The circulation of the blood and other writings*, trans. by Kenneth J. Franklin (London, 1963), 87.

13.   Harvey, *De motu cordis* (1628, ref. 9), 58; (1653, ref. 12), 80; (1976, ref. 5), 107.

14.   The heading of ch. 17 of *De motu cordis* is translated by Whitteridge as "The *hypothesis* of the movement and circulation of the blood is *proved* by those things which are to be observed in the heart and by those which are to be seen in anatomical dissection", p. 120 (my italics). The Latin text of 1628 has "Confirmatur sanguinis motus et circuitus ex apparentibus in corde, et ex iis, quae ex dissectione Anatomica patent", p. 64. The English translation of 1653: "The motion and circulation of the blood is confirm'd by those things which appear in the heart, and from those things which appear in Anatomical dissection", p. 93. "Aperta demonstratio" in *De motu cordis* (1628, ref. 9), 8: "Nec turpe putant mutare sententiam si veritas suadet et aperta demonstratio", is translated by Whitteridge as "They do not think it base to change their opinions if truth and *openly demonstrated proof* so persuade them", p. 7 (my italics). Here Whitteridge, by a small change from the 1653 translation of "open demonstration", has moved from the early seventeenth century anatomist to the modern scientist.

15.   Piccolomini stated that anatomy could supply the propositions for medical demonstrations (that is, for demonstrative argument rather than anatomical demonstrations). He wrote that these anatomical propositions were similar to those notions drawn from geometry or to universally accepted ideas: "Quod autem ad demonstrationes de rebus medicis valeat, hinc constare potest, quod propositiones omnes, quae de partibus corporis aliquid enunciant, et quae inspectione et sensuum observatione, conficiuntur, sunt illae quidem, vel tanquam notiones illae, quae a geometris postulari solent, vel tanquam notiones communes, quae omnibus hominibus notae et in confesso sunt, ex quibus positis et concessis, ut pote manifestissimis et verissimis demonstrationes omnes ad medendi artem pertinentes, defluunt atque conficiuntur; quales sunt hae. Ex cerebri medulla, quae intra calvam conclusa latet, octo nervorum coniungia proficiscuntur. . . ." Piccolomini stressed that anatomical propositions were not only confirmed by sense but also that they were primary and indemonstrable (precisely the situation that, I feel, applies to Harvey's suppositions): "Et aliae pene innumerabiles sunt propositiones de partibus corporis humani, quae sensuum fide et testimonio confirmatae, omnibus sunt notae et indubitatae. Quare tanquam notiones communes habentur; Ex quibus *primis, veris, immediatis, notioribus*, conficiuntur demonstrationes, quas ars medica molitur et affert. Ad has enim tanquam ad principia firmissima, confugiendum erit, Ergo anatomes cognitio, hoc est, cognitio singularis corporis partium, et propositiones, quae de illis enunciantur, sensuum ope et constantia stabilitae ac confirmatae, sunt tanquam bases et fundamenta, medicarum demonstrationum conficiendarum. Ex quibus apte et concinne confici potest, anatomen, ex omnibus medicinae partibus, certissima esse et proportione quadam respondere mathematicis disciplinis" (my italics), Archangelus Piccolomini, *Anatomicae praelectiones* (Rome, 1586), 40–41. The claim of Renaissance anatomy to provide the foundation for the rest of medicine forms part of a paper in preparation.

16.   The relevant headings of the chapters are, ch. 9: "Esse sanguinis circuitum ex primo supposito confirmato"; ch. 10: 'Primum suppositum de copia pertranseuntis sanguinis e venis in arterias et esse sanguinis circuitum ab obiectionibus vindicatur et experimentis ulterius confirmatur"; ch. 11: "Secundum suppositum confirmatur"; ch. 12: "Esse sanguinis

circuitum ex secundo supposito confirmato''; ch. 13: "Tertium suppositum confirmatur, et
esse sanguinis circuitum ex tertio suppositum''.

17. Harvey, *De motu cordis* (1628, ref. 9), 43 and (1976, ref. 5), 78.
18. *Ibid.*
19. Harvey, *De motu cordis* (1628, ref. 9), 58: "Cum haec confirmata sint omnia et rationibus
et ocularibus experimentis, quod sanguis per pulmones et cor, pulsu ventriculorum
pertranseat, et in universum corpus impellatur et immittatur, et ibi in venas et porositates
carnis obrepat, et per ipsas venas undique de circumferentia ad centrum ab exiguis venis in
maiores remeet, et illinc in venam cavam, ad auriculam cordis tandem veniat. . . .
Necessarium est concludere circulari quodam motu in circuitu agitari in animalibus
sanguinem. . . .'' If one translates "confirmata" as "confirmed" (Willis, p. 68, "show")
rather than "proved" (Whitteridge, p. 107) then what Harvey has shown or confirmed is the
observed course of the blood which taken together makes up the circulation, rather than
demonstrating the theory of the circulation. It may be helpful to remember that the Greek
'apodeixis' (demonstration) could mean the showing or making public of something and it is
this sense that the anatomists, and I believe Harvey, retained. See J. Barnes, "Aristotle's
theory of demonstration", in *Articles on Aristotle*, ed. by J. Barnes, M. Schofield and R.
Sorabji, i (London, 1975), 78.
20. Harvey, *De motu cordis* (1628, ref. 9), 60 and (1653, ref. 12), 86.
21. Harvey, *De motu cordis* (1628, ref. 9), 60–61: "Sunt insuper problemata, ex hac veritate supposita,
tanquam consequentia, quae ad fidem faciendam, veluti a posteriore non sunt inutilia . . .''
and (1653, ref. 12), 86.
22. Harvey, *op. cit.* (ref. 11), 4–5, 8–9 and 12–13.
23. *Ibid.*, Introduction, xxxiv. The division into structure, action and use can be found in Vesalius
and the anatomists who followed him. Fabricius used the same schema, but complained that
Vesalius paid too little attention to action and use; he ascribed its origins equally to Aristotle
and Galen. The idea that parts may be either "containing, contained or causing the force for
movement" is derived, as Whitteridge notes p. 8, n. 1 and p. 12, n. 2 from Hippocrates and
adopted by Galen and cited by Bauhin. It is also present in Laurentius, *Historia anatomica*
(Frankfurt, 1602), 44.
24. See ref. 34 for whether Harvey's use of 'action' was original.
25. Caspar Bartholin joined Laurentius with Realdo Colombo and Vesalius as taking part in
"controversiis gravioribus'', Caspar Bartholin, *Anatomicae institutiones corporis humani*
(Wittenberg?, 1611), Preface, 8* recto; and Jean Riolan referred to him as "doctissimus" in
his *Anthropographia* (Paris, 1618), 54.
26. Laurentius, *op. cit.* (ref. 23), 24–27.
27. *Ibid.*, 38–39.
28. Aristotle, *Metaphysics*, 981a24–982a4.
29. Jerome J. Bylebyl has discussed Cremonini's attack on anatomy in "The school of Padua:
Humanistic medicine in the sixteenth century", in C. Webster (ed.), *Health, medicine and
mortality in the sixteenth century* (Cambridge, 1979), 363–5.
30. *Ibid.*, 363. Also Cesare Cremonini, *Apologia dictorum Aristotelis de origine et principatu membrorum
adversus Galenum* (Venice, 1627), 51, where Cremonini states that anatomy is not an art *per se*
but is for the use of another art.
31. Cremonini, *Apologia*, 49.
32. Laurentius, *op. cit.* (ref. 23), 41.
33. Jerome Bylebyl, "*De motu cordis:* Written in two stages? Response", *Bulletin of the history of
medicine*, li (1977), 140–50, has pointed this out. In this interesting article Bylebyl justifies his
view that *De motu cordis* was originally written as two separate treatises, one dealing with the
heart and the other with the circulation. He points to a switch in methodology from Galenic
anatomical discussion of the action of the heart in the earlier 'treatise' to an Aristotelian

methodology in the later, where Harvey concentrates "on the purely factual demonstration. Second, by basing his factual case on the proof of a series of propositions Harvey seems to be trying to conform to the ideal of a 'necessary or scientific demonstration' as propounded by Aristotle in the *Posterior analytics*. And third, the further distinction between 'necessary' and 'probable' arguments is also one that is quite characteristically Aristotelian" (p. 147). However, this is to misunderstand Aristotle; for the *premisses* as well as the conclusion of a demonstration are necessary (*Posterior analytics*, 74b5–75a17), they are also indemonstrable (*Posterior analytics*, 71b25–71b34). This was known in the Renaissance, see Laurentius and Piccolomini (refs 27, 15 above); and Montanus wrote that demonstration should be used in 'scientia' but not in the arts which dealt with actions and particulars "quia demonstratio ex necessariis est, concluditque necessaria, maxime igitur in scientiis requiritur" (I. B. Montanus, *Medicina universa* (Frankfurt, 1587), 12). If one has to 'prove' the suppositions of chapters 9–13 they cannot be indemonstrable and necessary. Induction, rather than demonstration might have been used by Harvey — he favoured it in the preface of *De generatione* — but in *De motu cordis* he did not use it. Finally, I should point out that Harvey saw the circulation as being the action of the heart (see ref. 36). Harvey, in other words, was still in the second part of *De motu cordis* thinking in terms of action as he had done in the first part and, as Montanus pointed out, Aristotelian demonstration was inappropriate for actions; whilst, as I have shown above, anatomical demonstration was appropriate for action in the same way as it was for structure. (I should emphasize that my comments here do not affect Bylebyl's other arguments for the two-treatise view of *De motu cordis*.)

34. Laurentius, *op. cit.* (ref. 23), 24. That Laurentius felt that action could be observed from the motion of the parts rather than inferred from structure lessens Bylebyl's claims for Harvey's originality. See Bylebyl, *op. cit.* (ref. 33), 146 where he writes: "Now it certainly represents a profound change to give accounts of 'actio' and 'usus' that are based on observed 'motus' rather than observed 'structura' and this substitution epitomises the change in physiological method with which Harvey is so closely identified. Nevertheless, strictly from the viewpoint of anatomical reportage the change is not so radical since 'vivorum dissectio' was traditionally included with simple 'dissectio' as parts of 'Anatomia'." It seems, however, that not only was vivisection included in anatomy but that the possibility of observing 'actio' from 'motus' was put forward before Harvey — of course Harvey put this into practice more extensively than anyone before him.

35. Laurentius, *op. cit.* (ref. 23), 43.

36. For Bylebyl's views see ref. 33. Harvey, *De motu cordis*, 58 (ch. 14) wrote of the perpetual motion of the blood "et hanc esse actionem sive functionem cordis". It might be objected that "sive functionem" means that Harvey was uncertain whether he was talking of action or purpose. However, 'functio' was used by Harvey interchangeably with 'actio' and had the same meaning. See Harvey, *op. cit.* (ref. 11), 22–23 where he discusses first the action of the parts and then their uses: "1. Action [*actio*] is active movement whose performing is called function [*functio*]. . . . 2. The uses. . . ." Harvey used *actio* and *functio* in tandem when discussing the action of the lung, *ibid.*, 284–5: "The action [*actio*] of the lung is therefore double and consists in movement . . . [and] in alteration that is concoction, and this I call a public action [*actio publica*]", and 290–1: "That the lungs have some public office [*publicam functionem*] . . . it is evident that concoction is the second function of the lungs [*esse secondam functionem*]. Their chief function is movement [*Praecipua functio motus*] and their principal part, first and foremost, is constituted by the bronchi. According to the opinion of the physicians, both movement and concoction are the actions of the lungs [*Actio*]." That Harvey wrote of the action and function of the lungs interchangeably and did not take *functio* to mean purpose is made even more certain by his going on to discuss, separately, the *utilitates vel usus* of the lungs. Another passage in the *Anatomical lectures* showing the identity of meaning of action and function is in pp. 124–7. Perhaps more significant is the heading of chapter 5 of *De motu*

cordis, "Cordis motus actio et functio", but in the chapter itself only *actio* is mentioned so that *functio* must have meant the same as *actio* for Harvey, otherwise we should have had a separate section in the chapter devoted to *functio*. Chapter 5 of *De motu cordis* is also interesting in that it parallels chapter 14; one of the actions of the heart in chapter 5 being the transmission and propulsion of blood through the arteries to the extremities ("et una actio cordis est ipsa sanguinis transfusio, et in extrema usque, mediantibus arteriis propulsio"), *De motu cordis*, 1628 (ref. 9), 30. This supports the view that what Harvey was doing in chapters 9–13 was indeed to demonstrate or show the *action* of the heart, in other words the transmission of blood to the extremities and its circulation back again, and that he had not moved from a consideration of action in the first part of *De motu cordis* to a demonstrative proof in the second as Bylebyl states.

37. Whitteridge, *op. cit.* (ref. 1), 19.

38. Harvey, *Exercitationes anatomicae* (London, 1661), 180–1. English translation, *Two anatomical exercitations concerning the circulation of the blood* (London, 1653), 67–68.

39. Harvey, *Two anatomical exercitations* (ref. 38), 87, and *Exercitationes anatomicae* (ref. 38), 181.

40. The Latin of the whole passage is as follows: "Si nihil admitteretur per sensum sine rationis testimonio, aut contra quandoque rationis receptae dictamen, jam nulla essent problemata disputanda. Si non certissima per sensum fides foret, eaque ratiocinando stabilita (ut in suis constructionibus Geometri solent) nullam perfecto admitteremus scientiam: quippe, ex sensibilibus de sensibilibus demonstratio rationalis Geometrica est. Ad cujus exemplar, abstrusa et a sensu remota, ex apparentibus manifestioribus et notionibus innotescunt. Melius multo Aristoteles nos admonet (lib. 31 de gener. anim.) de generatione Apum disputans; 'rationi fides adhibenda', inquit, 'si quae demonstrantur, conveniunt cum iis, quae sensu percipiuntur, rebus: quae cum satis cognita habebuntur, tum sensui magis credendum quam rationi' ", *Exercitationes anatomicae* (ref. 38), 182. The second sentence could be translated as "If our faith through sense were not most certain, and if faith were to be established/assured by reasoning (as the geometricians usually do in their constructions) we would admit no science at all". Willis translated the sentence as "Had we not our most perfect assurances by the senses and were not their perceptions confirmed by reasoning, in the same way as geometricians proceed with their figures, we should admit no science of any kind (Harvey, *The works* (ref. 9), 131). However, 'si' governs both clauses, otherwise Harvey would have written 'nisi'. If my translation is correct then Harvey would be saying that knowledge established by reasoning alone would not be knowledge, which is a radical view but consonant with the context. However, of six classicists consulted, the vote was three to two with one abstention in favour of the rendering in the main text of this paper. The 1653 translation tends to support my translation in this footnote: "If our most certain authors were not our senses, and these things were to be established by reasoning, as the geometricians do in their frames, we should truly admit of no science", p. 69.

41. Harvey, *Two anatomical exercitations* (ref. 38), 69.

42. *Ibid.*, 71.

43. *Ibid.*, 74. The Latin reads "Denique hoc est, quod enarrare et patefacere, per observationes et experimenta conabar, non ex causis et principiis probabilibus demonstrare, sed, per sensum et experientiam, confirmatam rederre, anatomico more, tanquam majore authoritate, voluin", *Exercitationes anatomicae* (ref. 38). 187.

44. Harvey, *Two anatomical exercitations* (ref. 38), 70: "A man that is not expert in anatomy, in so far as he cannot conceive the business with his own eyes and proper reach, in so far is thought to be blind to learning, and unfit; for he knows not truly anything concerning which an anatomist disputes. . . ." See also p. 68.

45. See Karl Popper, *Objective knowledge* (Oxford, 1973), 102–7 and *passim*.

46. Harvey, *De motu cordis*, 1653, *2 verso; 1628, 5: "Meam de motu et usu cordis et circuitu sanguinis sententiam E.D.D. antea saepius in praelectionibus meis Anatomicis aperui novam: sed iam

per novem et amplius annos multis ocularibus demonstrationibus in conspectu vestro confirmatam, rationibus et argumentis illustratam."

47. Harvey, *De motu cordis* (1628, ref. 9), 6: "e vobis plurimos et fide dignos appellare possum testes, qui dissectiones meas vidistis et ocularibus demonstrationibus eorum quae hic ad sensus palam assevero, assistere candide et astipulari consuevistis."

48. Caspar Bauhin, *De corporis humani fabrica* (Basel, 1590), Preface, second page.

49. Harvey, *De motu cordis* (1653, ref. 12), 57–58; (1976, ref. 5), 86.

50. Harvey, *De motu cordis* (1653, ref. 12), 58–59; (1628, ref. 9), 47–48.

51. The recent scandals in America of false experimental results and the delay in discovering them are an indication of this.

52. On Harvey's own books see William Harvey, *Disputations touching the generation of animals*, trans. with introduction and notes by Gweneth Whitteridge (Oxford, 1981), 16–17: "Give me leave, therefore, gentle Reader, to whisper in your ear that what things soever I discuss in these my Disputations touching the generation of animals, you weigh them in the exact scale of experience, and no further give them credit than you perceive them to be most securely bottomed by the most faithful testimony of your own eyes."

53. Harvey, *De motu cordis* (1628, ref. 9), 8.

54. See *Letter to the Grand Duchess Christina* and also *The assayer*: "Philosophy is written in this grand book, the universe, which stands continually open to our gaze". Galileo added that the language of the book was mathematics. Galileo, *Discoveries and opinions of Galileo*, trans. with introduction and notes by Stillman Drake (New York, 1957), 177–216 and 237–8. For Paracelsus's use of the Book of Nature theme see W. Pagel, *Paracelsus* (Basel, 1958), 56–57.

55. Bauhin, *op. cit.* (ref. 11), a3 verso, Ad Lectorem: "non solum ex lectione Veterum et Recentiorum, sed ex ipso naturae libro ex Dissectionibus plurimis."

56. On the dating of *De generatione* see Robert G. Frank Jr, *Harvey and the Oxford physiologists* (Berkeley, 1980), 34–37. Frank does not explicitly discuss the dating of the Preface. Also C. Webster, "Harvey's *De generatione*: Its origins and relevance to the theory of circulation", *British journal of the history of science*, iii (1967), 262–74.

57. Whitteridge has argued forcibly that the *Second letter to Riolan* was written before the first and before Riolan's *Encheiridium* (1649) and was originally written as a general defence of *De motu cordis*, Whitteridge, *op. cit.* (ref. 1), 186–8.

58. Harvey, *op. cit.* (ref. 52), 8.

59. *Ibid.*, 9.

60. *Ibid.*, 9.

61. Bauhin, *op. cit.* (ref. 11), a4 verso, Ad Lectorem: "attamen ut clarum fiat omnibus, Hippocratem Aristotelem et maxime Galenum, in studio hoc Anatomico consumatissimos esse: et quo ostendamus liquido nos dependere ab eorum auctoritatibus, quantum quidem veritas permittit et ubi oculi non solum mei, sed recte quoque videntium contrarium non docent. (Amicus enim Hippocrates, amicus Aristoteles, amicus Galenus, sed magis amica VERITAS)." The sentence in brackets is a version of a scholastic tag going back ultimately to an ancient life of Aristotle and deriving from *Nicomachean ethics*, 1096a13–17 and Plato's *Republic*, x, 595. See H. Guerlac, "Amicus Plato and other friends", *Journal of the history of ideas,* xxxix (1978), 627–33. Guerlac wonders when the aphorism started to include Aristotle instead of, or as well as, Plato and Socrates, the earliest that he has found is Charleton in 1654. Bauhin would therefore interest him as coming earlier. Vesalius called Galen "after Hippocrates the prince of medicine" but he criticized Galen for errors in human anatomy — over two hundred, and praised those who "put more faith in their not ineffectual eyes and reason than Galen's writings". At the same time, Vesalius saw his job as not only to correct Galen's errors but also to bring to posterity an understanding of those books of Galen requiring the aid of a teacher. C. D. O'Malley, *Andreas Vesalius of Brussels 1514–1564* (Berkeley, 1965), 317, 321 and 323, trans. from A. Vesalius, *De humani corporis fabrica* (Basel,

1543), *2 recto, *3 verso and *4 recto. The point is that Vesalius was writing with one eye on Galen all the time, whilst Harvey wanted to write without constant reference to the past.

62. Argentarius wrote of the practice of stitching books together from the opinions of other men rather than using our own reason and senses, Argentarius, *In artem medicinalem Galeni commentarii tres* (Mondovi, 1566), 9. This is echoed in Harvey when he writes that he is not concerned with other men's opinions (Letter to Dr Argent) and in the Preface to the *Generation of animals* (ref. 52), 16: "Hence it is that sophisters and half-knowing men, pillaging other men's discoveries, boldly arrogate them to themselves. . . ."

63. Harvey, *op. cit.* (ref. 52), 20.

64. *Ibid.*, 10.

65. I am grateful to Dr Andrew Cunningham for reminding me of this. He should not be held responsible for the views that follow.

66. Strictly speaking, for Aristotle, knowing anything requires a grasp of causes. See Aristotle, *Aristotle's posterior analytics*, trans. with notes by Jonathan Barnes (Oxford, 1975), notes 96–97, and G. Patzig "Erkenntnisgrunde, realgrunde und erklarungen (zu anal. post. A13)" in E. Berti (ed.), *Aristotle on science: The Posterior analytics* (Padua, 1981), 143–56.

67. On Aristotle's view that knowledge of causes was the end of philosophy see *Metaphysics*, 981b13–982a7.

68. Harvey, *op. cit.* (ref. 52), 10; Aristotle, *Physics*, 184a16–184a25.

69. Harvey, *op. cit.* (ref. 52), 10.

70. On induction and demonstration in the *Posterior analytics* see refs 8 and 10.

71. See Pagel, *William Harvey's biological ideas* (ref. 1), 35. Dr Pagel kindly referred me to Bonaventure, *Sententiae*, II, dist. 24, p. 2, art. 2, quaest. 1, and Thomas Aquinas, *Summa theologica*, I, quaest. 84, art. 6. The opinion can also be found in Averroes's *Tahafut al-Tahafut*, trans. from the Arabic with introduction and notes by Simon Van Der Bergh (London, 1978), 354, where Averroes quoted al-Ghazali to the effect that "According to us nothing inheres in the intellect but what inheres in the senses". The tag derives from Aristotle, *De anima*, 432a7.

72. Bauhin, *op. cit.* (ref. 11), a3 verso, argued that reason as well as sense is necessary when discussing the use of organs as opposed to their structure: "Verum non sufficiebat hac notasse, nisi particularum omnium usus et cuius nomine conditae et creatae sint, esset perspectus: quare usum subiunximus qui non solum a sensu desumendus, licet is praecedere debeat, sed et ratione confirmandus: nil enim ut habet Philosophus 2 [corrected to 3 in later edns] de anima, est in sensu, quod non prius fuerit in intellectu: cuius nomine Medicus artifex sensatus nominatur."

73. Aristotle, *Posterior analytics*, 97b30 had written that particulars are easier to define than universals as ambiguities escape detection more easily in the latter.

74. Harvey, *op. cit.* (ref. 52), 10.

75. *Ibid.*, 11.

76. Zabarella, *Opera logica* (Cologne, 1597), 994, *In duas Aristotelis libros posteriores analyticos commentarii* writes: "Mihi videtur cum multis discendum esse, Aristotelem notare differentiam inter sensum et sentire: nam sensus, id est ipsa sentiendi facultas respecit obiectum universale, ut visus colorem, sed non hunc colorem." See Aristotle, *Posterior analytics*, 100a17.

77. Harvey, *op. cit.* (ref. 52), 11.

78. Significantly, Harvey did not consider how by 'nous', the mind or intuition, we grasp the universal from the particulars. Sanctorius following the traditional interpretation of the end of the *Posterior analytics*, had written that no number of particulars can lead to a universal conclusion, it has to be grasped by the 'light of the mind', Sanctorius, *Methodi vitandorum errorum omnium qui in arte medica contingunt* (Venice, 1603), 188v–189r. Perhaps Harvey was silent on the matter as it would have given the mind a function independent of the senses. On this see also ref. 91 and text.

79. Harvey, *op. cit.* (ref. 52), 11.
80. See Aristotle, *Posterior analytics*, 100a1–100a10; also *Metaphysics*, 980a25–981b9.
81. Harvey, *op. cit.* (ref. 52), 12.
82. See N. R. Hanson, *Patterns of discovery* (Cambridge, 1965), 11–19.
83. Pagel, *William Harvey's biological ideas* (ref. 1), 32 cites Aristotle, *Posterior analytics*, 87b28 which is translated by Barnes in his version of the *Posterior analytics* (Oxford, 1975), 46: "Nor can one understand through perception. For even if perception is of what is such and such, and not of individuals, still one necessarily perceives an individual and at a place and at a time, and it is impossible to perceive what is universal and holds in every case."
84. See Aristotle, *Posterior analytics*, 100b6–100b13, understanding and comprehension are 'always true'.
85. Harvey, *op. cit.* (ref. 52), 13.
86. Andreas Vesalius, *Fabrica*, *4 recto. Archangelus Piccolhominus, *Anatomicae praelectiones* (Rome, 1586), To the reader, 2nd–3rd pages, wrote of the need for realistic drawings. Andreas Laurentius, *Historia anatomica*, 24–25 wrote that pictures were not altogether vain and futile because they could communicate hitherto unknown information and could make good a lack of cadavers. Laurentius concludes, however, that nothing can replace the actual practice of dissection.
87. Harvey, *op. cit.* (ref. 52), 13.
88. *Ibid.*, 13, my italics.
89. Aristotle, *Posterior analytics*, 100a4–100a10.
90. Harvey, *op. cit.* (ref. 52), 15.
91. *Ibid.*, 15.
92. Harvey in practice often made reason appear to follow necessarily from observation. See Pagel, *William Harvey's biological ideas* (ref. 1), 41 and 41, n. 77 for loci and also see ch. 11 of *De motu cordis* on ligatures. The paradox of seeing reason both as separate from the senses and as derived from the senses originates, of course, from Aristotle and his reaction to Plato.
93. Harvey, *op. cit.* (ref. 52), 16.
94. *Ibid.*, 13, "solid and certain knowledge" requires frequent observations.
95. See ref. 84.
96. Colombo in his chapter on the lungs in *De re anatomica* had placed his experiments on pulmonary blood flow after the traditional sections of structure, action and use; in other words he did not integrate them into the traditional format of the anatomy books. This was not a problem for Harvey as he was not writing a traditional anatomy text book.

IV

Making sense of health and the environment in early modern England

Meanings of health and illness

Most of the chapters in this volume concentrate on medicine, its theories, organization, relations with the state and its general place in society. It is clear from them that 'medicine' has to be taken in a very wide sense, and its history is not just that of a limited, elite group of practitioners but encompasses many other groups in society (for instance the patients of the previous chapter). What is also obvious is that the ways in which health and illness were made sense of extend well beyond any single account of the theories of medical practitioners. In early modern England (1550–1750) some aspects of life which today are strongly 'medicalized' (under the control of doctors and medicine) were then less influenced by medicine, especially that of the elite or 'learned' medicine of the university-trained physicians. Childbirth and death were two such important events. Conversely, we might expect that the environment, the context in which all the stages of life took place, would not be related very closely to health in this period. After all, it was in the nineteenth century that the hygienic and sanitary revolutions took place, and it might seem that only in recent years has the environment been valued in its own right. However, in early modern England there were clear ways of making sense of the relationship between health and the environment. In this chapter I will first briefly sketch out an argument for putting the medical theories of this period into a social, economic and religious framework, and so lessening the sense that they are autonomous and separate from society. This will make it easier to understand how

Note : The editions of sixteenth- and seventeenth-century works that I have used are often later than the first edition.

childbirth and health, whose histories I also briefly discuss, were often placed into non-medical settings. The major part of the chapter deals with perceptions of health and the environment; less has been written on this and the topic deserves more extensive treatment. The emphasis will be on the ways in which meaning was given to significant aspects of health and illness.

Medical theories

Medical theories underwent radical change at this time. At the beginning of the period (1550) learned medicine, that is the medicine taught in the universities and practised by the Fellows of the London College of Physicians, was based on the classical authority of Galen and described the body in humoral, qualitative terms. At the end of the period (1750) Galenic medicine was in decline and had been replaced by chemical and mechanical explanations of the body. During the Civil War and Interregnum Paracelsian medicine, with its stress on chemical explanations of disease and chemical remedies, and with its radical opposition to Galenic learned medicine, became popular with the sectarian reformers of medicine. They felt that it provided the appropriate aetiological and therapeutic body of knowledge (its roots being popular rather than traditional and learned) for a new type of Christian, charitable medicine that would be available to all, especially the poor.[1] Politics and medicine were clearly connected. However, the most radical change in medical theory was produced by 'the scientific revolution' of the seventeenth century when a new natural philosophy (later called physics) and chemistry replaced the Aristotelian world of the four causes, four qualities and four elements (the four humours of the body being the analogues to the elements that made up the world).[2] This 'new science' was based on the idea that the world and the body were alike made from particles of matter of different sizes, shapes and motions. Although the theoretical shift appears to be very radical, for medicine this was less so. In the last three decades of the seventeenth century and during most of

[1] See Charles Webster, *The Great Instauration: Science, Medicine, and Reform 1626–1660* (London, 1975); for a revisionary view see Peter Elmer 'Medicine, Religion and the Puritan Revolution', in Roger French and Andrew Wear (eds.), *The Medical Revolution of the Seventeenth Century* (Cambridge, 1989), pp. 10–45.
[2] Put simply the four causes were the material, formal, efficient and final cause. A statue, for instance, was made of material (marble), it was given form (the formal cause) by a sculptor (the efficient cause) who had a purpose in mind (the final cause). The four qualities were hot, cold, dry, moist; in combination they produced the elements, water (moist and cold), earth (dry and cold), air (moist and hot), fire (hot and dry). The humours were phlegm (moist and cold) blood (moist and hot), yellow bile (hot and dry), black bile (dry and cold).

Health and the environment in early modern England

the eighteenth century there was a proliferation of new theories –
iatrochemical, iatromechanical, iatromathematical – but they did not
improve life expectancy nor did they produce better cures than the old
Galenic ones. Indeed, a case can be made that most of medicine remained
unchanged.[3] For instance, many therapeutic procedures such as the use
of bleeding, cupping, purging, the emphasis on diet and regimen (which
was especially present in learned medicine) retained their popularity
throughout the period; the one major change being that chemical
remedies came increasingly to the fore. Moreover, the existence of a
large number of empirics at the end of the seventeenth century who used
a variety of theories, often mixing Galenic with newer chemical and
mechanical ones, indicates that medical theories often were employed
more as a means of gaining patients (the appeal of traditional scholarly
learning, the attraction of the latest most fashionable philosophy) than
for any desire to identify any 'truth'.[4] The changing theories of medical
practitioners are most appropriately placed within the changing
commercial structure of the medical market place as described in the
previous chapter. If political and commercial considerations influenced
the type of medical knowledge that practitioners chose, then this is an
indication that medical theories of whatever type did not enjoy an
autonomous existence as 'objective' knowledge independent of society,
and that claims for their universal acceptance would fail.

   There is, in fact, much more to the meaning of health and illness than
the story of how learned medical theories changed. In the early modern
period, professional medicine with its strong claims to authority and
monopoly in medical matters had not come into existence, the types of
knowledge that could be used to make sense of health and illness went
beyond medicine to include magic, witchcraft and religion as well as lay
or folk medical knowledge. The decline in magic throughout the
seventeenth century, which has been traced by Keith Thomas in his
magisterial *Religion and the Decline of Magic*, and the secularization that
occurred after the Restoration of Charles II in 1660 meant that magical
and religious explanations of illness became less widespread. For instance,
the Anglican establishment of the Restoration attacked the 'enthusiasm'

[3] See Andrew Wear, 'Medical Practice in the late Seventeenth and early Eighteenth-Century
England: Continuity and Union', in R. French and A. Wear (eds.), *Medical Revolution*, pp. 294–320.
One new effective remedy was Chinchona bark (later 'quinine') which was used for fevers (it
worked against malaria); this was a plant and not a chemical remedy.
   [4] On empirics see Roy Porter, 'The Language of Quackery in England 1660–1880', in P. Burke
and R. Porter (eds.), *The Social History of Language* (Cambridge, 1986), pp. 73–103; Roy Porter,
Health For Sale. Quackery in England 1660–1850 (Manchester, 1989).

of the religious sects that flourished during the Civil War and in the Interregnum. Therefore recourse to God to explain physical illness as providential or madness as possession became suspect.[5] Such explanations were still used amongst non-conformist groups such as Quakers through the eighteenth century, but overall significant changes did occur in the non-medical meanings given to health and illness.

Birth and death

Two aspects of the life cycle, birth and death, which today are strongly medicalized, at the start of the period were very much in lay and religious hands, but as we come to the end of the seventeenth century the medicalization of birth increased and later it did for death as well. Adrian Wilson has shown[6] that in the early seventeenth century birth was an all female ceremony orchestrated by the midwife who was accompanied by the pregnant woman's friends and neighbours, the gossips. Men were excluded from the house during the birth. Only when there was a complication during labour was a male practitioner brought in and then normally only to extract or dismember the dead foetus.[7] At the end of the seventeenth century and the beginning of the eighteenth men became increasingly involved in delivery. Men midwives such as William Giffard claimed that their knowledge of anatomy enabled them to 'touch', and explore, the womb and to reposition the foetus to ensure that it would be born alive.[8] Additionally, in the early eighteenth century the public became aware of the use of the forceps (they had been

[5] See the conclusion of Michael MacDonald's, *Mystical Bedlam* (Cambridge, 1981) where he argues that the period from the Restoration to the end of the eighteenth century was a 'disaster for the insane.' Also Michael MacDonald, 'Religion, Social Change and Psychological Healing in England 1600–1800', in W. J. Shiels (ed.), *The Church and Healing* (Oxford, 1982), pp. 101–25; David Harley, 'Mental Illness, Magical Medicine and the Devil in Northern England, 1650–1700', in French and Wear (eds.), *Medical Revolution*.

[6] Adrian Wilson, 'Participant or Patient? Seventeenth Century Childbirth from the Mother's Point of View', in R. Porter (ed.), *Patients and Practitioners: Lay Perceptions of Medicine in Pre-Industrial Society* (Cambridge, 1985), pp. 129–44; but see also his 'The Ceremony of Childbirth and its Interpretation', in Valerie Fildes (ed.), *Women as Mothers in Pre-Industrial England* (London, 1990), pp. 68–107, where he rejects his former interpretation of childbirth as a rite of passage, he now sees it as an example of the 'world turned upside down' and as reinforcing the cohesion of women's culture.

[7] See the essays by Adrian Wilson, 'William Hunter and the Varieties of Man-Midwifery' and by Edward Shorter, 'The Management of Normal Deliveries and the Generation of William Hunter', in W. F. Bynum and Roy Porter (eds.), *William Hunter and the Eighteenth-Century Medical World* (Cambridge, 1985), pp. 343–69 and 371–83 respectively.

[8] See William Giffard, *Cases in Midwifery* (London, 1734). Giffard constantly contrasted his knowledge of anatomy and technique with the lack of it in the midwives whose mistakes, he claimed, he was constantly being brought in to correct.

Health and the environment in early modern England

a secret of the Chamberlen family throughout the previous century). Although forceps were not employed by all men midwives, female midwives were particularly discouraged from using them and this further downgraded their status. By the middle of the eighteenth century, men increasingly took charge of normal deliveries (though female midwives still delivered the majority of women) as well as being brought in as a matter of course for complicated deliveries. Historians are not agreed on the reasons why the childbirth scene changed from a female social ceremony (together with female expertise) to a male technical operation. Some feminist historians have seen the changeover as a deliberate male takeover of a female activity, as an attempt to have male control of all of medicine, an attempt which makes the female midwife subservient to the male practitioner and which begins the process whereby men assert the right, through claims of education and technological expertise, to control and manipulate women's bodies.[9] Other interpretations have pointed out that women themselves began increasingly to prefer male midwives and that fashion was important in getting male midwives accepted. In commercial eighteenth-century England a 'trickle-down' effect occurred whereby the elite levels of society influenced those lower down, and geographically as London led, the provinces followed.[10] The acceptance of male midwives is seen to fit this process. Additionally, the rational and scientific ethos of the eighteenth-century Enlightenment, in which the ideas of the natural were changing and the body was seen increasingly as a machine, may have allowed the presence of the men midwives to become more acceptable, since they claimed a superior knowledge and technical skill which was not possessed by women midwives. This is a point that appears to have been accepted by women. (Or, perhaps, as some women writers at the time implied, women preferred men to women.)[11]

None of the interpretations is completely satisfactory, all of them have been placed into larger interpretations with limited concrete evidence of

[9] See B. Ehrenreich and D. English, *Witches, Midwives and Nurses* (New York, 1973) and their, *Complaints and Disorders: the Sexual Politics of Sickness* (New York, 1974); Jean Donnison, *Midwives and Medical Men. A History of Interprofessional Rivalries and Women's Rights* (London, 1979).
[10] See, for instance Adrian Wilson, footnotes 6 and 7 above; Roy Porter, 'A Touch of Danger: the Man-midwife as Sexual Predator', in G. S, Rousseau and R. Porter (eds.), *Sexual Underworlds of the Enlightenment* (Manchester, 1988), pp. 206–32; Dorothy and Roy Porter, *Patient's Progress. Doctors and Doctoring in Eighteenth-Century England* (London, 1989), pp. 172–7; for the view that the man midwife represented a positive gain in health terms see E. Shorter, *A History of Women's Bodies* (London, 1983).
[11] See Sarah Stone, *A Complete Practice of Midwifery* (London, 1738), pp. xi–xii, on the 'finish'd assurance' of 'young Gentlemen-Professors'.

why women altered their choice over who delivered them. Nevertheless, it is clear that the meaning of childbirth changed.

Death also was a largely non-medical ceremony in the sixteenth and in the first half of the seventeenth century.[12] There were differences at the deathbed between Protestant and Catholic countries. For instance, the Catholic anointing with holy oil, the giving of the sacraments and the deathbed confession were viewed as Papist superstitions by many Protestants who believed the age of miracles was past.[13] But both religions insisted that a priest or minister should be in charge at the deathbed, the medical practitioner having departed when it was clear that no more could be done medically.

The process of dying was part of social life. Family and friends were present together with the minister to give the dying person encouragement at the moment when the temptations of the devil were at their greatest, and when the powers of good and evil fought for the soul of the dying. To help the dying meet the challenge books explaining the art of dying (*Ars Moriendi*) had been published from the Middle Ages onwards. Additionally, the dying had to give outward signs that they had died well. They were in a sense actors, who by showing calmness, rationality, fortitude, faith, forgiving their enemies and welcoming death and the chance of making the transition to heaven died 'a good death'. These actions gave the onlookers hope and expectation that the dying person had gone to heaven.[14] The public and religious nature of the

---

[12] On the history of death see Phillipe Ariès, *The Hour of our Death* (London, 1983); Michel Vovelle, *La mort et l'occident de 1300 à nos jours* (Paris, 1983); David E. Stannard, *The Puritan Way of Death* (New York, 1977); Gordon E. Geddes, *Welcome Joy, Death in Puritan New England*, Studies in American History and Culture; no. 28 (Ann Arbor, 1981); John McManners, *Death and the Enlightenment* (Oxford, 1981).

[13] William Perkins, the puritan theologian, condemned the anointing with holy oil as 'this greasy sacrament of the Papists' writing that 'anointing of the body was a ceremony used by the Apostles and others, when they put in practise this miraculous gift of healing which gift is now ceased', William Perkins, *A Golden Chaine* (London, 1612), p. 501. For a discussion of puritan attitudes in England to death see Andrew Wear, 'Puritan Perceptions of Illness in Seventeenth Century England', in Porter (ed.), *Patients and Practitioners*, pp. 55–99, especially pp. 64–70.

[14] John Donne in his 'Sermon of Commemoration of the Lady Danvers, Late Wife of Sir John Danvers, 1627' expressed the conventional actions expected of the dying: 'And in that forme of Common Prayer, which is ordain'd by that Church ... she joyn'd with that company, which was about her death-bed, in answering to every part thereof, which the Congregation is directed to answer to, with a cleere understanding, with a constant memory, with a distinct voyce, not two houres before she died ... Wee lost the earthly Paradise by death then; but wee get not Heaven, but by death, now. This shee expected till it came, and embrac't when it came. How may we thinke, shee was joy'd to see that face that Angels delight to looke upon, the face of her Saviour, that did not abhor the face of his fearfullest Messenger, Death? Shee shew'd no fears of his face, in any change of her owne; but died without any change of conternance or posture; without any struggling, any disorder; but her Death-bed was as quiet as her Grave.' John Hayward (ed.), *John Donne, Complete Poetry and Selected Prose* (London, 1929), pp. 574–5. For a discussion of the death-

Health and the environment in early modern England

deathbed was far different from today's medicalized death, which in western countries often takes place in medical institutions such as hospitals. The emphasis on the welcome transition from this world to the other world and its rational performance also militated against trying to concentrate on extending the last moments of life or on deadening the agonies of death.

The religious stress upon dying appears to have lessened in the second half of the seventeenth century. The Anglican Jeremy Taylor wrote that the struggle between good and evil did not occur in a special way at death but throughout life.[15] As Enlightenment ideals came to emphasize this present life, the existence of an after world was sometimes doubted. Thus, at least for parts of elite society, the religious meaning of death was lessened. John McManners has emphasized in his *Death and the Enlightenment* that most classes of society in France, the focus of his study, still saw death in religious terms. England, with its larger middle class was likely to have had a more extensive secularization of death, even though the process was not as thoroughgoing as some of the French *philosophes* would have hoped. In the latter half of the eighteenth century some doctors remained at the deathbed and 'managed' death, using opiates to deaden pain.[16] But in doing so they reduced both the independence of the dying and their role in the process of dying. If religious imperatives determined the ideal death in the sixteenth century, by the end of the eighteenth century the medicalized death was beginning to take shape. Again, this alteration reflects and confirms the decline of religion and the process of secularization which encouraged a medicalization of life and death.

The recent interest in the history of birth and death owes much to the present day concerns in western society with the way medicine controls the process of giving birth and of dying. Another modern-day concern is with the way our environment shapes our health. This topic was also of interest for the early modern period, though in this case, the forces of religion and of secularization were less evident. Despite attempts at sanitation and street cleaning, despite the ordinances controlling food markets, stinks and overcrowding, England at this time was often preceived as crowded, dirty, smelly and unhygienic. Probably many

bed and the behaviour expected of the dying 'actor' see A. Wear, 'Puritan Perceptions of Illness in Seventeenth Century England', and 'Interfaces: Perceptions of Health and Illness in Early Modern England', in Roy Porter and Andrew Wear (eds.), *Problems and Methods in the History of Medicine* (London, 1987), pp. 230–55.

[15] Jeremy Taylor, *Holy Living and Dying* (London, 1650, 1651).

[16] Dorothy and Roy Porter, *Patient's Progress*, pp. 144–52.

people were used to this but we rarely hear from them.[17] Many others, however, thought that this environment posed a danger to health and pictured a healthier alternative. I will first discuss how the environment and people were related at a general level, and then I shall consider how the environment was seen to affect health.

Health and the environment

England was perceived by the English, or at least by English eulogists as the best possible environment for English people. William Harrison in *The Description of England* (1577) and William Camden in his *Britannia* (Latin first edition, 1586) both agreed, at a time of intense national feeling, that the country was situated in the most temperate climate in the world, being neither too hot nor too cold.[18] As Camden put it 'Britaine is seated as well for aire as soile, in a right fruitful and most milde place.'[19] Harrison also argued that the English were taller, stronger, whiter and more courageous than those nearer the equator who were more feeble, delicate, fearful and blacker.[20] The way in which the connection was made between a country and its people was not an objective account, but often involved large doses of propaganda and patriotism.

From the point of view of health, the opinion was often expressed that the country in which one was born was the best and most healthy to live in, a view in keeping with the contemporary growth of the nation-state. A person's constitution or humoral balance was influenced by the constitution of the country of their birth. There was, therefore, an intimate correspondence between the two. William Vaughan, the Welsh writer and unsuccessful colonist of Newfoundland, asked in his *Directions for Health* 'What is the best Ayre?'. He replied:

[17] The physician Henry Brooke was one person who was satisfied with the environment. In *YΓIENH, Or A Conservatory of Health* (London, 1650), pp. 67–8 he wrote that many men not of the strongest constitution lived long and without sickness, 'amidst noysom and unpleasant Smells, as Oyl-men, Sope-boylers, Tallow-Chandlers' and those who dealt with 'Dung, cleaning of Common-shores and Jaxes' came to no harm 'because of the familiarity that by long use is begotton between such Smells and their Natures'. Brooke also robustly decried the too sensitive sensibilities of those who made themselves ill with the fear of imaginary dangers: 'However 'tis best for them that are any thing Healthful not be over -solicitous in the choice of Aire ... for they do thereby very much deject Nature, and opinionate themselves into Sickness. Such Imaginations keep the mind in continuall doubts and perplexities, and make us sickly, out of a fear of being sick.

[18] William Harrison, *The Descripton of England*, ed. George Edelen (Ithaca, NY, 1968), pp. 428–9; William Camden, *Britannia, or a Chorographical Description of ... England, Scotland and Ireland* (London, 1637), p. 2.   [19] Camden, *Britannia*, p. 2.

[20] Harrison, *Description of England*, pp. 445–6.

Health and the environment in early modern England

That which is a mans usuall soyle, and Countries ayre is best. This by the Philosophers is approved in this principle: 'Every mans naturall place preserveth him which is placed in it'. And by the Poet confirmed: 'Sweet is the smell of Countries soyle.'[21]

The enterprise of colonizing America forced people to articulate their ideas of how to judge whether a place was healthy or not, and the evidence from the North American colonies provides a good insight into how the environment and health were related. The many letters, pamphlets and books which gave optimistic accounts of Newfoundland, New England and Virginia written at the end of the sixteenth and the first half of the seventeenth centuries in the course of trying to attract prospective colonists and setting their minds at rest about the unknown frequently referred to the idea that a person's country of birth was most healthy for them. In the *Planter's Plea* (1630), a tract encouraging the development of the New England settlement, the writer extolled the air of the colony. Air, 'the very food of life' as Richard Whitbourne the promoter of Newfoundland had put it,[22] was probably the most important of all the characteristics that were considered when judging the healthiness of a place. *The Planter's Plea* stated:

No country yields a more propitious ayre for our temper [constitution], than New-England, as experience hath made manifest, by all relations: manie of our people that have found themselves alway weake and sickly at home, have become strong and healthy there perhaps by the dryness of the ayre and constant temper of it which seldome varies suddenly from cold to heate as it doth with us: so that Rhumes are very rare among our English there.[23]

The relationship between bodily constitution and the land was thus even better in New England than back home in Old England.

The connection between people and their country of birth was used in other contexts. When English writers such as Nicholas Culpeper in the mid seventeenth century argued for cheap medicines which could be collected locally from fields and used by the poor, or like William Harrison extolled home-grown remedies simply on a nationalistic dislike of anything foreign,[24] they drew upon this view of how people were related to their country of birth. Additionally, Culpeper referred to

---

[21] William Vaughan, *Directions for Health*, 5th edn (London, 1617), p. 4.

[22] Richard Whitbourne, *A Discourse and Discovery of New-Found-Land* (London, 1622), in Gillian T. Cell (ed.), *Newfoundland Discovered*, Hakluyt Society (London, 1982), p. 165.

[23] *The Planter's Plea*, in Peter Force (ed.), *Tracts and Other Papers Relating Principally to the Origin, Settlement and Progress of the Colonies of North America*, 4 vols. (New York, 1836–47; reprinted New York, 1947), II, tract 3. p. 13.   [24] Harrison, *Description of England*, pp. 266–8.

IV

God's providence and wisdom in the creation in having provided not
only food, but also appropriate remedies to cure the diseases of one's
native country. This was a common sentiment amongst writers who
were concerned with charity. In his *School of Physick* (1659) Culpeper
wrote:

As the Earth is called the Mother of all things, not because it bringeth them forth
onely, but yieldeth them perpetual nourishment, so is the Country of all people
so then named, the Parent of all parents. Then by Nature's laws, all things being
abundantly ministered unto us for the preservation of Health at home in our
own Fields, Pastures, Rivers etc, how can the Wisdom of God, and his Goodness
stand with the absence of Medicines and Remedies necessary for the Recovery
of Health, the need being as urgent of the one as the other...it followeth
necessarily that the Medicine should be as ready for the sick, as meat and drink
for the hungry and thirsty: which except it be applied by the Native Country,
cannot else be performed.[25]

Culpeper added that animals are given 'knowledge of Medicines to help
themselves, if haply disease [occur] among them; neither out of India nor
Arabia, but from their very haunt', and much more is given to us, 'the
Lords of all Creatures'.[26]

Ideas about health and illness often reflect the different intentions of
specific social groups. Most learned physicians, educated in the
universities and charging high fees, would have been hearty prescribers
of expensive foreign drugs. However, outside of London and one or two
large towns, such physicians were few on the ground, and, in any case,
were too expensive for most people.[27] As Roy Porter has pointed out in
the previous chapter, the medical market place was composed of family
members, neighbours, ministers and their wives, together with the wives
of country gentry who might all give advice and treatment for free and
practitioners such as wise women, uroscopists, astrologers, empirics and
apothecaries who normally charged low fees. The ethos of much of
medical practice was that it was demotic and open to all. Because of this
ethos, the self-sufficiency appeal of native herbs for native diseases had
added force, especially in the context of charity for the poor. The
biographical sketch of Culpeper produced soon after his death stated:

[25] Nicholas Culpeper, *School of Physick* (London, 1659), p. 7.
[26] *Ibid.*, p. 8. Culpeper was drawing upon, sometimes word for word, Timothie Bright's *A
Treatise Wherein is Declar'd the Sufficiencie of English Medicine* (London, 1580).
[27] See Margaret Pelling and Charles Webster 'Medical Practitioners', in Charles Webster (ed.),
Health, Medicine and Mortality in the Sixteenth Century (Cambridge, 1979), pp. 164–235 who show
that although medical graduates were few, the number of medical practitioners of all sorts was high.
Also Doreen G. Nagy, *Popular Medicine in Seventeenth Century Medicine* (Bowling Green, Ohio,
1988).

Health and the environment in early modern England

To the poor he prescribed cheap but wholesome Medicines; not removing, as many in our times do, the Consumption out of their bodies into their purses; not sending them to the East Indies for Drugs, when they may fetch better of their own Gardens.[28]

The countryside and the city

The link between people and their environment (their native land) that has been discussed so far, treated both the country and its people as undifferentiated. What was different was other peoples, other countries and their climates, and foreign illnesses and remedies. Not only was the doctrine used for patriotic propaganda purposes (implying a sense of belonging and of excluding), and for expressing a political view about medicine, but it also had a moralizing aspect where categories such as natural and unnatural came into play. For instance, Thomas Tryon, a fervent exponent of vegetarianism in the later seventeenth century, deplored the use of exotic drugs as a sign of the degeneration of society from its pure natural state.[29]

The environment, however, was not always seen as an undifferentiated whole, to be patriotically idealized if it was one's own country or to be suspiciously sniffed at if foreign. When people came to look at England in detail they saw many different types of environment.

The major distinction between town and countryside, which was current amongst writers on health and the environment as well as in literary culture, forms the backbone of the rest of the chapter. The countryside was perceived to be much healthier than towns or cities. This view is confirmed by modern historical demography. The population of London, which had grown from 120,000 in 1550 to 490,000 by 1700, would have declined over this period if it had not been for the continued influx of people from the countryside that made up for the drain on the city's population caused by its high mortality.[30] This was realized by John Graunt whose *Natural and Political Observations ... upon the Bills of Mortality* (1662) was the first study of population demography. It was based on a quantitative analysis of the weekly bills of mortality compiled by London parish clerks which gave numbers and causes of death. The book's numerate approach was very much in

[28] In Culpeper, *School of Physick*, sig. C4.
[29] Thomas Tryon, *The Way to Health, Long Life and Happiness* (London, 1697), pp. 382–8.
[30] See R. Finlay, *Population and Metropolis: the Demography of London 1580–1650* (Cambridge, 1981) and Roger Finlay and Beatrice Shearer 'Population Growth and Suburban Expansion', in A. L. Beier and Roger Finlay (eds.), *The Making of the Metropolis. London 1500–1700* (London, 1986), pp. 37–6c.

keeping with the 'new science' of the Royal Society, and it also marks the start of the endeavour of relating deaths and types of death to environmental causes in a quantitative way. Nevertheless, Graunt's ideas of the environmental factors causing illness and death were traditional.

On the population of London Graunt noted that between 1603 and 1644 burials (363,935) exceeded christenings (330,747) and he concluded:

From this single Observation it will follow, that London should have decreased in its People; the contrary whereof we see by its daily increases of Buildings upon new Foundations, and by turning of great Palacious Houses into small Tenements. It is therefore certain, that London is supplied with People from out of the Country, whereby not only to supply the overplus differences of Burials above mentioned, but likewise to increase its Inhabitants according to the said increase of housing.[31]

Graunt discussed the reasons for this imbalance between London and the countryside. He wrote that the number of breeders (women of childbearing age) was fewer in London than in the countryside.[32] But he also believed that London itself was less healthy than the country, though those who were 'seasoned' (whose bodies had adapted over time to the environment of London) could live long:

As for unhealthiness, it may well be supposed, that although seasoned Bodies may, and do live near as long in *London*, as elsewhere, yet new-comers and Children do not: for the *Smoaks*, *Stinks* and close *Air*, are less healthful than that of the Country; otherwise why do sickly Persons remove into the Country-Air? And why are there more old men in Countries than in London, per rata?[33]

Graunt indicted both the pressure of people and the air they breathed:

I considered, whether a City, as it becomes more populous, doth not, for that very cause, become more unhealthful: and inclined to believe, that London now is more unhealthful than heretofore; partly for that it is more populous, but chiefly because I have heard, that sixty years ago few Sea Coals were burnt in London, which are now universally used. For I have heard that Newcastle is more unhealthful than other places, and that many People cannot at all endure the smoak of London, not only for its unpleasantness but for the suffocation which it causes.[34]

Thomas Short, one of Graunt's eighteenth-century successors, whose demographic studies ranged across England, also believed that high population densities caused ill health. A sense of the suffocating closeness of towns helped to explain the figures from the parish registers:

[31] John Graunt, *Natural and Political Observations ... upon the Bills of Mortality* (London, 1676), pp. 57–8. [32] Graunt, *Observations*, p. 62. [33] *Ibid.*, p. 63. [34] *Ibid.*, p. 94–5.

Health and the environment in early modern England

The closer Towns and Villages stand, the more pent-up the Houses, the lower and closer the Rooms, the narrower the Streets, the smaller the Windows, the more numerous the Inhabitants, the unhealthier the Place. This is evident from several Towns in our Tables.[35]

Graunt did not believe that London's air produced barrenness in the same way as it produced a greater degree of death and disease than was found in the countryside (though he did blame London for its greater adulteries and fornications which 'do certainly hinder Breeding').[36] But, like many early modern writers, he made the connection between the body and the mind, and wrote that city life could produce psychological barriers to natural activities:

The minds of men in *London* are more thoughtful of business than in the country, where their work is corporal Labour and Exercises; All of which promote Breeding, whereas Anxieties of the mind hinder it.[37]

The countryside was the norm, from which urban living was an unnatural departure that incurred additional health risks. The health advice books, of which a very large number were printed in this period,[38] structured the relationship between health and the environment by means of the traditional 'six non-naturals' (air, food and drink, sleep and waking, retention and evacuation, exercise and rest, and the passions). These books were aimed at sedentary readers such as merchants, clerics and the studious, and they extolled the virtues of country air, food and exercise. (What the illiterate, who comprised the majority of the population thought about health remains largely a blank: the history of how people perceived health and the environment in this period is based on evidence from the literate.) Works such as Thomas Cogan's *Haven of Health* (1584) and the English translation of Leonard Lessius' *Hygiasticon* (1634) emphasized that country people took a lot of exercise and were generally longer lived. As Cogan, a physician and a Fellow of Oriel College, Oxford, put it:

Husbandman and Craftsmen for the most part doe live longer, and in better health than Gentlemen and learned men, and such as live in bodily rest.[39]

The country gentleman could live in the countryside, benefit from

---

[35] Thomas Short, *New Observations on City, Town and Country Bills of Mortality*, London 1750, ed. Richard Wall (London, 1973), p. 65.   [36] Graunt, *Observations*, pp. 63–4.

[37] *Ibid.*, p. 64.

[38] See Paul Slack 'Mirrors of Health and Treasures of Poor Men: the Uses of the Vernacular Medical Literature of Tudor England', in Charles Webster (ed.), *Health, Medicine and Mortality in the Sixteenth Century* (Cambridge, 1979), pp. 237–73.

[39] Thomas Cogan, *The Haven of Health* (London, 1636).

country air, yet suffer the same ills as his town counterpart. As well as country air, it was the way of life associated with the country, hard labour, a meagre diet and a lack of luxury which produced health. The well-to-do part of society, those 'increasing the wealth of the kingdom' (just under half the population in Gregory King's calculation for 1688),[40] was being advised that the poorer part of the population, if it lived in the countryside, was healthier than they were.

William Bullein in the *Government of Health* (1558) wrote in dialogue form:

JOHN. I have found verie much disquietnes in my body, when my servants and labouring familie have found ease and yet we are partakers of one aire.
HUMPHREY. The cause why thy labouring servants in the field at plough, pastures, or woode, have such good health, is exercise labour, and the disquietness commeth partly of idleness and lack of travail [work], which moderately used, is a thing most sovereign in nature.[41]

What John's labouring servants thought about their master's way of life compared to their own we do not know; the illiterate remain silent, but the equation of health with the poorest sections of society can be interpreted as an implied justification for doing nothing about their condition of life, and fits that strand of sixteenth and seventeenth-century English social policy which held that there was no necessity to ameliorate the lot of the poor.[42]

The distinction between the healthy countryside and unhealthy towns and cities was made throughout the early modern period, and many people felt that they could express opinions with some authority about health and the environment. Much of the knowledge was traditional, based on long experience or on authorities such as Galen. Sometimes it was founded on personal observation and experience, which through the sixteenth and seventeenth century was being given increasingly high status in subjects like astronomy, medicine and natural philosophy and was taken to be a guarantee of truth. This view was also current in society at large. It was used by American settlers when they tried to convince their readers back in England of the truth of the claims about

[40] Cited by Peter Laslett, *The World We Have Lost – Further Explored* (London, 1983), pp. 32-3, Laslett cautions against the accuracy of King's figures, p. 298 note 4. Keith Wrightson, *English Society 1580–1680* (London, 1982), p. 148, finds King's results of value: 'in [his] opinion at least half of his countrymen in 1688 were scarcely able to simply provide an adequate maintenance for their families. The poor had emerged as a massive and permanent element in English society.'

[41] William Bullein, *Government of Health* (London, 1591), p. 31v.

[42] See Paul Slack, *Poverty and Policy in Tudor and Stuart England* (London, 1988) for a discussion of the underlying attitudes of government to the poor and their relief.

Health and the environment in early modern England

the health and riches to be found in the new lands. One writer asserted that the temperate nature of the New England climate was 'made manifest by experience, the most infallible proof of all assertions'.[43] A leading puritan, Francis Higginson, writing back to England to prospective immigrants took care to stress not only that as a preacher he could not lie, but that he reported nothing unless he had:

seen it with my own eyes and partly heard and inquired from the mouths of very honest and religious person(s), who by living in the country a good space of time had had experience and knowledge of the state thereof and whose testimonies I do believe as myself.[44]

Anyone could be an authority about health and the environment, because anyone could draw upon personal experience and upon traditional knowledge. This mirrors the way in which anyone could set up as an authority in the medical market place of the time.

Despite the possibility of individual differences of opinion there was a consensus as to the topography of health and illness that held, on the whole, for most of the early modern period. What constituted healthy places, airs and waters was generally agreed upon, and everyone believed that healthy places meant healthy bodies. In 1576 William Lombarde had commented in his *A Perambulation of Kent* that Romney Marsh was sparsely populated because 'most men be yet still of Porcius Cato his minde, who held them starke madde, that would dwell in an unwholsome Aire.'[45] (Modern historical demographers also agree that low-lying marsh ground produced a higher death rate.)[46] Tobias Venner, the Bath physician, in his book on regimen, *Via Recta ad Vitam Longam* (1628), wrote at length on the relationship between health and low-lying places:

Therefore he that desireth to live a long and healthy life, must dwell in an eminent and champion country, or at least, in a place that is free from muddy and waterish impurities: for it is impossible, that a man should live long and healthily in a place, where the spirits are with impure ayre daily affected.[47]

Marshy air produced nearly all 'the diseases of the braine and sinews, as

---

[43] G. Mount (pseudonymous), *An Historicall Discoverie and Relation of the English Plantations of New England* (London, 1627), sig. D2v.
[44] Everett Emerson (ed.), *Letters From New England. The Massachusetts Bay Colony, 1629–1638* (Amherst, 1976), p. 30.
[45] William Lambarde, *A Perambulation of Kent* (London, 1576), p. 159.
[46] Mary Dobson, '"Marsh Fever": A Geography of Malaria in England', *Journal of Historical Geography* 6 (1980), 359–89, and *idem*, 'The Last Hiccup of the Old Demographic Regime: Population Stagnation and Decline in Late Seventeenth and Early Eighteenth-Century England', *Continuity and Change*, 4 (1989), 395–428.
[47] Tobias Venner, *Via Recta ad Vitam Longam* (London, 1628), p. 8.

Crampes, Palsies etc. with paines in the joynts; and to speake all in a word, a general torpidity both of minde and body'.[48] Venner elaborated on how the mind was affected, 'those living in eminent and champion Countrys' were 'witty, nimble, magnanimous and *alta petentes*'. However he warned:

the contrary is seene in low and marish places: for there, the Inhabitants, by reason of the evilnesse of the Ayre, have grosse and earthy spirits, whereof it is, that they are for the most part men, *humun tantum sapientes*, dull, sluggish, sordid, sensual, plainly irreligious, or perhaps some of them, which is little worse, religious in shewe, external honest men, deceitfull, malicious, disdainfull.

From this stance of environmental determinism Venner advised, in conclusion that 'all such as are ingenious, generous, and desirous of perfection, both in minde and body, that they endeavour by all means, to live in a pure and healthy Ayre'.[49]

In the second half of the seventeenth century a more distinctly 'scientific' style of reporting on the climate, health and natural history of a place began to emerge. The new Baconian and Royal Society ideology of exactness and exhaustiveness in observation can be discerned in reports such as John Clayton's letters to the Royal Society 'of several observables in Virginia' (1688), John Ray's *Observations …made on a journey through part of the Low Countries, Germany, Italy and France* (1673), Hans Sloane's *A Voyage to the Islands of Madera, Barbadoes, Nieves, St Christopher's and Jamaica, with the Natural History of the last* (2 vols. 1707, 1725), William Hillary's *An Account of the Principal Variations of the Weather, and the concomitant Epidemic Disease, as they appeared at Rippon and the circumjacent Parts of Yorkshire from the Year 1726 to the End of 1734* (1740), and Thomas Short's *New Observations on City, Town and Country Bills of Mortality* (1750).

Nevertheless, despite the new style of writing, little had essentially changed from the early seventeenth century. Thomas Short no longer agreed that England had the healthiest climate in the world,[50] but he did concur that the countryside was the healthiest place in which to live. He wrote that he had begun with the country registers:

as a rural life was the first State of Man and as it is still the healthiest, and affords the truest and most innocent Pleasures: For there (except in great, rich, or opulent Men's Houses) still remains such Vestiges of Virtue, Sobriety,

---

[48] *Ibid.*, p. 3.   [49] *Ibid.*, p. 9.   [50] Short, *New Observations*, pp. 1–2.

Health and the environment in early modern England

Regularity, Plainness, and simplicity of Diet as bears some small Image or Resemblance of the primeval State.[51]

Short used information from parish registers of births, marriages and deaths to draw epidemiological conclusions which were not much different from those of a hundred or more years before that had been based upon common experience and tradition. Short concluded from his data that:

Dry, open Situations meanly elevated, neither like Beacons on the Tops of lofty Mountains, nor like Reeds in the marshy Vallies, are above all others (*caeteris paribus*) the healthiest; for such Habitations have a free, pure, open Air...[52]

The unhealthiest places were:

Low Habitations, especially on stiff Clay, rotten Earth, or near a Level with the sea, great Rivers, Marshes, Lakes or putrid standing Waters. These are worst of all; for their Air is always moist, gross, and loaded with Exhalations often putrid [53]

There was also a stream of advice on creating the best environment. This could involve, for instance, the siting of a house. Garvase Markham, in his *The English Husbandman* (1635) which was addressed to a newly prosperous group in English society, advised:

let not your house be too neere great Rivers or Brookes, they may smile in Summer, but they will be angrie in Winter, and it is better to have them wash your Grounds than wet your house, Besides they oft vomit forth ill ayres, and are in their owne natures Aguish and unwholesome.[54]

Robert Burton wrote in the *Anatomy of Melancholy* (1621) that:

A clear air cheers up the spirits, exhilarates the mind; a thick, black misty, tempestuous, contracts, overthrows. Great heed is therefore to be taken at what times we walk, how we place our windows, lights and houses, how we let in or exclude this ambient air.[55]

How far anyone acted on such advice is unclear. When the mortality in Jamestown, Virginia, became too great, plans were made to move the settlement to high ground away from its marshy air which was blamed for the deaths. Such action at this time was rare. Romney Marsh, despite its reputation, was not deserted. Lambarde noted that it was 'famous throughout the Realme, as well for the fertilitie and quantitie of the

[51] *Ibid.*, p. 1.   [52] *Ibid.*, p. 13.   [53] *Ibid.*, p. 19.
[54] Gervase Markham, *The English Husbandman* (London, 1635), p. 22.
[55] Robert Burton, *The Anatomy of Melancholy*, ed. Floyd Dell and Paul Jordan-Smith (New York, 1938), p. 435.

soile...' and that 'it offered Wealth without healthe'.[56] If a place was economically attractive then its reputation for ill health was ignored. This was certainly the case with the most populous place in England, London.

As we have seen, too many people in one place could, it was believed, be a cause of disease and death (an idea which also finds approval today). The authorities were aware of the dangers of overcrowding. A royal proclamation of 1580 tried to limit new buildings in London and to prevent more than one family living in a house (like others of its kind it was unsuccessful). The proclamation argued that disease, especially plague, could spread in crowded conditions:

Where there are such great multitudes of people brought to inhabit in small houses, whereof a great part are seen very poor, and they heaped up together, and in a sort smothered with many families of children and servants in one house or small tenement, it must needs follow (if any plague or popular sickness should by God's permission enter amongst those multitudes) that the same would...spread itself and invade the whole city and confines, as great mortality should ensue to the same.[57]

Despite the fear of plague, despite the acknowledged higher risk of disease and death, people still flocked to London from the healthy countryside and the city grew inexorably. As today, knowledge about

[56] Lambarde, *A Perambulation of Kent*, p. 158. William Strachy's account of the healthiness of Jamestown in 1610, the need to settle on a hill and the analogy with England illustrates some of the points of the chapter so far: 'True it is, I may not excuse this our Fort, or James Towne, as yet seated in some what an unwholesome and sickly ayre, by reason it is in a marish ground, low, flat to the River, and hath no fresh water Springs serving the Towne, but what wee drew from a Well sixe or seven fathom deepe, fed by the brackish River owzing into it, from whence I verily beleeve, the chiefe causes have proceeded of many diseases and sicknesses which have happened to our people, who are indeede strangely afflicted with Fluxes and Agues; and every particular season (by the relation of the old inhabitants) hath his particular infirmity too, all which (if it had bin our fortunes, to have seated upon some hill, accommodated with fresh Springs and cleere ayre, as doe the Natives of the Country) we might have, I beleeve, well escaped: and some experience we have to perswade our selves that it may be so, for of foure hundred and odde men, which were seated at the Fals, the last yeere when the Fleete came in with fresh and yong able spirits, under the government of Captaine Francis West, and of one hundred to the Seawards (on the South side of our River) in the Country of the Nansumundes, under the charge of Captaine John Martin, there did not so much as one man miscarry, and but very few or none fall sicke, whereas at James Towne, the same time, and the same moneths, one hundred sickened, & halfe the number died: howbeit, as we condemne not Kent in England, for a small Towne called Plumsted, continually assaulting the dwellers there (especially new commers) with Agues and Fevers; no more let us lay scandall, and imputation upon the Country of Virginia, because the little Quarter wherein we are set down (unadvisedly so chosed) appears to be unwholesome, and subject to many ill ayres, which accompany the like marish places.' William Strachy 'A true Reportorie of the Wreck and Redemption of Sir Thomas Gates, Knight; upon and from the ilands of the Bermudas: his comming to Virginia and the Estate of that colonie then...July 15. 1610', in 'Samuel Purchas, *Hakluytus Postumus or Purchas His Pilgrimes*, 20 vols. (1625; reprinted Glasgow, 1905), XIX, pp. 58–9.

[57] Cited in Lawrence Manley, *London in the Age of Shakespeare* (London, 1986), pp. 184–5.

Health and the environment in early modern England

health risks does not easily change people's behaviour when faced with the economic opportunity or the social magnet of the city.

Understanding knowledge about the environment

Medical theories came and went in the early modern period – Galenic humouralism, alchemy, iatrochemistry, chemistry, iatromechanism. The changes are easy to discern. Tobias Venner rationalized in a traditional Galenic manner that marshy air was bad 'for impure, grosse and intemperate ayre doth corrupt the spirits and humours'.[58] Over a hundred years later Thomas Short was urging parents living in towns or cities to place their children in the countryside, if they could. He justified his argument by using the mechanical and chemical language of his time which had replaced that of the humours. The town's or city's

Atmosphere is loaded, and has its Spring lessened by sulphurous, and other Steams, so as it cannot duly inflate and distend the Lungs, nor compress the sanguinous Vessels, cool the Blood, nor communicate fresh Fewel to it, for the City Air is full of perspired Matter, discharged from both dead and living animal bodies, and other noxious Matter; Matter as well from diseased as healthy Bodies, and many insensibly convey the Seeds of several Distempers with the unhealthy State of those Juices they exhaled from.[59]

By and large both humoral and mechanical writers agreed on the facts of the case – city air was bad – but they explained why this was so in different ways.

There were, however, other ways of understanding the relationships between health and the environment apart from the learned theories of medicine, chemistry and natural philosophy. How did early modern society judge whether an environment (or food and drink) was bad? People used their senses: smell, for instance, was very important.[60] Not only could smell indicate that something was healthy or unhealthy, but smells were employed in an active manner to maintain health and to keep out disease. In times of plague bunches of sweet-smelling flowers or herbs were carried to counter the foul-smelling vapour or miasma (infectious air) coming from places like cesspits that was believed to cause plague. Thomas Muffet, in his *Health's Improvement* (1655) published fifty-one years after his death, advised that plague air was to be corrected with 'good fires, and burning of Lignum Aloes, Ebony, Cinamon bark, Sassaphras and Juniper. Burn also the piths of Oranges, Citrons and

---

[58] Venner, *Via Recta*, p. 8.   [59] Short, *New Observations*, p. 63.
[60] For a slightly later period see Alain Corbin, *The Foul and the Fragrant* (Leamington Spa, 1986).

Lemons, and Myrrh and Rosen; and the poorer sort may perfume their chambers with Baies, Rosemary, and Broom itself.'[61]

More generally, Robert Burton extolled the virtues of 'artificial air' as a way 'to correct nature by art', this was 'to be made hot and moist, and to be seasoned with sweet perfumes, pleasant and lightsome as may be; to have Roses, Violets, and sweet smelling flowers ever in their windows, Posies in their hand'.[62] John Evelyn in his *Fumifugium* (1661) outlined a grandiose scheme to counteract London's foul air which he believed came from the burning of sea coal and from the stench of church yards, charnel houses, chandlers and butchers.[63] A mass of sweet-smelling trees, bushes and plants would be planted to surround and vivify London.[64] Evelyn argued that London's air 'carries away multitudes by languishing and deep Consumptions, as the Bills of Mortality do weekly inform us', and that 'almost half of them who perish in London, dye of phthisical and pulmonic distempers; That the inhabitants are never free from Coughs and importunate Rheumatisms, spitting of Impostumated and corrupt matter, for remedy whereof, there is none so infallible, as that in time, the Patient change his Aer, and remove into the Country'.[65]

Behind such a scheme seems to lie the smells and images of the paradisical garden and of exotic worlds. The Dedication to Charles II of the *Fumifugium* was perhaps hyperbolic and other worldly even for its own time, but this was still an age of strange new worlds. Evelyn explained that he wrote:

'to render not only Your Majesties Palace, but the whole City likewise of the sweetest and most delicious Habitations in the World; and this with little or no expense; but by improving those Plantations which Your Majesty so laudably affects in the moyst, depressed and Marshy grounds about the Town...upon every gentle emmission through the Aer, should so perfume the adjacent places with their breath, as if by a certain charm, or innocent Magick, they were transferred to that part of Arabia, which is therefore styl'd the Happy, because it is amongst the Gums and precious spices.[66]

[61] Thomas Muffet, *Health's Improvement* (London, 1655), p. 25. Muffet added, p. 26: 'But here a great question ariseth, whether sweet smels correct the pestilent aire, or rather be as a guide to bring it the sooner into our hearts? To determin which question I call all the dwellers in Bucklers Berry in London to give their sentence: which only street (by reason that it is wholly replenished with Physick Drugs, and Spicery and was daily perfumed in the time of the plague with pounding of Spices, melting of gums, and making perfumes for others) escaped that great plague brought from Newhaven, whereof, there died so many, that scarce any house was left unvisited.'
[62] Burton, *Anatomy of Melancholy*, p. 436.
[63] John Evelyn, *Fumifugium or the Inconvenience of the Aer and Smoak of London Dissipated* (London, 1661), pp. 56, 21. [64] *Ibid.*, pp. 24–5. [65] *Ibid.*, 12–13.
[66] *Ibid.*, sig. A3r.

Health and the environment in early modern England

This language of sweet sensation should not be dismissed merely as the effusions of a keen gardener (Evelyn was the gentleman-gardener of Sayes Court where he had retreated to during the Interregnum, and was to write treatises on forest and fruit trees). The enterprise of bringing the country into the city is still with us in the shape of public parks and gardens and in the ethos of the suburban garden. Moreover, Evelyn rightly used as evidence of a longing for the countryside and its health the common practice of the ill and convalescent of travelling into the countryside for a change of air and to escape the diseases of the city.

Behind the idea of *rus in urbe* lay, I think, the Garden of Eden,[67] the paradisical garden where the smells of the plants were the most fragrant. and where there was neither death nor disease. In a sense, paradise was the absolute measure against which all other environments were measured. The power of Christianity in this period made the Garden of Eden a potent symbol, but paradise had also the functional role of representing perfection in a society which lacked today's instruments and scales that give us our measure of objective degrees of impurity (as for chemicals or bacteria in water).

The ideal perfection of paradise was not attainable on earth by human art. As John Parkinson put it in the title page of his botanical work the *Paradisi in Sole Paradisus Terrestris* (1629), 'who wishes to compare art with nature and our parks with Eden, without wisdom measures the stride of the elephant by the stride of the mite and the flight of the eagle by that of the midge'. Nevertheless, Thomas Short noted that the 'rural life' still bore 'some small image or Resemblance of the Primeval State'. Perfection did not now exist, but we could still glimpse in the countryside what it had been like. There were different opinions on whether the pale images of paradise to be found on earth were creations of nature or of man. Virgin America was often likened to paradise, and the noble savage, the Indian, enjoyed the good health appropriate to such a place.[68]

On the other hand, nature could be seen as hostile with demi-paradise having to be worked for. The cartographer, John Norden, in his

---

[67] For a much wider cultural context to the perception of the environment, gardens, paradise and the treatment of animals see Keith Thomas, *Man and the Natural World. Changing Attitudes in England 1500–1800* (Harmondsworth, 1984), which is the standard work on the subject. Also Raymond Williams, *The Country and the City* (London, 1985).

[68] See H. C. Porter, *The Inconstant Savage, England and the North American Indian 1500–1660* (London, 1979); C. Clacken, *Traces on the Rhodian Shore* (Berkeley, 1976). Peter Hulme, *Colonial Encounters. Europe and the Native Caribbean 1492–1797* (London, 1986).

IV

Surveiors Dialogue (1610) discussed the different types of agricultural land in England. He felt that if left to nature even:

the fairest pastures, and greenest meadows, would become in short time, over-grown with bushes, woods, weeds and things unprofitable, as they were before they were rid and cleansed of the same by the industry of man, who was inioyened that use and travaile to manure the earth, which for his disobedience should bring forth these things.[69]

After the Fall there could be no natural paradise, though it could be hoped and worked for. In the *Dialogue* the 'Surveyor' speaks of 'Tandeane' in Somerset as 'the paradise of England' which is a product of its natural fruitfulness but also of its people doing 'their best by art and industry' and 'they take extraordinarie paines in soyling, plowing and dressing their lands'.[70]

Paradise might be perceived for a while in the *terra nova* of America with its noble savages and its gardens of Eden until epidemics, famine and the need to shape the land, and to take the Indian's lands changed the perception of both land and Indians to hostile and unpleasant entities. Paradise could also be found in a vestigial form in the countryside whether in its natural state or as something to be worked for, never reached perhaps but distantly approached by art and industry. In a sense the Fall ensured that the environment, like man and woman, would always be tainted and unhealthy to some degree.

Paradise and the Fall is a useful way of showing how the perception of the countryside as healthy had its counterpart in the revealed truth of religion. The story of the Fall also gave a Biblical origin for the need for curative medicine to counteract newly arrived death and disease. The means to ameliorate the consequences of the Fall were given by God to man but they likewise could not restore the original situation. Tobias Whitaker, a Norwich and London physician, wrote in 1638 in a work extolling the health-giving virtues of wine:

for had Adam never sinned, yet must his body have been preserved and maintained by diet, which is part of physick. But after his fall so violated his equall temper [constitution] that as then he became subject to mortalitie and naturall decay. Then came in the necessity of medicine and ever since for this necessitie sake, hath the Almighty commanded an honour to be given to the Phisician for he heath created him an Angell of mercy.[71]

The environment was not merely a place where people lived, whether

---

[69] John Norden, *The Surveiors Dialogue* (London, 1610), p. 184.
[70] *Ibid.*, pp. 191–2.
[71] Tobias Whitaker, *The Tree of Humane Life or The Bloud of the Grape* (London, 1638) sig. A 3r.

Health and the environment in early modern England

in cities, on mountains or in swampy land. From it came food and drink. Just as a healthy environment provided healthy people, so too a healthy environment was thought to produce healthy plants and animals and pure water, and hence health-giving food and drink. Mrs Ann (possibly Aphra) Behn's poem in support of Thomas Tryon's call for vegetarianism pointed to the example of Adam and the long-lived Patriarchs who did not eat meat, but it also evoked the golden-age environment of 'Christal Streams' and 'plenteous Wood' which provided 'harmless drink and wholsom food'.

> In that blest golden Age, when Man was young,
> When the whole Race was vigorous and strong.
> When Nature did her wonderous dictates give,
> And taught the Noble Savage how to live.
> When Christal Streams and every plenteous Wood
> Afforded harmless drink and wholsom food;
> ... E'er that ingratitude in Man was found
> And ev'ry Age produced a feebler Race,
> Sickly their days and those declin'd apace, ...
> Give us long life and lasting Vertue too:
> Such were the mighty Patriarchs of old
> Who in God in all his glory did behold,
> Inspir'd like you [Tryon], they Heavens
>   Instructions show'd
> And were as Gods amidst the wondring Croud;
> Not he that love th' Almighty Wand cou'd give
> Diviner Dictates, how to eat and live
> And so essential was this cleanly Food,
> For Man's eternal health eternal, eternal good,
> That God did for his first – lov'd Race provide
> What thou, by God's example, best prescribed ... [72]

The allusion to paradise gave a benchmark for judging the health of the environment and its products, but it was of little use in the practical daily business of deciding which products one should select to eat and drink. Ideas of cleanliness and dirt, of the natural and unnatural, of light and darkness, of movement and sluggishness underlay many of the descriptions of healthy and unhealthy food and drink. These are to be found in the health advice books of the time and judging from the large numbers written there was a market for them amongst the literate section of the population.[73] The link between medicine and food is still a strong one today (diet and heart disease, cancer etc.); in the early

[72] In Thomas Tryon, The Way to Health, sig. A 4r.   [73] See note 38 above.

modern period advice on how to judge not only the healthiness but also the goodness or freshness of water, fish and meat was prominent. Effective official inspection of food and analysis of water was developed in the nineteenth and twentieth centuries. Consumers in the early modern period had to judge for themselves. Moreover, medicine was closely connected to cooking. A Hippocratic view had been that internal medicine was a specialized form of dietetics and that preparing food was analogous to preparing medicines.[74] Sixteenth- and seventeenth-century manuscript collections of medical prescriptions or recipes often included recipes for food, and as Thomas Cogan put it 'the learned Physition ... is, or ought to be a perfect cooke in many points'.[75]

Animals were judged to be healthy (hence to be healthy food) in the same way as humans. As the husbandman working in the fields was thought to be healthier and longer lived than the city merchant or student so animals and fish coming from the wild were equated with health and cleanliness. Thomas Venner wrote that eating fish produced 'much grosse, slimie superflous flegme' which in turn could cause gout, bladder stone, leprosy, scurvy and other skin diseases. He advised great care in the choice of fish 'as that it be not of a clammie, slimie, neither of a very grosse and hard substance ... neither of ill smell and unpleasant savour'. Venner considered what conditions produced the healthiest fish:

Wherefore of sea-fish, that is best which swimmeth in a pure sea, and is tossed and hoysed with winds and surges: for by reason of continuall agitation, it becometh of a purer, and lesse slimie substance, and consequently of easier concoction [digestion], and of a purer iuyce.[76]

Similarly fresh-water fish was best:

Which is bred in pure, stonie or gravelly rivers, running swiftly. For that which is taken in muddie waters in standing pooles, in fennes, mores and ditches, by reason of the impuritie of the place, and water, is unwholesome ...[77]

The concepts (and language) can be found in a number of writers. Sir Thomas Elyot in the sixteenth century had written in his best-selling *Castell of Health* (1534):

The best fish after the opinion of Galen is that which swymmeth in a pure sea and is tossed and lift up with wynds and surges. The more calme that the water

---

[74] A point made in the Hippocratic treatise *On Ancient Medicine*.
[75] Cogan, *Haven of Health*, p. 112.
[76] Venner, *Via Recta*, p. 69; see also Cogan, *Haven of Health*, p. 161.
[77] Venner, *Via Recta*, p. 70.

Health and the environment in early modern England

is, the worse the fish. They which are in muddy waters, do make much fleume and ordure, taken in fennes and dyckes be worst.[78]

Just as fish could be polluted, so could water. The best water was that which came from rain water or from fountains or springs, and flowed swiftly. William Vaughan indicated that good water was known 'By the clearnesse of it. That water is best which is light, transparent, agreeable to the sight, Christalline, and which runneth from an higher to a lower ground'. (He also added that 'some use to try [test] water by putting a clean Napkin in it and if any spots appeare upon the same they suspect the goodnesse of the water'.)[79] Bad water was found in standing pools, marshy ground; river water could also be of poor quality, if, as Venner wrote, 'it be polluted by the mixture of other things, as it commeth to passe in Rivers, that run thorow marish places, or neere unto populous Townes and Cities: for then, by reason of all manner of filth running, or cast into them, they become very corrupt and unwholesome'.[80] Venner added that it was up to the inhabitants of towns to find and to select wholesome river water which 'runneth with a full streame upon gravell, Pebble-stones, Rockes, or pure earth: for that water, by reason of the purity of the place, motion, and radiant splendor of the Sun is thinner, sweeter and therefore more pure and wholesome'.[81]

There are some common factors underlying these types of explanation. There was a holistic approach to the environment and its products. Not only did the environment affect living things and its own substances such as water, but the explanations used to make sense of the environment and plants and animals were often the same. As we have seen above, motion was a common key to the healthiness of fish and of water. Cogan expressed this in explicit terms:

For the flowing water doth not lightly corrupt, but that which standeth still: Even so bodies exercised, are for the most part more healthfull, and such as bee idle more subject to sicknesse.[82]

---

[78] Sir Thomas Elyot, *The Castell of Health* (London, 1580), p. 32v
[79] Vaughan, *Directions for Health*, pp. 25–6. Burton, *Anatomy of Melancholy*, p. 397, described the sensory qualities of good water: 'Pure, thin, light water by all means use, of good smell and taste, like to the air in sight, such as is soon hot, soon cold ...'
[80] Venner, *Via Recta*, p. 10.   [81] *Ibid.*, p. 11.
[82] Cogan, *Haven of Health*, p. 2. Lack of exercise was often thought to lead to disease. Sir Richard Hawkins gave as one of the causes of scurvy 'the want of exercise also either in persons or elements, as in calmes. And were it not for the moving of the Sea by the force of windes, tydes and current, it would corrupt all the world'. He advised 'to keepe the company occupied in some bodily exercise of worke, of agilitie, of pastimes, of dancing, of use of Armes; these helpe much to banish this imfirmitie'. 'The Observations of Sir Richard Hawkins, knight, in this Voyage into the South Sea, An. Dom. 1593', in Purchas, *Hakluytus Postumus* xvii, pp. 76–7.

IV

More general and unifying types of explanation were also used. The earth itself could be seen anthropomorphically, to be cared for in the same way as people. John Norden described the land in terms of hot, dry, cold and moist, the four qualities that made up both the world and the body,[83] and he advised the farmer to give the best care to his land:

For land is like the body, if it bee not nourished with noutriture and comforted and adorned with the most expedient commodities, it will pine away, and become forlorne, as is the minde that hath, no rest nor recreation waxe the lumpish and heavy.[84]

Farmers also treated the illnesses and hurts of their animals in ways that mirrored the medical practice that was applied to humans. Henry Best, a farmer from Elmswell in Yorkshire, wrote about the health of sheep in his manuscript Farming Book (1641). One entry has:

It is usuall with sheepe, and especially with hogges and lambs, to fall blind by reason of an humour that falleth out of the head into the eyes, whereby groweth (as it weare) a scumme over the stine [the cornea] of the eye. Many Shepheards will undertake to cure this by bloodinge them in the wykes of the eyes with a penne-knife, but the only way is to take ground-Ivy-leaves and to chewe them in your mouth, and to take the leafe with your finger after yow have sucked the Juice from it. This Juice you are to spurte into the eye morninge and eveninge, or if you will, thrice a day.[85]

A humoral explanation, use of bleeding, and disagreement about remedies was typical of medical practice for people. The use of the same types of theories and practices for animals as for people must have helped to produce a sense of interrelatedness. A sense which, for the link between humans and the environment, was formally expressed in the quasi-philosophical belief that the microcosm (the body of man) was a miniature version of the macrocosm (the greater world of the universe), and that events in the latter affected the former.[86]

Moreover the unity between the environment, living organisms like plants and animals and humans was expressed in the food cycle. Animals

---

[83] Norden, Surveiors Dialogue, p. 196. [84] Ibid., p. 76.
[85] David Woodward (ed.), The Farming and Memorandum Books of Henry Best of Elsmwell 1642, British Academy Records of Social and Economic History, New Series VIII, 1982. In the sixteenth century William Turner argued that medicinal baths should be made in Bath for animals in addition to those for humans. William Turner, The Rare Treasor of the English Bathes, in Thomas Vicary, The Englishmen's Treasure (London, 1586). p. 108.
[86] A small illustration of this is in Henry Whitmore, Febris Anomala Or, The New Disease that Now Rageth Throughout England (London, 1659) at p. 126 where the author notes that the new disease begun 'to visibly abade and slacken; which if I mistake not was about the latter end of November, when the cold weather begun to break forth, which on a sudden growing sharp made in the microcosm, the body of man a change as well as in the macrocosm'.

Health and the environment in early modern England

were what they ate, and we in turn were what we ate of them. As Cogan put it: 'Such as the food is, such is the blood: and such as the blood, such is the flesh.' [87] He went on to argue that our health depends on what we eat. This also applied to animals:

Yet the goodnesse of the pasture helpeth much to the goodnesse of the milke: for ill pastures made ill milke, and good pastures made good milke: for such as the food is such is the bloud and such as the bloud is, such is the milke.[88]

Given the view that there was a close union between all the parts of the organic and inorganic worlds it is not surprising that specific ideas such as the healthiness of motion were applied to a wide range of objects and creatures. At the level of these specific ideas there was a perceived dichotomy between town and country, short life and long life, the unhealthy and the healthy, the stultifying and the fresh, the stagnant and the moving, dark and light, crowded and uncrowded, the tame and the wild, ('unhealthy places in the countryside' could be substituted for town or city in the first pair of opposites). These were not merely opposing pairs of ideas, but towns, for instance, could be associated with one part of each pair, with tameness, bad stagnant air or water, darkness and smoke, overcrowding, bad health etc. That such contrasts really were current is clear from the example of the pig.

Swine's flesh was looked on with some suspicion, but it was believed to be healthy if the pig had been allowed to roam in the wild and to eat natural foodstuffs. Cogan wrote:

Also better [to eat] of a wilde swine than of a tame, because as Galen saith, the flesh of swine fed at home is more full of superflous moysture for want of motion, beside they live in a more grosse ayre than those that live wild. But our use in England is for the most part to breed our swine at home, except it be for the time of mast falling, for then they feed abroad in the woods, which kinde of feeding in my judgement is most wholesome: wherefore brawne, which is of a bore long fed in a stie can in no wise be wholesome meat, although it be young. For beside that it is hard of digestion (as common experience proveth) it must needs breed ill iuce in the body, considering the want of motion and grosse feeding thereof for which course we use commonly to drinke strong wine with brawne to help digestion.[89]

Thomas Fuller in his *History of the Worthies of England* (1662) praised 'Hampshire Hoggs' as producing the best bacon because:

Here the swine feed in the Forrest on plenty of Acorns (mens meat in the Golden, Hog's food in this Iron Age); which going out lean, return home fat,

---

[87] Cogan, *Haven of Health*, Epistle Dedicatory.   [88] *Ibid.*, p. 176.   [89] *Ibid.*, p. 133.

without either care or cost of their owners. Nothing but fulness stinteth their feeding on the mast falling from the Trees, where also they lodge at liberty (not pent up, as in other places to stacks of Pease), which some assign the reason of the fineness of their flesh.[90]

Thomas Muffet agreed that the pig was especially nourishing 'if he feed abroad upon sweet grass, good mast and roots; for that which is penn'd up and fed at home with taps droppings, kitchin offal, soure grains and all manner of drosse cannot be wholsom'.[91] And Thomas Tryon at the end of the century held a similar view: 'That Bacon and Pork, which is fed with Corn and Acorns and have their liberty to run, is much sweeter and wholsomer, easier of digestion and breeds better blood than that which is shut up in the Hogg-sties, such Bacon for want of motion becomes more of a gross phlegmatic Nature'.[92]

The idea that fresh air, fresh food and freedom to move were good for pigs (and for men and women) remained the same despite changes in theoretical perspectives, and these ideas can also be found today amongst the 'green' or environmental movements as well as amongst many other groups. A characteristic of such 'natural' ideas is that they were generalized enough to be applicable to many different types of situation. Thomas Muffet, for instance, wrote about the fattening of fowl and he united the view that lack of exercise produced unhealthy food with another basic concept (already referred to) that there is a close connection between the qualities (psychological as well as physical) of the bodies that we eat and our own:

But here a question may be moved, Whether this penning up of birds, and want of exercise, and depriving them of light, and cramming them so often with strange meat, makes not their flesh as unwholesome to us as well as fat? To which I answer that to cramb Capons, or any bird and to deprive them of all light, is ill for them and us too: for though their body be puffed up, yet their flesh is not natural and wholsom; witness their small discoloured and rotten livers; whereas Hens and Capons feeding themselves in an open and clean place with good corn have large, ruddy and firm livers...[do not feed them] in a coope or close roome, for then the aire and themselves will smell of their own dung, but in a cleane house spacious enough for their little exercise; not in a dark place, or stitching up their eyes, for that will cause them to be timerous, or ever sleepy; both which are enemies to their bodies, and consequently ours.[93]

[90] Thomas Fuller, *The History of the Worthies of England*, 2 vols. (London, 1811), I, p. 400.
[91] Thomas Muffet, *Health's Improvement* (London, 1655), p. 68.
[92] Tryon, *The Way to Health*, p. 67.
[93] Muffet, *Health's Improvement*, pp. 43-4. Thomas, *Man and the Natural World*, p. 189 cites this in part when discussing the perceived cruelty of poultry farming.

Health and the environment in early modern England

Despite the great changes that have taken place in medical ideas, many views about the healthiness of the environment and its products have remained largely unchanged. In a sense, they express the aspirations of certain parts of society: condemnation of present-day developments and a yearning for a natural world whose attributes – clean, light, spacious allowing motion, uncrowded etc. – are still viewed today, unquestioningly, as good and positive characteristics. Perhaps an anthropologist would use such attributes, and the pairs of opposites listed earlier, as evidence from which to construct a picture of the type of society that created them. A historian of medicine, after cautious caveats about the limited currency of such ideas, can note that early modern England possessed a well-articulated body of knowledge about the health of the environment. At a time when cities and towns were growing in size and in unhealthiness a set of values was present which acted as a counter weight, which some of the literate classes, at least, could refer to even if they did not always act on them. (Though as Philip Curtin has shown in his study of mortality in the tropics, the mortality of European armies declined when some of these ideas such as siting camps on hill stations, good ventilation, clear water were put into practice in the nineteenth century.)[94]

I would like to thank Lindsay Granshaw, Roy Porter and Phillip Wilson for their helpful comments on this chapter.

[94] Philip Curtin, *Death by Migration. Europe's Encounter with the Tropical World in the Nineteenth Century* (Cambridge, 1989).

V

Religious beliefs and medicine in early modern England

Social history of medicine, influenced perhaps by attempts to focus on 'history from below' and by critiques of modern scientific medicine, has taken on a much broader view of medicine and its practitioners. Rather than focusing only on great doctors and discoveries and on elite practitioners it now studies popular and quack medicine, and the views of patients, and conceives its subject as health and illness in its social, political and economic aspects as well as in its medical and demographic contexts. As part of this change, the relationship between religion and medicine in the early modern period has received increased attention.[1]

In some ways, religion in the early modern period fits easily into the perspective of the social history of medicine. For instance, religious sentiments and beliefs about illness were widespread amongst clergymen who wrote diaries. There is ample material from diarists such as Ralph Josselin, the minister at Earls Colne in Essex, or Henry Newcombe, a Non-conformist clergyman preaching in Manchester,[2] who were concerned to give a daily account of their dealings with God and His with them,[3] to construct a picture of the patient's view of medicine and religion, although obviously the patient involved is a special type.

The fact that some ministers like Richard Napier and Richard Baxter[4] also acted as healers and medical practitioners has allowed medical historians to place religion in the early modern 'medical marketplace' which has been the object of attention.[5] The medical marketplace has been a valuable organising concept that has helped to make sense of the large number of different kinds of medical practitioner in early modern England. Although the term and the concept emerged in the Reagan and Thatcher years and during the ascendancy of market economics, it should be seen as having connotations that go beyond the purely economic. Ministers and gentlewomen gave free medical services for the spiritual benefits to be gained from such charity; and in a more general sense there was an exchange market where friends and family members offered each other their favourite medical receipts, and sometimes medical care, within a context of social and family ties.

Other traditions of historiography have also helped to shape historians' view of the relationship between religion and medicine. The fierce emotions associated with the religious, political and nationalist self-consciousness of many sixteenth- and seventeenth-century Protestants have been echoed by historians such as Christopher Hill, Patrick Collinson and Keith Thomas,[6] and the English Protestant tradition appears to have influenced medical historians towards seeing the relationship between medicine and religion in sectarian and political terms. More generally, the wish of medical historians to give priority to social and political interests is found in the work of historians of science and intellectual historians who have been concerned with integrating their fields with general history, while moving away from the self-contained discipline of the history of ideas where ideas often seemed to exist autonomously, separate from society as in the Platonic world of forms.[7] Such approaches have helped to create something closer to a 'total history' of medicine, and one that is much better integrated with the social and political events of the time.

A caveat can be entered, however. It can be difficult to incorporate structural analysis in the new social history of medicine: for instance, the similarities in the Christianity of Catholics and Protestants are often ignored by English historians in favour of a stress upon their differences. This is to set aside not only much theology held in common, including many of the teachings of the Bible, but also the shared culture and tradition of the Latin-based university curriculum which allowed the learned to recognise each other across Europe. The difficulty for the historian wishing to point out such structural similarities is that the differences were often more explicit in the consciousness of people at the time whilst similarities were more implicit.

In this essay I will discuss in an introductory and general way how, at the level of religious doctrine, we can speak of a relationship between religion and medicine. It should provide some of the conceptual framework to a world of practice in which medicine and religion often interacted, though at times this might be at the level of exhortation and rhetoric as, for instance, in the case of plague or in the treatment and care of the sick poor[8] which the learned physicians tended to avoid. It points out the similarities between Catholic and Protestant views on religion, medicine, and illness and then focuses on differences, specifically on how Calvinist doctrines were used by the elite university-trained 'learned physicians' to bolster their authority against their competitors. The essay ends by briefly discussing how some learned physicians argued that the Christian doctrine on the charitable care of the sick poor could be limited and could not be used to justify unlearned medical practice.

General background

Christianity offered both an explanation for illness and a cure. Illness was often viewed in the sixteenth and seventeenth centuries as God-given. Plague, for instance, was considered to be one of the most devastating signs of God's power. This was the time when God or his angels aimed their plague darts at whole communities. Both Catholics and Protestants produced communal responses.[9] Their precise nature could differ. Catholics often paraded the bones of the town's patron saint round the town's boundaries in solemn procession, or prayed to St Roch the plague saint. Protestants would have days of communal prayer and humiliation directed at God alone and not at the saints, the worship of saints being condemned as a Catholic superstition.

The agreement between Catholics and Protestants seen from a present-day point of view appears greater than the differences and, though at the time the differences had for many greater force, the basic relationship between Christianity, illness and medicine was contained in doctrines from the Bible and from the early Church Fathers upon which both Catholics and Protestants agreed. Prayer, pleading for divine mercy, was Christianity's remedy for an illness that was viewed as God's punishment or as a trial of one's faith.

At the individual level, there was a similar connection between illness, sin and God. The association between the illness of an individual and God's will was greater perhaps for Protestants, especially Calvinists, for whom God's providence showed itself in the happenings of their everyday lives. The sense of being completely in God's hands which permeated Protestant thinking was underpinned by the reliance on faith alone for salvation and by the denial of the Catholic emphasis on good works. The latter gave the individual a sense of controlling his or her own destiny, the former left a person at the mercy of God's providence; and the onset of illness was one sign of God's providence. The remedies were prayer and repentance, and were common to both sides of western Christianity. For Catholics, they were channelled through the mediation of the Church and its sacraments. Protestants practised a more direct and personal form of praying that sought communication on a one-to-one level between the sick person and God.

There were similarities between Protestants and Catholics in their approach to illness not only at the general level but also in detail. Continuities across time are striking. For instance, in the fourteenth-century preacher's hand-book, the *Fasciculus Morum*, composed in England and extensively copied, there occur some of the standard expressions that have been taken as being peculiarly Protestant: illness was perceived to be the chastisement of God, who as a loving father used the rod of illness to correct an erring child; extended medical metaphors were used to explain how spiritual illness could be healed; and Christ was depicted as the good physician:

we must know that for our spiritual sicknesses Christ comes as a good physician to heal us. Christ acts like a physician in the following way. A doctor investigates the condition of the sick person and the nature of his sickness by such methods as taking his pulse and inspecting his urine. Thus when Christ visits a sinner, he first enlightens him with his grace to understand himself and his own sin, so that he may repent of his sins and shun them; Jeremiah 3: 'See your ways and know what you have done'. Second, after diagnosing the sickness he gives the sick person a diet as he requires and prescribes what he should eat and what he should avoid; this means that Christ teaches to avoid the occasions of sin and to seek the occasions for practicing the virtues. Third, after he had prescribed and worked out a diet, he gives the sick person some syrup, an electuary, or some other medicine against this sickness to expel it; that is, Christ gives him contrition of his sins, which is made from bitter herbs... of it is written: 'Your drink will be bitter'. Fourth, when the sick person is healed, he warns him against relapsing and teaches him how to live, so that he fosters in him a good intention to live a good life. Christ further heals us in many additional ways as if from physical illness.[10]

Underlying all the forms of prayer and of ceremonies was the fact that Christ was, as innumerable texts put it, the physician of both the body and the soul. The healing of the sick, the blind, the lame, the casting out of devils to cure madness, and the ultimate cure of all, that of raising Lazarus from the dead, all illustrated that Christ was the only real physician. The Church quickly made use of the image of Christ the Physician, and the early Church Fathers, as Darrel Amundsen has shown, described Christ as the Great Physician, the *verus Medicus, solus Medicus, ipse et medicus et medicamentum* – Himself both the physician and the medication.[11] Catholics and Protestants alike saw Christ as a physician. And it is the fact that Christ himself had healed as well as the claim of Christ to be the saviour of the world that gave added credence to the prayers of the sick.

Despite the differences discussed below, Catholic and Protestant teaching on illness had much in common. The differences have been too often exaggerated. For instance, in Keith Thomas's magisterial and influential *Religion and the Decline of Magic*, sixteenth- and seventeenth-century Protestant views of Catholicism have been accepted and used by Thomas as correct characterisations of Catholicism. This has the result that we are presented with a negative picture of a 'superstitious' and magical Catholic Church very different from the Protestant Churches. Recently, however, Valerie Flint has produced a convincing counter to the view of a superstitious medieval Church by showing how non-Christian magic was selected and integrated into Christianity for well-thought-out and positive reasons.[12]

The relationship between medicine and religion received, as might be expected, more attention from religious than from medical writers. Medical writers did not feel constrained by religious teaching or think that they were in conflict with it, and they tend to be silent on the relationship between medicine and religion. It is true that from the Middle Ages onwards men such as John of Salisbury deployed the trope of physicians as atheists and greedy, money-grabbing atheists at that;[13] John Ford in the *Lovers Melancholy* (1629) reiterated a traditional view of the physician which was at variance with the ideal type, 'the grave physician', constructed by the learned physicians:

Thou art in thy religion an Atheist, in thy condition a cur, in thy diet an epicure, in thy lust a goat, in thy sleep a hog; thou takest upon thee the habit of a grave physician, but thou art indeed an impostorous empiric. Physicians are the cobblers, rather the botchers, of men's bodies; as the one patches our tattered clothes, so the other solders our diseased flesh. [1.2.129-35][14]

But there was little obvious conflict up to the sixteenth century between Christianity and the secular medicine of Hippocrates and Galen. Part of the reason must lie in the assimilation of Christianity and Aristotelian philosophy (and with it Galenic medicine) in the Middle Ages, as well as in the compromise made at an early stage by Christian writers such as Clement of Alexandria (c.150-c.220), Origen (c.184-c.253), Basil (c.329-379), Jerome (c.345-c.419), John Chrysostom (c.349-407), and Augustine (c.354-c.430) who accepted that God in his mercy had placed herbs and other medicines on earth for use by man (and also by physicians), and that through the action of God's will, especially when a prayer was made before treatment, the medicines ('God's means' as sixteenth- and seventeenth-century English Protestants called them[15]), would work. In this way medicine was formally incorporated into religion. But the possibility that God could heal directly, of his own will, was always present and accepted.

In a more specifically theological sense, the interest of religious writers in illness and medicine stems not only from the example of Christ the Physician and the recognition that Christianity was a healing religion, but also from the perception that the body and the soul were closely connected and that Christianity dealt with the transition from life to death and hence to the next world, a transition when the body and soul were separated.[16] This was given concrete expression by both Catholics and Protestants who insisted that the authority of Christianity to manage this transition was paramount over the claims of medicine, and thus excluded physicians from the dying person's bedside in favour of priests and ministers.

But in their concepts, as opposed to their actions, clergymen could not avoid using medical or natural-philosophical terms when discussing the transition from this life to the next world through death. There was a constant ambiguity and sense of connection between the bodily and the spiritual that often led to the use of such terminology by both Catholics and Protestants (and of medical metaphors in general as in the *Fasciculus Morum*), especially as religious writers would have been exposed to it while studying at university.

For instance, Henry King (1592-1669), Bishop of Chichester, who was a conservative Calvinist, one of the godly who stayed within the Church of England, clearly shared in the learning of the orthodox, Galenic physicians. On the question of how Christ rose from the dead, King made use of Galenic conceptions of digestion as he attempted to make the supernatural understandable in terms of natural processes:

Three daies he lay in Earth, like sleeping Samson in the lap of Delilah, *Linteis involutus*: manicled and *bound with linnen cloathes*, as you reade in the Gospell. He might truly say, *Cinxerant mee funes Mortis*: The snares or cords of Death compassed me; but *it is impossible for him to be holden with those cords* (saith another Scripture). And therefore, *loosing the sorrowes or Bands of Death* (so the Syriack reades it), he came out. His incorruptible body lay indeed like a dangerous surfet in the Stomacke of Earth, which was unable to digest it or by assimilation to turne it into its own substance, as by that common chyle of putrefaction ordinary courses convert into Earth; and therefore it must needs cast Him up againe, or perish by that distemper.

And cast Him up it did, as Egypt ejected Israel, laden with their owne spoiles.[17]

Medical metaphors have recently been studied by David Harley with an emphasis on Protestant sectarian interests; here I would like to add some structural and theological points to his account.[18] The use of medical and physical metaphors to explain the inexplicable or the supernatural was part of the Catholic and Protestant preachers' general use of language whereby the more familiar things of this world help to make understandable those of the spiritual and miraculous world.

The ambiguous connection between the physical and spiritual realms, which allowed for medical metaphors as well as many others drawn from everyday life, can be illustrated in questions concerning the physical location of hell. Despite being on a supernatural plane, the physicality of hell and its ability to torment the body, as if it was a living body, created a supernatural-natural dualism analogous to that of the duality of soul and the body in this world. Hell, as King put it, created 'the Paine of Losse and the Paine of Sense, One to torment the Soul the other the Body'. It worked on both spiritual and physical levels. Its fire and its geographical location were alike ambiguous, lying in either the spiritual or physical realms:

When I have said this, no man's curiosity (I presume) will expect a more punctuall Description of this *Summum Malum* – Highest Degree of Evill; Or desire to be resolved what kinde of Fire it is, whether Materiall or Immateriall; What Place it hath, whether in the Body of the Earth, or in the Aire; What Intermissions, what Duration.

I am not so well skilled in the Chorography and Mappe of Hell, as those that undertake both to dispute and Define these things... What this Gehenna is, Tertullian will sufficiently resolve: *It is a Treasure of Fire which will breake out at the last Day*. That this fire *differs from that culinary Fire which serves our use*, there is no controversie. That there shall bee a difference in the Torment, wee may boldly pronounce for Truth: For as all shall not bee regarded with equall degree of Beatitude, so neither shall all Sinners bee punished alike. Adultery, and Theft, and Murther, meet in one and the same Center Hell, but the Theefe and the Murtherer shall not burne alike.[19]

The life of the damned in hell was also double-faced, being both immortal and this-worldly, and its description stretched language to its limits:

All *Epithets* are too narrow to comprehend, all language too light to expresse the weight of those Torments, all Arithmeticke too little to calculate the duration of them. It is *Mors sine Morte, Finis sine Fine, Defectus sine Defectu*: An Immortall Death, a dying yet never determining Life, an Endlesse End, a Plenty of all Misery, but Dearth of all Comfort. The Punishment of Hell is a torture that kills not, A Judgement that executes eternally, but never finishes the execution. 'Tis an everlasting Calenture, a Disease under which the Body ever languishes, but never impaires.[20]

Christian teaching on topics such as the living death of hell, the changing (in Catholic belief) of bread and wine into flesh and blood, and most significant of all, the dual nature of Christ, both God and man, shows that at the heart of Christianity lay a close interconnection between this world and the next, with much of Christian theology being, of course, concerned to express the links between the two. Medicine and natural philosophy provided a linguistic bridge between the two worlds. Medicine with its hope of the cure of the body could also by extension be used in discussions of the cure of the soul. Likewise illness with its connotations of bodily corruption was a ready metaphor for descriptions of sin and the soul's corruption. In a sense, medical metaphors and theories served as resources that dovetailed well with Christian teaching. King could write of 'the Literall Plague of Disease and Noysome Pestilence or the Metaphoricall Plague of Sinne; Dangers of the Body or of the Soule'. Perceived reality also underpinned the preachers' link between the literal and metaphorical, for physical illness and especially plague was seen as having both physical and spiritual causes and remedies, and at the same time the soul's cure could heal the body. The dramatist Thomas Dekker wrote of the plague of 1603:

Only this Antidote apply,
Cease vexing heaven, and cease to die,
Seeke therefore (after you have found
Salve naturall for the naturall wound
Of this Contagion) Cure from thence
Where first the evill did commence,
And that's the Soule: each one purge one,
And *Englands* free, the Plague is gone.[21]

Medical metaphors were by no means the only ones used. Images drawn, for instance, from warfare, the social structure of society, or the happenings of everyday life, were constantly employed to make real and familiar moral teachings and descriptions of the next world. The end result was that if religion had in theological terms incorporated medicine into itself, and thus put medicine under its authority, yet the linguistic base that underpinned its teachings owed more than a little to medicine and the secular world.

If we turn from the way medical metaphors were used by Christian preachers to the specific issue of how English ministers gave advice to the sick, it appears that the spiritual significance of sickness was stressed. Sickness was spiritualised and the redemptive side of Christianity was made to appear more significant than medicine, at least initially, for often the healing, quasi-medical side of religion would also emerge. Today illness and dying have been 'medicalised' and are clearly within the ambit of physicians' authority, but in the seventeenth century the attempt to bring dying, and to some extent illness, within the scope of religion was part of the concern of Christianity to govern all aspects and stages of life.

For instance, the sixteenth-century English Protestant Thomas Becon (1512-1567) stressed the spiritual use of illness. It could punish one's sins or try one's faith. His focus was religious, with little concern for medical matters. In the *Prayer for them that are Sick*, he points out that those that are most sinful are often not visited with illness, but that in the end they will receive the eternal pains of hell; but that if God wills the salvation of someone then he may make them ill:

> O Jesu, the Saviour of the world, and the true Physician both of the body and of the soul, we are not altogether ignorant how detestable a thing sin is in thy sight, how greatly thou abhorest them that commit iniquity... Some that thus ungodly behave themselves thou sufferest to go forth still in their beast-like manners, without correction or punishment to live in pleasure and wantoness upon the earth, to nourish their hearts as in a day of slaughter, to sowe their belly as their God and voluptuously to spend their days without all fear of thee, that at the last they, being altogether nousled in voluptuousness and dying without repentance (for the sorrows, plagues, punishment of the wicked begin at their death) may with that rich and beast-like glutton be tormented forever in hell-fire. For convenient it is that they, which in this world live all in pleasure, do in another world receive their pains.[22]

So, if people are healthy it is not necessarily the case that they have not sinned, but that perhaps they have sinned too much (a point which might have served to console those that were ill).

Becon does go on to state that sickness has a positive role; it can mean that the sick person is not lost forever to hellfire but may, through sickness, gain salvation. Sickness, as many religious writers taught, can punish and subdue the sinner to the will of God:

> Again some that walk inordinately, and contrary to the rules of thy holy law, thou, tendering their salvation, visitest them with sickness and punishest their bodies with the loving rod of thy correction, that they may no longer be proud, cruel, and fierce against the spirit, whose servant and bond-slave the body of right ought to be, but rather be obedient and serviceable, that it may from henceforth not so much as once lust against the spirit: and by this means thou mercifully callest them (which as wandering sheep have so long strayed abroad) home again unto thy sheep-fold.[23]

Becon makes the point that those whom God loves, those he punishes, and that 'sickness and adversity is sent from thee unto the children of men for their great profit and singular commodity'.[24] Sickness thus had a clear spiritual function, leading the sinner to repentance. Yet, the hope of physical cure and healing from God was always present.

Becon ended his *Prayer* by uniting the spiritual and the physical dimensions of illness:

> O Lord, it is *not* thy property alway to chide, alway to be angry, neither to deal with us according to our sins... Be thou therefore, O most merciful Saviour, a physician to such as are diseased either in body or soul, and, after this thy loving correction, restore unto them the benefit of health, both corporally and spiritually.[25]

At a general level, it seems as if religious writers by spiritualising illness, by stating that medicines and physicians were put on earth by God, and by constant allusion to Christ the physician of body and soul, as well as by their use of medical metaphors in sermons, were incorporating medicine and illness into religion as befitted the dominant ideology of the time – rather than being concerned with the content of medicine. It is also worth remembering that the Anglican Church had its own ceremonies for the sick: the 'visitation of the sick' and 'the communion of the sick' which were set out in great, and on the whole, unchanging detail in the various books of common prayer from 1549 to 1662. Apart from the anointing of the sick person contained in the 1549 prayer book but omitted from 1552 onwards, the ceremonies used no spiritual medicine except prayer; on the other hand, they made no mention of the power of God's means, of physical remedies. From the moment that the clergyman entered the sick person's house and was enjoined to say 'Peace be in this house, and to all that dwell in it' and then to kneel in the sick person's presence, religious sentiments were dominant and references to medicine were absent. The strict order and ritual into which the themes of repentance, God's mercy, the hope of recovery through Christ, and illness as a test of a Christian's faith and as a chastisement of God, were interwoven in the visitation of the sick, had no counterpart in medicine; although medical writers since the time of Hippocrates' *Decorum* had given advice on how to visit a patient, there was no sense of medicine's providing a ritual order to challenge that of the Church in the way that perhaps modern hospitals and clinics do. The specific instance of the Anglican ritual for the sick indicates that the Church could at times ignore medicine when dealing with illness.

The primacy of religion was also stressed when the patient was given advice on the relative importance of religion and medicine. Andrew Boorde, a Carthusian who in 1534 conformed to Protestantism, stressed in his medical hand-book *The Breviary of Helthe* (1543) that religion should come first, in both the patient's thoughts and actions:

I do advertyse every sicke man and al other men the wiche hathe any infyrmitie... to pacify him selfe... and to fix his harte and mynd in christes death and passion and to call to his rememberance what paines, what advesyte, and what penury and povertye Christ dyd suffer for us. And he that can thus pacyfy him selfe, and feele his owne payne in Christs passion shall mitigate his paynes and angiushe be it never so great.[26]

Both Catholics and Protestants emphasised that if the patient was to summon outside help, the priest or minister was first to be called and then the physician. Catholics gave specific priority to making a confession without which they believed that the soul was in peril of hell, but Protestants also believed in the necessity of calling on a minister, or God Himself, if death might be imminent. Boorde advised:

V

And then if the patient will have any councell in physicke. Fyrste let him call to him hys spyrytuall phisician which is his goostly father, and let him make his conscience clene and that he be in perfyte love and charite, and yf he hath done any wronge let him loke to it... Then let the pacient provyde for his body, and take councell of some expert phisician howe and in what wyse the body may be recovered of his infyrmitie, and then to commyt his body to the industry of his physician.

Although Boorde gave priority to religion, in his *persona* as physician he stressed the need for the patient to obey the medical practitioner and so avoid the sin of self-destruction.

And at all tymes redy to followe the wyll, mynd and counsell of his physicion, for who soever will do the countrary saynt Augustine saythe 'Seipsum interimit qui precepta medici observuare non vult' that is to say. He doth kill himself that doth not observe the commandment of his phisicion.[27]

Physicians did not usually concern themselves with the substance of religion. There are, of course, exceptions. Religion and medicine was integrated in a very personal way by Sir Thomas Browne. Less exceptionally, medical writers often brought in religious considerations when discussing plague and to a lesser extent syphilis, or when differentiating between physical madness and spiritual possession.[28] They might write in a perfunctory and conventional way that a remedy worked with God's help, but at the bedside there was usually no mention of a religious ceremony associated with medical treatment, unless a minister-physician was involved. The surgeon William Clowes in his treatise on syphilis of 1585 did none the less set out a prayer to:

The heavenly Physician that hast not only provided but also profered to miserable man, the wholesome medicines of health... We beseech thee make us diligent in searching, careful in using, and faithful in practising and applying of those remedies, that thou has taught us. Blesse our labours, we beseech thee, that thy power giving force to these medicines, they may bee effectuall to the removing the griefes of thy people.[29]

Because of his subject Clowes was able to give vent to a great deal of moral judgement (the lower orders got syphilis because of their sexual sins and depravity, the respectable could suffer from it without sexual contact) and the prayer is part of the moral ethos of Clowes's text. If Clowes was not typical of medical writers, yet Robert Burton in the *Anatomy of Melancholy* shows that the ideal practice which united religion and medicine was known:

We must use prayer and physick both together: and so no doubt but our prayers will be available, and our physick take effect. 'Tis that Hezekiah practised, Luke the Evangelist; and which we are enjoined, not the patient only, but the Physician himself. Hippocrates, an heathen, required this in a good practitioner, and so did Galen, and in that tract of his, regarding Times and Manners, 'tis a thing which he doth inculcate, and many others. Hyperius, speaking of that happiness and good success which all Physicians desire and hope for in their cures, tells them that it is not to be expected, except with a true faith they call upon God, and teach their patients to do the

V

like. The council of Lateran decreed they should do so; the Fathers of the Church have still advised as much. Otherwise, as the Prophet Jeremy denounced to Egypt, *In vain shalt thou use many medicines, for thou shalt have no health.*[30]

However, as we shall see, certain Protestant doctrines did become relevant to some of the learned physicians.

Religion and the learned physician's monopoly

From the point of view of the university-trained, learned English physicians, the Protestant religion provided a useful rhetorical resource in their struggles against their competitors in the largely unregulated medical marketplace of sixteenth- and seventeenth-century England. The Protestant Reformation produced new doctrines which could be used to justify physicians' claims to a monopoly of practice, and it also reiterated previous Catholic praise of the classical knowledge that formed the cognitive basis of the physicians' assertion that their medicine was best.

A critical issue that divided Catholics and Calvinists concerned the question of whether priests could, through the sacraments, the laying on of hands, and anointing with holy oil, still heal miraculously as had Christ's disciples. Calvin, of course, denied any miraculous power in general to the sacraments. As part of this attack he denied the continued gift of healing to anyone other than God, and also denied that any physical material or even touch had miraculous powers. Whenever Calvin discussed a healing miracle in his commentaries on the Gospels, he repeated the point that Christ could have healed without the physical laying on of hands. His word or nod alone would have been enough.[31] On the healing of Simon's mother-in-law of a fever, Calvin stressed the symbolic nature of the laying on of hands, and that Christ's healing was not for bodily health but for the spiritual purpose of enlightening the sick and to prove his divinity.

It was a more sure and notable proof of divine power to remove a grievous disease in a moment, and at a single touch. Though he could have done it with a nod alone… My interpretation simply is that Christ laid his hands on the sick to commend them to the Father, and to win them grace and deliverance from their diseases.[32]

Concerning 'the purpose of healing their diseases', Calvin wrote:

They in their bodies felt the Grace of Christ, but we must look to the end in view, for it would be preposterous to tie ourselves to a fading benefit [life], as though the Son of God were a physician of the body… He gave light to the blind in order to show Himself to them as the light of the world. He gave life back to the dead, that He might prove Himself to be the resurrection and the life; similarly with the lame and paralysed.[33]

Calvin was clearly trying to move away from the ceremonial nature of the miracle and from the emphasis on Christ the physician healing the body, to the underlying spiritual motives.

Calvin interpreted in a similar way the passage in Mark VI: 12-14 ('And they went out, and preached that men should repent, and anointed with oil many that were sick, and healed them') which was used by Catholics to justify the ceremony of anointing the sick with oil. He denied that physical means, whether of touch or oil, could have any miraculous power, nor, he added, could the oil have been a kind of medicine. The argument, of course, was related to Calvin's refutation of the real power of the sacraments and his affirmation of their merely symbolic status.

> Therefore I consider this [the oil] to have been a visible symbol of spiritual grace which testified that the healing of which they were the ministers came from the secret power of God... But what a perverted aping of the apostles it is to invent in the Church a ceremony of anointing the sick! This is quite clear from the fact that the gift of healing that Christ bestowed on the apostles was not an inheritance for them to hand down to their descendants, but a seal of the preaching of the Gospel for that occasion. And today the ignorance of the Papists is too ridiculous: they claim that their stinking unction, which precipitates the half-dead to their graves is a sacrament.[34]

In the *Institutes of the Christian Religion* Calvin developed at length his denial of the present-day efficacy of extreme unction and he also made the point that although St James wished all sick persons to be anointed (James V: 12) 'these fellows smear with grease not the sick but half-dead corpses when they are already drawing their last breath, or (as they say) *in extremis*. If in their sacrament they have a powerful medicine with which to alleviate the agony of diseases, or at least to bring some comfort to the soul, it is cruel of them never to heal in time'.[35]

The whole tenor of Calvin's argument was against the Catholic Church or its priests having any miraculous power of healing. As he put it, the age of miracles was past. The emphasis on God as the only being who could now heal miraculously meant an end to the original compromise which allowed religious and medical healing to exist side by side. For Calvinists, no living individuals could heal miraculously through the power of God. The healing miracles that Augustine noted as being performed in his time after the physicians had failed were no more, indeed in the eyes of Calvinists they had never taken place.[36] A result of this was that learned physicians could assert from the authority of religious doctrine that some of their competitors who claimed a God-given power of healing, or God-given knowledge of medicine, were bogus.

An allied issue was what kind of physician Protestants should recommend. This was certainly a topic related to religion, for ministers often stressed that people had a duty to take care of their body's health, the temporal house of the soul. (Luther wrote that failure to do so was a form of self-murder.)[37] Calvin clearly supported learned medicine. Unlike Luther he did not emphasise the atheistic nature of classical learning, nor did he call, like Luther, for a reform of the universities and the replacement of Aristotelian philosophy with a greater emphasis on the scriptures.[38] The Lutheran position, though, was not one of outright condemnation of classical learning for, as Sachiko Kusukawa has brilliantly shown, Melanchthon at Wittenberg developed Aristotelian and especially Galenic doctrines for Lutheran

theology,. and taught Galenic anatomy to divinity students – to show God's creative wisdom and the nature of the house of the soul.[39] For Calvin, the classical
writings were to be admired for their truths, which came from God.

> Shall we say that the philosophers were blind in their fine observations and artful description of
> nature? Shall we say that those men were devoid of understanding who conceived the art of
> disputation and taught us to speak reasonably? Shall we say that they are insane who developed
> medicine, devoting their labour to our benefit? What shall we say of all the mathematical
> sciences? Shall we consider them the ravings of madmen? No, we cannot read the writings of the
> ancients on these subjects without great admiration. We marvel at them because we are com-
> pelled to recognise how pre-eminent they are. But shall we count anything praiseworthy or
> noble without recognising at the same time that it comes from God?[40]

This acceptance of classical learning, the learning of the establishment, is reiterated in Calvin's discussion of God's workmanship and wisdom in creating the
world and human beings. The unlearned can grasp God's workmanship through
their eyes, but 'men who have either quaffed or even tasted the liberal arts penetrate with their aid far more deeply into the secrets of divine wisdom'.[41] Calvin's
approval of the established university subjects is made explicit for medicine when
he writes that Galen had demonstrated most perceptively God's workmanship:
'likewise, in regard to the structure of the human body, one must have the greatest
keenness in order to weigh with Galen's skill, its articulation, symmetry, beauty
and use'.[42] Calvin's praise of God's workmanship and of the classical university
learning which often expounded upon it can be found in Catholic and Protestant
writers alike.[43] He and they were heirs to the medieval accommodation of pagan
classical learning with Christianity. However, if one wished to reject the learning
of the universities then the pagan and heretical nature of its classical basis could
be emphasised, as in Luther's discussion of Aristotle or, in England, in the early
Paracelsian work of Richard Bostocke. Bostocke stressed in 1585 that Aristotle and
Galen were atheists who had asserted the eternity of the world; they had not only
denied the immortality of the soul, but had also excluded God's direct action on
earth by their emphasis on secondary causes.[44] The material was always there for a
Christian rejection of classical learning, despite the synthesis of the Middle Ages.
Calvin, however, clearly approved of classical, establishment learning, in the same
way as he approved of secular magistrates. It can be concluded that Calvin also
approved of the learned (Galenic) physicians. He certainly appears familiar with
their technical terminology – he mentioned, for example, the difference between
leprosy and elephantiasis, and the different pains produced by chronic and acute
paralysis, and he knew of the optic nerve.[45]
    In England William Perkins, the late sixteenth- and early seventeenth-century
Calvinist divine, also approved of learned physicians. He advised the sick to avoid
wise men and women or charmers, he attacked uroscopy and empirics, and littered
his texts with references to Galen and to the learned tradition in medicine. He
wrote that 'speciall care must be had to make choice of such Physicians as are

V

knowne to bee well learned, and men of experience, as also of good conscience and good religion. For as in other callings, so in this also, there be sundry abuses which may indanger the lives and the health of men'. Perkins went on to set out the example of uroscopists as one such abuse.[46] Together with advice on how to choose a good physician came warnings on whom to avoid. Perkins and other Protestant writers took a strong stand against magical remedies and attacked cunning men and women, or white witches, as real wizards and witches. In this way those who might be thought to have the gift of healing were tainted with witchcraft. Perkins condemned the 'use of such meanes as have no warrant' such as 'all charmes or spels' and he wrote that

these unlawfull and absurd meanes are more used and sought for of common people than good physicke. But it stands all men greatly in hand in no wise to seeke foorth to enchanters, and sorcerers, which indeed are but witches and wizzards, though they are commonly called cunning men and women. It were better for a man to die of his sickenesse, then to seeke recovery by such wicked persons.[47]

Henry Holland, a Puritan minister and medical practitioner, in his *An Admonition Concerning the Use of Physick* (1603) concluded from the denial of God-given (or Catholic) healing that it was the learned physician who was God-given. 'Now then the gift [of healing] ceasing... the learned physician [is] the comfortable and ordinary means which God hath left unto us in nature as long as the World endureth' and he quoted in support the famous text of Ecclesiasticus XXXVIII: 10: 'honour the physician with that honour that is due unto him for the Lord hath created him'. Thomas Dekker, more generally, placed the learned physicians, amongst whom he included Paracelsians, into the framework of godly learning. He referred to them as God-given, gathering the herbs that God had placed on earth to cure diseases, and as being far superior to empirics. Yet, his own medicines culled from religion were, he wrote, superior to those of the great medical authorities. Dekker, who showed in his writings a close knowledge of medical matters, had clearly absorbed the sentiments both of the learned physicians and of ministers, and he saw no conflict between the two. Rather, Dekker indicated that the former were well integrated into religion, though spiritual remedies of ministers were more efficacious.

Is Sickness come to thy doore!... Make much of thy Physitian: let not an Emperick or Mounti-bancking Quacksaluer peepe in at thy window, but set thy Gates wide open to entertaine thy learned Physitian: Honour him, make much of him. Such a Physitian is Gods second, and in a duell or single fight (of this nature) will stand brauely to thee. A Good Physitian, comes to thee in the shape of an *Angell*, and therefore let him boldly take thee by the hand, for he has been in Gods garden, gathering herbes: and soueraine rootes to cure thee; A good Physitian deales in simples, and will be simply honest with thee in thy preseruation... yet... I will aduenture to Minister Physicke, and Salues to any one, that in this time, is troubl'd with the *Sicknesse*: and my Patients in the end, shall confesse: That *Gallen, Hyppocrates, Paracelsus*, nor all the great Maisters, of those Artes, did never lay downe sounder prescriptions. And heere come my Medicines martching in.

Art thou (in this visitation) stricken with Carbuncles, Blaynes, and Blisters, Is thy body spotted all over... Be rulde by me, and take this receipt; Trust to it, for it cur'd a King of Israel. Cry out with *David*, O Lord! Chastize me not in thy wrath, for thine Arrowes haue lighted vpon mee.[48]

English learned physicians, who in the sixteenth and early seventeenth centuries denounced all other practitioners, at times used the authority of the new religious doctrines. They attacked those who claimed to have the gift of healing or knowledge of medicine from God. The Salisbury physician John Securis argued in his defence of learned medicine of 1566 that

god doth not geve the gyfte of healing to any wicked people, but only by a special privilege to those only that be of a most pure, sobre and holy lyfe, as we reade of the apostles, and some of the Prophetes. And as sanct Paul saythe in the first epistle, the 12th chapter to the Corinth[ians]. To some is given the gyfte of healing by the holy ghost. So that to hele by this maner of meanes, is not commonly to use herbes, roots or other drougs bought at the poticaries shop, or to take any money or other reward for the healynge. For this kynde of healing is the mere gift of God workynge in those (to whome it pleaseth God to geve it) withoute any laboure or studye. We heare of none nowe a days that hathe thys gyfte of nature (I meane of God) savynge only the Kynges of England, and the Frenche Kynges, whyche... have a special gift to heale the Kyngs evil.[49]

Securis probably had in mind the statute of 1542, which elsewhere he attacked explicitly. This Act had allowed people with God-given rather than learned knowledge of remedies to practise in a limited way. These were, as the Act put it, 'divers honest persons... whom God hath imbued with the knowledge of the nature, kind and operation of certain herbs, roots and waters, and the using and ministering of them to such as been pained with customable diseases'.[50] The Act denounced the rapacity of surgeons and contrasted it with the charitable practice of the unlearned healers. As we shall see, learned practitioners often felt they had to counter claims of charitable practice when they fulminated against competitors such as charitable gentlewomen or pastor physicians. Such competitors, and many others of lower social status, often combined medicine with other work or callings.

In his commentary on Paul's Epistle to the Corinthians, Calvin had explained the verse 'Let every man abide in the same calling wherein he was called' (1 Corinthians VII: 20). Calvin did not believe that this instruction had to be rigidly adhered to, but he condemned the unreasonable, restless and disorderly movement from one position to another. In other words, the doctrine of calling was tied to the necessity for social order. Calvin wrote that Paul

does not lay it down, that each person must remain in a certain way of life, once he had adopted it; but on the other hand, he condemns the restlessness which prevents individuals from remaining contentedly as they are, and his advice is: 'let the shoemaker stick to his last', as the old proverb has it.[51]

The next verse: 'Art thou called being a servant? care not for it: but if thou mayest be made free, use it rather', reinforces the connection between calling, social order and hierarchy. The slave or servant should not be anxious, that is 'care', about being a slave, and Calvin wrote 'from that we infer, not only that there are, by the providence of God, distinct stations and classes in society, but also that His word directs us not to ignore them'.[52] Although Calvin wrote that 'it makes no difference to God what a person's means of livelihood is in this world since differences in this respect do not destroy harmony in religion',[53] he often saw calling as a lesser form of election and in relation to the calling to the Church, saw it as ordained by God. Of himself he wrote 'we ought to believe that it is entirely the gift of God and not the fruit of our own efforts that we have been called to govern his Church'. Calling thus had for Calvinists connotations of social order and of being part of God's plan for the individual. Logically, a healer who claimed the God-given gift of healing would seem to have had a calling rather like Calvin's which was 'not the fruit of our own efforts', rather than the calling of the learned physician which, according to Securis, required study and 'labor and peinful diligence with a long time'.[54] However, the sense of healing as a natural rather than as an acquired skill, as a providentially given calling, was challenged by the Protestant belief that the age of miraculous healing was past and by the denial that people could have two callings, which often was the case with healers.

Calvin's doctrine of calling was one amongst many arguments including lack of learning, dangerous practice, and accusations of witchcraft, deployed by medical practitioners against their competitors. As in Calvin's formulation, social disorder and not keeping to one's calling were often associated with each other.

Calvin's doctrine of calling could be used for monopolistic ends by elite medical practitioners. William Clowes, who became sympathetic to Paracelsians and was as fierce in his condemnation of empirics as the Galenic physicians, in 1585 attacked

this beastly broode following: which doe foresake their honest trades wherunto God hath called them and do daily rush into Phisicke and Chirurgerie. And some of them be Painters, some Glasiers, some Tailors, some Weavers, some Joiners, some Cutlers, some Cookes, some Bakers and some Chandlers etc. Yea, now a daies it is to apparant to see how Tinkers, Tooth-drawers, Pedlers, Ostlers, Carters, Horse-gelders and horse-leeches, Ideots, Apple-Squires, Broommen, bawds, witches, coniurers, South-saiers and sow gelders, Roages, Rat-catchers, Runagetes and Procters of Spitelhouses, with such lyke rotten and stincking weeds, which do in town and Countrie, without order, honestie, or skil daily abuse both Physick and Chirurgerie having no more perseverance, reason or knowledge.[55]

This rhetoric echoes the pervading fear of wandering beggars and vagabonds, who were perceived as dangerous to the settled order of society, and who were constantly attacked in print as well as by the Poor Laws. The practice of such healers appeared to Clowes as unlearned and empirical and he condemned it in terms which had been employed by Galen, by the subsequent tradition of learned medicine, and by Paracelsians to castigate opponents 'as a certain blind practise, without wisdom or judgement, and most commonly useth one remedie for all diseases, and one waye of curing to all persons'.[56] The social and professional condemnations reinforced each other and the doctrine of calling helped to link the parts of Clowes's diatribe.

The Northampton physician John Cotta, writing in 1612, also used Calvin's denial of the continued existence of the gift of healing, when he attacked 'pastor physicians' who practised medicine. In addition, like Clowes, he had recourse to Calvin's doctrine of keeping to the calling that God had bestowed on an individual to argue that clergymen should keep to their task and not meddle in that of others. Cotta wrote of ministers who practised medicine:

Their master saint Paul teacheth every man to walk within his owne calling, and not to be busy stragling in others... I know the gift of healing in the Apostles was the gift of God in his grace and speciall favour and allowance unto them for those times; but it was in them a miraculous and divine power consecrated unto an holy end: but in these times it is an acquired faculty.[57]

In other words, medicine is acquired, learned; Cotta would add, preferably in the universities, and clergymen should keep out of medicine, though the learned physician can also be a godly one.

Cotta's fellow Northampton physician, James Hart, wrote in the Epistle to the Reader of the *Arraignment of Urines* (1623), which Hart based on Peter van Foreest's attack on uroscopy, that parsons should not intrude into the calling of medicine. The ministry was a calling with work enough, and Hart added that the age of religious miraculous cures was past:

Is it not apparent that many of our Parsons and Vicars in this kingdome, as though they were of the secret counsell of Aesculapius... have like usurpers intruded upon other mens right? Now that the preaching of the word... and practising of Physicke are in the word of God two seuerall distinct callings I think cannot be denied. And in the second place... whosoever will conscionably performe the worke of the Ministery as hee ought, shall therein finde worke enough without meddling with the health of the body... As for the curing of Disease, it was both miraculous and lasted but for a time, they [Christ's disciples] being as free from covetousness and pecuniary traffique, as ours at this time are addicted to the same. The holy Apostle Paul willeth every man to abide in the same calling (not callings) wherein hee was called.[58]

Calvin's intellectual preferences and religious doctrines were therefore useful resources in bolstering the claims of the learned physicians, and in attacking not only healers who claimed divinely given powers, but also clergymen who practised medicine. The secular tendency that many have seen in Calvinism seems again apparent, if we interpret such doctrines as limiting the scope or ambit of religion. Such an interpretation is, of course, paradoxical since Calvinists claimed that God's power directly affected all aspects of human life. The crucial point concerns the direct power of God, for, as expressed by Calvinists, it eliminated the power of the saints and of many ceremonies and sacraments, and the Church and its clergy also lost a great deal of the divine influence previously ascribed to them. Such devolved power had been integrated into the fabric of social behaviour, and ranged from the processions of the bones of a patron saint through a town, to christenings and burials. Calvinists moved to reduce the diffusion of divine power to individuals, ceremonies, and institutions, and instead to concentrate it only on God. The denial of contemporary divine healing and the disapproval of pastor physicians are two small aspects of this tendency. If for Calvinists divinity was more sharply and powerfully represented by God, yet for them the power of divinity was no longer immanent in society – and to that extent one can talk of a process of secularisation. Of course, the picture is not so black and white. Protestant patients still believed in healers with the gift of healing, and Anglican church services never completely lost the sense of the divine. Nevertheless, it could be argued that Protestants had helped to create the conditions for a secular world, including a more secular medicine, and that this was realised after the intense religious fervour associated with Protestantism declined in its extent and its political influence.

Religion, medicine and charity

One aspect of religion which had always sat awkwardly with learned medicine was that of Christian charity. The learned physicians were expensive and could appear uncharitable. William Clowes took care to advise the young surgeon 'not [to be] to covetous for money, but a reasonable demander, being good unto the poore, let the rich pay therefore'.[59] Henry Holland pragmatically recognised that the learned physicians were not for the poor:

Let the Rich seeke for the godly, wise and learned Physician, and take heede of wicked ignorant bold Empyricks, which kill many men… And let the poorer sort with good advise and counsell (if they can have any) use Master Phares medicines in his short but learned Treatise of the Pestilence, which hee wrote of purpose for the benefit and comfort of the Poor.[60]

The charitable care of the sick was taught by Christianity as one of the six (later seven) corporal works of mercy (Matthew XXV: 35-6: 'for I was an hungred, and ye gave me meat: I was thirsty, and ye gave me drink: I was a stranger and ye took me in: Naked, and ye clothed me: I was sick and ye visited me: I was in prison, and ye came unto me'). It was unique to Christianity, being unknown as a general practice or doctrine in the classical world. After the Reformation in England and the closure of the monasteries and many of the hospitals and almshouses which had looked after the sick poor, charitable care still continued. Noblewomen and gentlewomen such as Lady Margaret Hoby and Lady Grace Mildmay[61] often acted as medical practitioners to the poor, as might clergymen like Richard Napier, or their wives, such as Mrs Elizabeth Walker who 'made herself mistress… in physick and chirurgerey to assist the neighbours of the parish'.[62] At the town and parish level, poor rates and private charitable bequests helped to provide medical treatment and care for the sick poor. Although the central government had, by the beginning of the seventeenth century, produced through the Poor Laws a uniform legislative basis for such care across the country, it was put into effect in diverse

V

ways locally, with churchwardens and church congregations acting as local ad-ministrators.[63] The charitable and the rate-based care of the sick poor was firmly embedded in the English Church and state, and was seen as a moral and social duty by some of the better-off members of society. To attack those who practised the charitable treatment of the sick poor was to attack a centuries-old custom, sanctioned by Church and society and continued in different guises after the Reformation.

Medical works on medicine for the poor such as that referred to by Clowes were evidence not only of a concern for the poor on the part of some medical practitioners, but of a rich-poor divide in which the learned physicians were seen as affordable only by the rich. In their attack on their unlearned competitors some learned physicians also attacked the charitable care of the sick, ignoring both the charitable imperative of Christianity, and the fact that the poor in any case could not afford learned physicians – such was their wish to eliminate competitors and to have only one type of medical knowledge and practice. John Cotta, who was probably a Puritan, opposed the argument that a clergyman should cure the sick poor out of a sense of private, individual charity, with one drawn from public policy and law.

It is indeed a deed of mercie to save and helpe the sicke and a worke of charitie to advise them for their health and ease; but the common good and public weale and the law for both do inhibit the doing of every good by every man, and both do limit and refraine it unto some speciall and select sort of men for necessary causes, and respects unto good government and policie and for avoiding confusion which is the ruine of publicke weales. Shal then Divinitie teach and allow for public deeds, ends and respects of charitie and mercie, to break publicke edicts, to transgress lawes, to condemme magistracie, to confound and disturbe good order?[64]

Cotta drew upon the potent rhetoric of good order enjoined by the state and by Calvinism to argue his case. As he wrote, 'it is manifest that this fluctuation of these men between two callings is offensive to God, scandalous unto religion and good men, and injurious unto commonweales'.[65] But, much more prosaically, he saw 'pastor physicians' as competitors, eager to get the credit for cures that proper physicians had nearly achieved. Cotta told the story of a 'Pastor Physician led by a secret ambition of stealing the praise of such a cure who in 1611, after the patient was getting better by means of a course of Galenic therapy, advised instead "aurum potabile"' (a remedy of the chemists whom the learned physicians ferociously attacked). The patient acquiesced in this as it seemed to make him feel better ('now measuring his good by his ease'). In the process 'he studiously and contin-ually defiled his Physition, and with evill clamours filled all the corners of the country'. Of course, the patient subsequently got worse and had to have recourse to 'other learned Physitions but useth them by uncertaine fits, as his owne conceit induced, and with reserveation of his sole happinesse, and best security in Aurum potabile'.[66] Ignorant competitors, dangerous treatments, and disobedient and credulous patients were the staple characters for stories that argued for medical monopoly. James Hart echoed Cotta. Social order was more important than the charity of pastors:

Their colourable excuse of doing good to their neighbours is to small purpose: for then were it lawfull for every man to meddle with another mans profession, then might the Lawyer become a Physitian, the Physitian a Divine and the Divine all three... But God is the God of order, not of confusion; and never did allow of this confused chaos of callings.[67]

Two years later Hart in another treatise on uroscopy attacked 'ignorant Empiricks, women and many other such' and he dismissed the claims of ministers to care for both the soul and the body: 'as for cleargie men they cannot be ignorant, that they ought to be employed about businesses of an higher nature. And if they will have a care of the soules entrusted to them they need not trouble themselves with their bodies'.[68] Like Cotta he recounted the case of a patient damaged by 'a Parson-practiser'.[69]

The Calvinist godly in England stressed the God-given power of magistrates; they were conservative and until the Laudian changes they felt themselves to be part of the establishment and that they made up the real Anglican Church. The wish for a settled social order, with no masterless men or wandering beggars and with everyone in their own calling, could easily be used to argue for the suppression of wandering healers and pastor physicians and with it the charitable non-'professional' treatment and care of the sick poor.

However, it is unclear how coherent was this use of Calvinist teachings. The evidence comes from only a few sources and Calvinist arguments are intermixed with many others deploring the lack of learning and skill amongst competitors. In other words, Christian or Calvinist doctrines are not clearly demarcated. Also, attacks on the clergy practising medicine could be made without reference to Calvinist doctrines. James Primrose in his *Popular Errours* (1638, and English translation 1651) relied on the fact that few, if any, could adequately learn medicine in addition to religion, and that in any case the Councils of the Church forbade the clergy to practise medicine.[70]

There are some pointers, nevertheless, which would argue for the importance of religious arguments for learned practitioners. As William Birken has shown, physicians and clergymen often had close ties. Of the 67 physicians admitted to the status of Candidate and/or Fellow of the College of Physicians of London between 1603 and 1643, the social origins of 57 are known, and 17 of them came from clerical families.[71] In the same period, of the 635 university-educated physicians listed by John Raach[72] as practising outside London, Birken has found that out of the total of over 200 who were educated at Cambridge, up to 43 were also clergymen.[73] Despite this close association and the existence of some episcopal licensing outside London, the statutes of the College of Physicians barred clergymen from practising medicine.[74] The College's statute was, however, not rigidly enforced. In 1627 the perpetual curate of Thurlby in Lincolnshire was allowed to practise in London, whilst ten years later a mere deacon, Mr Pordage, was refused a licence.[75] How many ministers practised medicine in the first half of the seventeenth century whilst receiving a church stipend is, however, unclear. The closeness between medical practitioners and clergy probably gave added point to the attacks on pastor-physicians by medical writers, who may have seen them not only as taking away trade like the empirics, but also as intellectual rivals having a similar educational background. The use by physicians of arguments drawn from religion against pastor-physicians was to give some standing to the latter (something that was, in any case, inevitable given the importance of religion), in contrast to the total denigration of empirics. William Birken has argued that the College of Physicians in the early seventeenth century was Puritan, though not politically very radical.[76] It may be, and this is very hypothetical, that arguments drawn from Calvinist teaching fitted the Puritan world of some practitioners and were employed because they were believed in. If so, what initially looks like a self-interested attempt to separate religion from medicine would have been viewed at the time as the implementation of a religious viewpoint, though with hindsight we may feel that such a viewpoint helped in a small way to create our secular world.

Conclusion

It is only in the 1640s in England, with the rise of sectarian groups and revolutionary thinking, that religious doctrines, mainly centred around charity, are actively used to argue for the reform of medicine, together, as Charles Webster has pointed out, with the possibility that clergymen could practise medicine on a nationwide basis.[77] This went with a rejection of Galenic learned medicine in favour of Paracelsian and chemical medicine. However, up to this time in England at least, Calvinism was used by learned physicians for essentially conservative purposes and rightly so, given the conservative nature (at least in a social sense) of Calvin's doctrines.

Christianity, whether used by religious writers discussing the place of medicine or using medical metaphors, or employed by medical men arguing for a monopoly of practice or for medical reform, appears to have had far greater authority than medicine. But the fact that clergymen had to employ medical metaphors suggests another conclusion: that Christianity could be remote from the experience of illness and suffering, and that preachers knew that to make Christianity relevant they had to bring medicine and the bedside into religious discourse. On balance, the first conclusion is the stronger, but something of the second was also present in the relationship between religion and medicine. The *modus vivendi* between learned medicine and Christianity extending from the Middle Ages to the time of Calvin was formally dominated by religion, yet it also allowed medicine to have its own relatively undisturbed space, and in hindsight it might be said that the seeds of secularism were present. Structurally, the use of medical and natural-philosophical terms to describe supernatural phenomena, although a sign at the time of a shared religious and medical-scientific culture, was to have significant implications for religion in the nineteenth and twentieth centuries as science and medicine chan-

V

ged. More immediately, in seventeenth-century England, Protestant beliefs paradoxically began to threaten Christianity's role as a religion that healed both the
soul and the body.

Notes

1. See for instance the essays in W.J. Sheils (ed.), *Studies in Church History*, no. 19, *The Church and Healing* (Oxford: Basil Blackwell for the Ecclesiastical History Society, 1982); R.L. Numbers and D.W. Amundsen (eds.), *Caring and Curing: Health and Medicine in the Western Religious Traditions* (New York: Macmillan, 1986); O.P. Grell and A. Cunningham (eds.), *Medicine and the Reformation* (London and New York: Routledge, 1993). See also A. Wear, 'Puritan Perceptions of Illness in Seventeenth Century England', in R. Porter (ed.), *Patients and Practitioners: Lay Perceptions of Medicine in Pre-Industrial Society* (Cambridge: Cambridge University Press, 1985), pp. 55-99; D. Harley, 'Medical Metaphors in English Moral Theology, 1560-1660', *Journal of the History of Medicine*, 48 (1993), 396-435.

2. On Josselin, see L.M. Beier, *Sufferers and Healers. The Experience of Illness in Seventeenth-Century England* (London: Routledge and Kegan Paul, 1987), pp. 182-210; for Newcombe, see Henry Newcombe, *The Diary of the Rev. Henry Newcombe*, ed. Thomas Heywood, Chetham Society vol. 18 (Manchester, 1849).

3. On religious autobiographies see P. Delany, *British Autobiography in the Seventeenth Century* (London: Routledge, 1969); on Puritan perceptions as seen through their diaries, see O. Watkins, *The Puritan Experience* (London: Routledge, 1972).

4. On Napier, see M. MacDonald, *Mystical Bedlam: Madness, Anxiety and Healing in Seventeenth-Century England* (Cambridge: Cambridge University Press, 1981), and on Baxter, see Wear, 'Puritan Perceptions', pp. 90-9.

5. Harold J. Cook seems first to have used the term 'medical marketplace', in his *The Decline of the Old Medical Regime in Stuart London* (Ithaca and London: Cornell University Press, 1986). It is now part of the common currency of social historians of medicine. Given its origin at a time when the British National Health Service was being put into the market-place and when free market philosophies had become the norm, perhaps English historians need to be somewhat cautious in applying the term to early modern English medicine lest they view the past in terms of the present too crudely or naively.

6. See for instance C. Hill, *Society and Puritanism in Pre-Revolutionary England* (London: Secker and Warburg, 1964); idem, *Change and Continuity in 17th Century England* (London: Weidenfeld and Nicolson, 1974); P. Collinson, *The Religion of Protestants: the Church in English Society 1559-1625* (Oxford: Clarendon Press, 1982); K. Thomas, *Religion and the Decline of Magic* (London: Weidenfeld and Nicolson, 1971).

7. Perhaps the classic example of such a study in intellectual ideas, which, despite its faults, was deservedly successful, was A.O. Lovejoy's *The Great Chain of Being* (Harvard: Harvard University Press, 1936).

8. See P. Slack, *The Impact of Plague in Tudor and Stuart England* (London: Routledge and Kegan Paul, 1985), and idem, *Poverty and Policy in Tudor and Stuart England* (London: Longman, 1988).

9. See C. Cipolla, *Faith, Reason and the Plague* (Brighton: Harvester Press, 1979); R. Palmer, 'The Church, Leprosy and Plague in Medieval and Early Modern Europe', in Sheils, *The Church and Healing*, pp. 79-99; B. Pullan, 'Plague and Perceptions of the Poor in Early Modern Italy', in T. Ranger and P. Slack (eds.), *Epidemics and Ideas* (Cambridge: Cambridge University Press, 1992), pp. 101-23; and Slack, *Impact of Plague*.

10. S. Wenzel (ed. and trans.), *Fasciculus Morum, A Fourteenth-Century Preacher's Handbook* (Pennsylvania: Pennsylvania State University Press, 1989), p. 255. On illness as a punishment, see pp. 139-41.

11. D Amundsen, 'Medicine and Faith in Early Christianity', *Bulletin of the History of Medicine*, 56 (1982), 326-50, at p. 331. See also G. Ferngren, 'Early Christianity as a Religion of Healing', *Bulletin of the History of Medicine*, 66 (1992), 1-15.

12. V.I.J. Flint, *The Rise of Magic in Early Medieval Europe* (Oxford: Clarendon Press, 1991), esp. her concluding remarks which are addressed to Keith Thomas: pp. 392-407. A study which challenges secularism as 'the norm' is C.J. Sommerville, *The Secularization of Early Modern England: From Religious Culture to Religious Faith* (Oxford: Oxford University Press, 1992).

13. John of Salisbury (*The Metalogicon of John of Salisbury*, trans. D.D. McGarry (Gloucester, Mass.: Peter Smith, 1971), Book I, chap. 4, p. 18), wrote of physicians: 'verily they have judged it unfitting, and foreign to their profession, to attend the needy and those who are either loath or unable to pay the full price. Their second maxim does not come, as I recollect, from Hippocrates, but has been added by enterprising doctors: "Take [your fee] while the patient is in pain". When a sick person is tortured by suffering, it is a particularly auspicious time for demanding one's price. For then the anguish of the illness and the avarice of the one affecting to cure it collaborate'.

14. I am grateful to Natsu Hattori of Trinity College, Oxford, for this quotation. It is cited by W. Birken, 'The Social Problem of the English Physician in the Early Seventeenth Century', *Medical History*, 31 (1987), 211.

15. See Wear, 'Puritan Perceptions', pp. 78-82. For a strong statement of the usefulness of local remedies placed on earth by God for local diseases, see Timothie Bright, *A Treatise: Wherein is Declared the Sufficiencie of English Medicines for Cure of all Diseases Cured with Medicine* (London, 1585). See also Laurent Joubert, *Erreurs Populaires au fait de la Medicine* (Bordeaux, 1578), pp. 13-14, 55-7.

16. On the religious management of dying, with its aim of achieving a 'good death', which stemmed from the medieval *Ars Moriendi*, see P. Ariès, *The Hour of our Death* (Harmondsworth: Peregrine Books, 1983); D. Stannard, *The Puritan Way of Death* (New York: Oxford University Press, 1977); C. Gittings, *Death, Burial and the Individual in Early Modern England* (London: Croom Helm, 1984); R. Houlbrooke (ed.), *Death, Ritual and Bereavement* (London: Routledge, 1989); M.C. O'Connor, *The Art of Dying Well* (New York: AMS Press, 1966).

17. M. Hobbs (ed.), *The Sermons of Henry King (1592-1669), Bishop of Chichester* (Cranbury, N.J.: Associated University Presses, 1992), p. 102.

18. Harley, 'Medical Metaphors'.

19. *The Sermons of Henry King*, p. 209.

20. Ibid.

21. Ibid., p. 111; Thomas Dekker, *Newes from Graves-ende* (London, 1604), in F.P. Wilson (ed.), *The Plague Pamphlets of Thomas Dekker* (Oxford: Clarendon Press, 1925), p. 102.

22. Thomas Becon, *Prayers and Other Pieces*, ed. J. Ayre, Parker Society (Cambridge, 1844), pp. 31-2.

23. Ibid., p. 32.

24. Ibid.

25. Ibid.

26. Andrew Boorde, *The Breviary of Helthe* (London, 1547), fol. A4^v.

27. Ibid., fol. A5^r.

28. See, for instance, the details of the Mary Glover case, which are ably described and documented by M. MacDonald, *Witchcraft and Hysteria in Elizabethan England: Edward Jorden and the Mary Glover Case* (London: Routledge, 1990); also D. Harley, 'Mental Illness, Magical Medicine and the Devil in Northern England, 1650-1700', in R. French and A. Wear (eds.), *The Medical Revolution of the Seventeenth Century* (Cambridge: Cambridge University Press, 1989), pp. 114-44. My impression that medical writers often made no reference to religion in the substantive parts of their texts is supported by Slack, *Impact of Plague*, p. 38: 'in many medical tracts reference to divine providence was a final caveat or an introductory formality

in an otherwise secular account of the origins of epidemic disease'.

29. William Clowes, *A Briefe and Necessarie Treatise, Touching the Cure of the Disease called Morbus Gallicus* (London, 1585), pp. 45ᵛ-46ʳ. The surgeon William Hall also included prayers in his medical writings: see his *A Most Excellent and Learned Worke of Chirurgie Called Chirurgia Parva Lanfranci* which contains his *An Historicall Expostulation: Against the Beastlye Abusers, bothe of Chyrurgie and Physycke* (London, 1565), which prints two prayers for the surgeon (fols. Eeeivʳ-Fffiᵛ).

30. Robert Burton, *The Anatomy of Melancholy*, ed. F. Dell and P. Jordan-Smith (New York: Tudor Publishing Co., 1983), p. 385.

31. D. Torrance and T. Torrance (eds.), *Calvin's New Testament Commentaries, A Harmony of the Gospels Matthew, Mark and Luke, 1*, trans. A.W. Morrison, 13 vols. (Grand Rapids, Mich.: W.B. Erdmans, 1989), I, pp. 162-3.

32. Ibid., I, p. 163.

33. Ibid.

34. Ibid., II, p. 1.

35. Calvin, *Institutes of the Christian Religion*, ed. J.T. McNeill and trans. by F.L. Battles, 2 vols. (Philadelphia: Westminster Press, 1960), II, pp. 1466-69 (Book IV, chap. 19, sections 18-21), quotation at p. 1468.

36. Augustine, *City of God*, Book XXII, chap. 8.

37. See Luther's *Plague Letter*. M. Luther, *Man vor den Sterben Fliehen Muge* (Wittenberg, 1527).

38. See Luther's tract 'To the Christian Nobility Concerning the Reform of the Christian Estate', in H.T. Lehmann (ed.), *Luther's Works*, vol. 44, ed. J. Atkinson, *The Christian in Society*, Part 1 (Philadelphia: Fortress Press, 1966), pp. 200-7.

39. S. Kusukawa, *The Transformation of Natural Philosophy. The Case of Philip Melanchthon* (Cambridge: Cambridge University Press, 1995).

40. Calvin, *Institutes*, I, p. 274 (Book II, chap. 2, section 14).

41. Ibid., p. 53 (Book I, chap. V, section 2).

42. Ibid., pp. 53-4.

43. For discussion of this see V. Nutton, 'Wittenberg Anatomy', in Grell and Cunningham, *Medicine and the Reformation*, pp. 11-32; for a more general discussion see the section on anatomy by A. Wear, 'Medicine in Early Modern Europe, 1500-1700', in L.I. Conrad et al., *The Western Medical Tradition* (Cambridge: Cambridge University Press, 1995), pp. 264-92.

44. R.B. [Robert Bostocke], *The Difference betweene the Auncient Phisicke, first Taught by the Godly Forefathers... and the latter Phisicke Proceeding from Idolaters, Ethnickes and Heathen as Galen and such other* (London, 1585), fols. Aiv-A6ᵛ.

45. Calvin, *Commentaries*, I, pp. 234, 248, and II, p. 39.

46. William Perkins, *Salve for a Sicke Man*, in *The Workes of that Famous and Worthy Minister of Christ... Mr William Perkins* (London, 1616), p. 505.

47. Ibid., p. 506. John Cotta, *The Triall of Witch-Craft* (London, 1616), pp. 60-1, wrote that 'wisemen' and 'wise-women' were either real sorcerers and witches, or impostors. Significantly, Cotta, like other writers, wrote of the Devil as the physician who surpassed all earthly physicians, but whose skill was a natural rather than a supernatural one (p. 59) and so was limited. Nevertheless, those who claimed the gift of healing like wisemen and wisewomen could be said to derive the gift from the Devil rather than from God: 'let us now lastly see... concerning the power of the Divell in curing disease, from whom all these inferiour Agents, Witches and Sorcerers do derive their power and skill' (ibid.).

48. Henry Holland, *An Admonition Concerning the Use of Physick* (London, 1603), pp. 49-50; Thomas Dekker, *London Loocke Backe at that Yeare of Years 1625, and Looke Forward upon this Yeare 1630* (London, 1630), in Wilson, *Plague Pamphlets*, pp. 188-9.

49. John Securis, *A Detection and Querisome of the Daily Enormities and Abuses Commited in Physic* (London, 1566), sigs. B4ᵛ-B5ʳ.

50. In J.W. Willcock, *The Laws Relating to the Medical Profession* (London, 1830), p. clxxvii.

51. *Calvin's New Testament Commentaries. First Epistle of the Apostle Paul to the Corinthians*, trans. J.W. Fraser (Grand Rapids, Mich.: W.B. Erdmans, 1989), p. 153.

52. Ibid.

53. Ibid., p. 155.

54. *Calvin's New Testament Commentaries. The Epistles of Paul the Apostle to the Galatians, Ephesians, Philippians and Colossians*, trans. T.H.L. Parker (Philadelphia: Westminster Press, 1988), pp. 20-1, on Galatians I:12. Securis, *A Detection*, sig. A3[v].

55. Clowes, *Briefe... Treatise*, p. 8[r].

56. Ibid., p. 8[v].

57. John Cotta, *A Short Discoverie of the Unobserved Dangers of Several Sorts of Ignorant and Unconsiderate Practisers of Physicke in England* (London, 1612), p. 88.

58. James Hart, *The Arraignment of Urines* (London, 1623), pp. A3[v]-A4[r].

59. Clowes, *Briefe... Treatise*, p. 42.

60. Holland, *An Admonition*, p. 53.

61. For a study of Lady Grace Mildmay, see L. Pollock, *With Faith and Physic. The Life of a Tudor Gentlewoman, Lady Grace Mildmay 1552-1620* (London: Collins and Brown, 1993).

62. [Anthony Walker], *The Holy Life of Mrs Elizabeth Walker* (London, 1690), p. 67.

63. See Slack, *Poverty and Policy*.

64. Cotta, *Short Discoverie*, p. 88.

65. Ibid., p. 89.

66. Ibid., pp. 92-3.

67. Hart, *Arraignment of Urines*, 'Epistle to Reader', p. A4[r].

68. James Hart, *The Anatomie of Urines...Or, the Second Part of our Discourse of Urines* (London, 1625), pp. A5[v] – A6[r].

69. Ibid., p. 110.

70. James Primrose, *Popular Errours* (London, 1651), pp. 10-18.

71. Birken, 'Social Problem', pp. 204-5.

72. J.H. Raach, *A Directory of English Country Physicians, 1603-1643* (London: Dawsons of Pall Mall, 1962).

73. Birken, 'Social Problem', pp. 207-8.

74. G. Clark, *A History of the Royal College of Physicians of London*, 2 vols. (Oxford: Clarendon Press, 1964-6), I, p. 385, prints the relevant statute from 1555.

75. Ibid., pp. 247-8. On clergy-physicians see also M. Pelling and C. Webster, 'Medical Practitioners', in C. Webster (ed.), *Health, Medicine and Mortality in the Sixteenth Century* (Cambridge: Cambridge University Press, 1979), pp. 165-235.

76. See Birken, 'Social Problem', and esp. his thesis, 'The Fellows of the Royal College of Physicians of London, 1603-1643: A Social Study' (unpublished Ph.D., University of North Carolina at Chapel Hill, 1977).

77. C. Webster, *The Great Instauration: Science, Medicine and Reform 1626-1660* (London: Duckworth, 1975), pp. 247-323.

VI

Puritan perceptions of illness in seventeenth century
England

Introduction

Not many historians so far have examined Puritan attitudes to physical
illness. A lot of the contextual spadework, however, has already been
done by social, cultural, political, religious and demographic historians.[1]
They provide the larger picture in which to place the subject and they
also help to illuminate related issues (for instance, the spiritualisation
of life, providence, the different shades of Puritanism, the material
conditions of society, etc.). Moreover, thanatology has recently
become popular.[2] As death was often the expected consequence of
illness in the seventeenth century, people's attitudes to it had a close
relationship to their perceptions of illness.

Attitudes to illness itself have been studied by Keith Thomas and

---

[1] See for instance: William Haller, *The Rise of Puritanism* (New York, 1938;
my edition Harper Torchbook, 1957); Perry Miller, *The New England Mind:
The Seventeenth Century* (Cambridge, Mass., 1967; 1st edn. 1939); C. Hill,
Society and Puritanism in Pre-Revolutionary England (London, 1964) (hereinafter
Society); Owen Watkins, *The Puritan Experience* (London, 1972); Lawrence
Stone, *The Family, Sex and Marriage in England 1500–1800* (London, 1979);
George Yule, *Puritans in Politics* (Appleford, 1981); E. A. Wrigley and R. S.
Schofield, *The Population History of England 1541–1871* (London, 1981); Keith
Wrightson, *English Society 1580–1680* (London, 1982); Peter Laslett, *The World
We Have Lost – Further Explored* (London, 1983) (hereinafter *Lost World*). This
is a small sample; the list is huge.

[2] For example: Philippe Ariès, *The Hour of our Death* (London, 1983); Michel
Vovelle, *La mort et l'Occident de 1300 à nos jours* (Paris, 1983); David
E. Stannard, *The Puritan Way of Death* (New York, 1977) (hereinafter *Death*);
John McManners, *Death and the Enlightenment* (Oxford, 1981); Gordon
E. Geddes, *Welcome Joy. Death in Puritan New England* (Studies in American
History and Culture No. 28, Ann Arbor, 1981); C. Gittings, *Death, Burial
and the Individual in Early Modern England* (London, 1984).

Alan Macfarlane.[3] Both bring out the importance of providence as a means by which Puritans made sense of illness. Thomas also provides an influential and important overview of cultural change in seventeenth century England that shows magic declining with a trend towards secularisation after the Restoration. It may be, as Jonathan Barry points out in this volume, that secularisation was not as rapid or as clear-cut as some historians, following Thomas, have imagined.[4] Also, more specifically, the case for providentialism may have been over-emphasised, and in this essay I shall spell out in detail the nature of the eclectic use of physical and religious explanations of illness.

Psychological illness in the seventeenth century has received some recent attention. Michael MacDonald has produced a brilliant study of the practice and the patients of Richard Napier, an astrological physician working at the beginning of the seventeenth century.[5] Napier's case notes cover thousands of patients, throwing light on medical practice and on the types of events and situations that produced psychological disorders in a wide range of people. However, MacDonald's work is of limited use for this essay. Mainstream Puritans did not approve of astrological medicine, and they certainly would not have conjured the Archangel Raphael as Napier sometimes did.[6] Furthermore, MacDonald is concerned with psychological rather than physical illness. Also, if the perceptions of the *patient* are to be the focus of study, it is not clear whether Napier's case notes can be safely used, for it is possible that patients' conversations were 'made sense of' by Napier.

Historical work on mental illness, however, does act as a point of reference for this essay's concern with physical illness. Elsewhere, MacDonald and others have described Puritan, Anglican and Non-conformist attitudes to mental illness in the pre- and post-Restoration period.[7] The Puritans should have been interested in the workings of

[3] Keith Thomas, *Religion and the Decline of Magic* (London, 1971) (hereinafter *Religion*); Alan Macfarlane, *The Family Life of Ralph Josselin* (Cambridge, 1970) (hereinafter *Josselin*).

[4] See below, note 9.

[5] Michael MacDonald, *Mystical Bedlam* (Cambridge, 1981).

[6] *Ibid.*, p. 210.

[7] As well as *Mystical Bedlam* see also MacDonald's, 'Religion, social change and psychological healing in England 1600–1800' in W. J. Sheils (ed.), *The Church and Healing* (Oxford, 1982), pp. 101–25; Thomas, *Religion*; D. P. Walker, *Unclean Spirits: Possession and Exorcism in France and England in the Late Sixteenth and Early Seventeenth Centuries* (Philadelphia, 1981); Roy Porter, 'The rage of party: a glorious revolution in English psychiatry?', *Medical History*, XXVII (1983), 35–50; H. D. Rack, 'Doctors, demons and early

the mind was natural, given Calvin's 'institutionalisation' of the believer's inner anxiety and his injunction to know and to be displeased with ourselves[8] (a recipe for guilt-laden self-analysis). Puritans put much effort into understanding mental processes, and it is no accident that the first chapter of Haller's *The Rise of Puritanism* is entitled 'Physicians of the Soul'. With the Restoration and the consequent dislike for 'enthusiasm'[9] in religion (already apparent in the 1650s and earlier in Robert Burton)[10] the healing role of religion in mental illness declined, though Nonconformists continued the practice of religious healing.

Can the history of physical illness be interpreted in the same way? Christopher Hill wrote of the 'spiritualisation of the household' to describe how the minutiae of family life came under the influence of religion.[11] Were the body and its illnesses spiritualised also? Certainly the body's perceived closeness to the soul would have made it a likely candidate. This essay will show, however, that among mainstream Puritans the spiritualisation of illness was only partially accomplished. More tentatively, the essay supports the view that post-1660s Anglicans moved to a more secular, rational view of illness, though Barry's paper warns us against easy generalisations.

Methodist healing', in W. J. Sheils (ed.), *The Church and Healing* (Oxford, 1982), pp. 137–52.

[8] Paul Delany, *British Autobiography in the Seventeenth Century* (London, 1969) (hereinafter *British Autobiography*), pp. 34–5, citing Calvin's *Institutes*, I, l, 1 and II, v, 19.

[9] An important work for the reaction to enthusiasm is M. C. Jacob, *The Newtonians and the English Revolution* (Hassocks, Sussex, 1976); Michael Heyd has a good article on enthusiasm, pointing out the nature of the opposition to it: 'The reaction to enthusiasm in the seventeenth century: towards an integrative approach', *Journal of Modern History*, LIII (1981), 258–80. See also Porter, 'The rage of party' and MacDonald, *Mystical Bedlam* and 'Religion, social change and psychological healing'. Christopher Hill finds the reaction to enthusiasm significant; see his *Some Intellectual Consequences of the English Revolution* (London, 1980), pp. 62–7. However, historians could be putting too much explanatory power on enthusiasm. Jacob's idea that the scientific laws of the later seventeenth century are the result of religious and political positions taken on enthusiasm relies too much on the imaginative use of analogies. Moreover, the social historian – unless a historian of elites and of professional society – must be unhappy at the limited extent of pro- and anti-enthusiasm ideas.

[10] MacDonald in his 'Religion, social change and psychological healing', p. 104, gives the impression (no doubt inadvertently) that Robert Burton associated religious melancholy mainly with strict Puritans ('giddy precisians'); sectarians did figure in his argument but, overall, the vast majority of Burton's examples and descriptions came from Catholic or pagan history.

[11] Hill, *Society*, pp. 443–81.

58

I take 'Puritan' to mean the 'godly' sort of people who up to the 1640s tended to conform and who were not openly hostile to the establishment though they wished for further reformation.[12] Moderate Puritans like William Perkins, Richard Greenham and William Gouge have been seen as shaping the mainstream of Puritan thought.[13] I have looked at their views and related them to the perceptions of illness of a generally later group of diarists and autobiographers who shared the same moderate views (after 1640 many would be Presbyterians). As they disliked Sectarians, Baptists, Ranters and Quakers as much as Papists, I have not discussed the more 'enthusiastic' healing miracles of the sects nor the material on religious healing in George Fox's *Journal.* Also left to one side are the radical Puritan reformers who, as Charles Webster shows, were concerned with changing the relationships between religion and medicine,[14] as they were more interested in institutional relationships than with how an individual should approach illness and death.

Finally, some comments are needed on the material that I am using. How individuals perceived illness can be discovered by looking at

[12] The definition of 'Puritan' and 'Puritanism' has produced a huge literature. See for example: Haller, *Rise of Puritanism*, pp. 18–20; Charles and Katherine George, *The Protestant Mind of the English Reformation* (Princeton, 1961); Michael G. Finlayson, *Historians, Puritanism and the English Revolution: The Religious Factor in English Politics Before and After the Interregnum* (Toronto, 1984) – the last two deny the existence of Puritanism; John F. H. New, *Anglican and Puritan, The Basis of their Opposition* (London, 1964); C. Hill, *Society*, pp. 13–29 gives a social as well as religious definition; J. Sears McGee, *The Godly Man in Stuart England: Anglicans, Puritans and the Two Tables, 1620–1670* (New Haven, 1976); William Lamont, *Godly Rule: Politics and Religion 1603–1660*, pp. 25, 93–7 (hereinafter *Godly Rule*); Peter Lake, *Moderate Puritans and the Elizabethan Church* (Cambridge, 1982), pp. 11–14. My own description has been influenced most by Haller, and the following: Claire Cross, *Church and People 1450–1660* (London, 1976); G. Yule, *Puritans in Politics* (Appleford, 1981), pp. 72–105; Basil Hall, 'Puritanism: the problem of definition', in G. J. Cumming (ed.), *Studies in Church History* (London, 1965), vol. 2, pp. 283–96. Hall writes 'before 1642 the "serious" people in the Church of England who desired some modification in Church government were called Puritans: after 1640 party names came increasingly into use, of Presbyterian, Independent and Baptist'; he goes on to point out that Presbyterians such as Baxter did not think of themselves as Puritans, who they associated with the time before 1640.

[13] Haller, *Rise of Puritanism*, pp. 49–82; H. C. Porter, *Reformation and Reaction in Tudor Cambridge* (Cambridge, 1959), pp. 216–26 (hereinafter *Reformation*); Lamont, *Godly Rule*, p. 42; Yule, *Puritans in Politics*, pp. 75–7.

[14] Charles Webster, *The Great Instauration* (London, 1975), pp. 245–323 (hereinafter *Instauration*).

diaries, autobiographies, 'lives' and letters. In seventeenth century England diary writing flourished. The cosmos of the Puritan diary centred on the individual and his or her personal communion with God, though Puritans were also intensely interested in the wider world. The Puritan was encouraged to keep a reckoning and judgement of his actions. John Dod wrote:

If we keep an assises at home in our own soules, and find ourselves guilty, and contemn ourselves, then shall not we be judged of the Lord: but because we deal very partially in our own matters, therefore is the Lord driven to help us, by laying his correcting hand some way or other on us.[15]

The diary became the vehicle for this confessional assessment, and seventeenth century England saw a great expansion in diary writing.[16] Isaac Ambrose wrote that the diarist 'observes something of God to his soul, and of his soul to God'.[17] John Fuller in his introduction to John Beadle's *The Journal or Diary of a Thankful Christian* used an accounting or trading metaphor:

A Christian that would be exact hath more need, and may reap much more good by such a journal as this. We are all but stewards, factors here, and must give a strict account in that great day to the high Lord of all our ways and of all his ways towards us.[18]

The Puritan diary, then, was written with an eye towards God. By noting 'God's ways towards us' as well as 'our ways', the diarist was constantly trying to discover evidence of the hand of God as it touched his life.

It is no surprise, therefore, that Puritan diarists should emphasise God's providence. Was a Puritan diary merely a formalism, a literary artefact written for religious reasons and bearing little relation to 'real life'? Although the diaries have to be used with caution, the writing of the diaries was part of the real life of the authors, and they contain enough width of daily experience to give us confidence that what was

[15] John Dod and Robert Cleaver, *Seven Godlie and Fruitful Sermons* (London, 1614), p. 44 (hereinafter *Seven Sermons*). The first six sermons are by Dod.

[16] On diaries see Watkins, *Puritan Experience*, which analyses Puritan perceptions through diaries and autobiographies. Haller, *Rise of Puritanism*, p. 38; Macfarlane, *Josselin*, pp. 3–11 who regrets the small use made of diaries by historians, though see now Linda Pollock, *Forgotten Children* (Cambridge, 1983).

[17] Isaac Ambrose, *Prima, The First Things in Reference to the Middle and Last Things* (London, 1674), p. 118. Cited by William Sachse in his edn of *The Diary of Roger Lowe* (London, 1938), p. 2 (hereinafter *Diary*).

[18] Quoted by Delany, *British Autobiography*, p. 64.

60

put down to God's providence was not merely a circumscribed part of the author's life. Yet it has to be remembered that this highly providentialist vision was relatively short-lived and limited mainly to Puritans, and many diaries were written by Puritan ministers who would naturally think in this way. In other words, although the religious ethos of Puritan diaries was for their authors normal and not artificial, for the historian, who puts them into an overall context, they may appear to have the aura of artificiality associated with any genre of writing.

The religious background

Religion had always been closely associated with illness, and Puritan interest in healing and illness was nothing new. Similarities between Catholic and Protestant views will often occur in this essay. However, there were differences. Protestants did not make Church processions, or offer prayers to saints or to their relics when seeking cure from community-wide or individual illness.[19] Calvin's emphasis on God and the Bible moved people away from the pantheon of minor Christian divinities. The structure, nevertheless, remained the same: communal and individual prayer was still offered to relieve physical ills.

More specifically, Puritans had a different view from Roman Catholics of the role of religion at the sick-bed. In Puritan eyes, the age of miracles had long since past, and in their attack on the superstitions of the Roman Church Puritans stated that the Catholic sacraments had merely a symbolic meaning without any real or material power. This meant that the Church could no longer heal. William Perkins, perhaps the outstanding Puritan writer at the turn of the century,[20] wrote that the Catholic rite of anointing the sick was an ineffectual imitation of that of the primitive Church:

The fifth of James is commonly alleged to this purpose, but the anointing there mentioned is not of the sa: :c kind with this greasy sacrament of the Papists. For that anointing of the bod; was a ceremony used by the Apostles and others, when they put in practise this miraculous gift of healing, which gift is now ceased. Secondly, that anointing had a promise that the party should recover his health, but this popish anointing hath no such promise,

---

19 See for instance R. Palmer, 'The Church, leprosy and plague in early modern Europe', in Sheils (ed.), *The Church and Healing*, pp. 79–100, and C. Cipolla, *Faith, Reason and the Plague* (Brighton, 1979).

20 Haller, *Rise of Puritanism*, p. 91; Yule, *Puritans in Politics*, pp. 75–6. For modern accounts of Perkins' life see Haller, *Rise of Puritanism*, pp. 64–5; W. Perkins, *The Works of William Perkins*, ed. I. Breward (London, 1970), pp. 3–131.

because for the most part the persons thus anointed die afterward without recovering; whereas those which were anointed in the primitive Church always recovered.[21]

The Reformation not only took the power of healing from the priest, it also took from him the power of judging and absolving men from sin (sickness and sin came together for 'by God's word...sickness comes ordinarily and usually from sin'[22]). All that was left for the reformed Church was, in Perkins' words, 'but a ministry of reconciliation',[23] where the minister tried to reconcile the sick-man to God.

The denial of the Church's God-like and miraculous power formed part of the 'disenchantment'[24] of the world and its consequent rationalism that gains momentum through the seventeenth century. Keith Thomas has charted this process, and, as with all pioneering efforts, his research can be modified. Although the rejection of the Church's role as an institution of divine power through which man's relations with God were mediated led to a direct and personal communion between the two, this does not mean that religion had ceased to be a third party. Puritans such as Richard Greenham, William Perkins and William Gouge emphasised the teaching role of the Church. At the same time, like any other didactic institution, religion needed authority. Through the century, many Puritans whether pre-1640 conformists, or later, Presbyterians or Congregationalists, believed in some level of organisation, and certainly in the specific calling of the ministry, and in the transcendent authority of the Bible to uphold them in their calling. How illness and death relate to the authority of the Church and to its teaching is discussed next.

Religion, illness and death

In the first half of the seventeenth century religion was a dominant system of thought.[25] Moreover, at the institutional level, Puritan

---

[21] William Perkins, *A Golden Chaine* (London, 1612), p. 501 (hereinafter *Chain*). The same passage in James was used by Baptists to justify their healing practices: see Thomas, *Religion*, p. 149.

[22] Perkins, *Chain*, p. 501.

[23] *Ibid.*, p. 500, citing II Corinthians 5: 18.

[24] See Heyd, 'The reaction to enthusiasm', p. 258. The word comes from 'Entzauberung' used by Max Weber in the essay 'Wissenschaft als Beruf'.

[25] Hill, *Society*, p. 32 writes, 'In the sixteenth and seventeenth centuries the Church had a monopoly of thought control and opinion forming. It controlled education; it censored books.'

ministers such as William Gouge[26] exuded a self-confident belief in their power to govern all aspects of men's minds. This belief in the right of a minister to control and influence behaviour had its mirror-image on the political stage from the Elizabethan to the Civil War period, where religion was a major influence. The power of religion also showed itself on a more local and intimate level, with consistory courts, and later Presbyterian and Congregational officials, punishing breaches of personal morality; and paralleling this policing was the belief held by clergymen that they had the right and duty to give advice ('practical divinity') on how individuals should live their lives.[27] This included guidance on how to be ill and how to die, and how to look after the sick.

Advice books set down the hierarchical relations and reciprocal duties between rulers and subjects, husbands and wives, parents and children, masters and servants, and it was in such a context that Puritan ministers stressed that looking after a sick wife, husband, child or servant was one of the duties of each member of a family.[28]

There were other more theological or theoretical reasons for the Church's interest in giving advice about health and sickness apart from the attempt at social education and control. At the level of the individual rather than of society, religious writers saw the body as God's workmanship: Robert Horne called it the Temple of God which

[26] See especially William Gouge, *Of Domesticall Duties* (London, 1622) (hereinafter *Duties*). On Gouge see Haller, *Rise of Puritanism*, pp. 67–9; Porter, *Reformation*, pp. 222–3.

[27] Haller, *Rise of Puritanism*, pp. 24–6; Porter, *Reformation*, p. 222, 'For Perkins, as for Aristotle, the family was a natural institution, "the seminary of all other societies", though "the only rule of ordering the family is the written word of God". By this rule he laid down the essentials of domestic justice: with particular chapters on the duties of husband and wife and son, and on to the relation of master and servant. This tradition of practical divinity was continued in William Gouge's...*Of Domesticall Duties*'; Hill, *Society*, pp. 443–81.

[28] Whether the sick were, in fact, looked after by their families is a difficult question to answer. Despite the small nuclear family of seventeenth century England where grown-up children left parents to form separate family units, it seems that few people lived in institutions and that widowers and widows rarely lived separately (7 and 14 per cent respectively in one study: Laslett, *Lost World*, pp. 295–6). Not surprisingly, no diarist that I have read, admits to having deserted a family member who was ill or dying (with the characteristic exception of Pepys who, when his servant Susan fell ill with an undiagnosed illness that might have been plague, sent her away to her mother: Samuel Pepys, *The Diary of Samuel Pepys*, ed. Robert Latham and William Matthews (11 vols., London, 1970–83), vol. 7, pp. 115–22 (hereinafter *Diary*); the illness proved to be an ague).

had to be kept pure and clean;[29] John Sym argued that failure to look after one's body was an indirect form of suicide.[30] The body had an appointed and natural span of life and it was man's duty to survive that span; Gouge, therefore, condemned 'the practise of gluttons, drunkards, unchaste and voluptuous persons, who to satisfy their corrupt humours, impair their health, pull diseases upon them and shorten their days'.[31] Perkins made it clear that the body could not be divorced from the soul, the secular from the divine, and he stated that the hold of God extended to this life and to our bodies:

Whereas our bodies are God's workmanship, we must glorify him in our bodies, and all the actions of body and soul, our eating and drinking, our living and dying, must be referred to his glory: yea we must not hurt or abuse our body, but present them as holy and living sacrifices unto God.[32]

A further reason for placing the body within the ambit of religion was that body and soul were taught to be intimately connected. The body was the instrument of the soul; if the body was impaired the soul could not express itself in this world:

the body of man is the organ or instrument whereby the soul works organically: and therefore, he that kills his own body destroys all those works, that the soul was to work in it, and which it cannot do without it.[33]

How far people took note of religious advice to look after their own health is unknown. Certainly the interest that religiously orientated diarists such as Ralph Josselin, Henry Newcome and Oliver Heywood had in their health can be explained not only in providential terms (illness or health being a mark of God's providence) but as a sign that they were heeding the advice to look after their bodies. That religious writers expected to be able to affect health practices is indicated by the sometimes quite detailed guidance that they gave on matters such as wet-nursing,[34] or on a husband's duty to satisfy his pregnant wife's 'longing', the want of which could result in her death or that of the child or both.[35]

There were other ways in which the Church and ministers entered

---

[29] Robert Horne, *Life and Death, Foure Sermons* (London, 1613), p. 25 (hereinafter *Life*). Horne was citing I Corinthians 6: 15, 19.

[30] John Sym, *Lifes Preservative Against Self-killing* (London, 1637), pp. 109–10 (hereinafter *Self-killing*).

[31] Gouge, *Duties*, p. 85.

[32] Perkins, *Chain*, p. 153.   [33] Sym, *Self-killing*, p. 81.

[34] See Thomas Becon, *The Catechism*, ed. J. Ayre for the Parker Society (Cambridge, 1844), pp. 347–8.   [35] Gouge, *Duties*, p. 399.

the world of illness and also of death, and at this point I want to concentrate on the latter. The death-bed scene constantly recurs in diaries, 'lives' and autobiographies. The similarity between its various enactments points to the fact that dying was a learnt procedure, part of the ceremonial of life. When dying one had to show evidence of piety (hence prayers and quotations from the Bible), a repentance of sin, and most importantly the mind had to be prepared to accept death, which was shown by exclamations of eagerness to enter Heaven. For example, John Angier described the death-bed scene of his wife:

they called me up, she being very ill, she then said Lord receive my spirit, into thy hand I commit my spirit, for thou hast redeemed it, come Lord Jesus, come quickly, make no tarrying he doth not yet come, will he not make hast?[36]

There was a whole genre of religious writing in the seventeenth century teaching people how to die (stemming from the medieval *ars moriendi*, the art of dying) and stressing the transitory nature of life. The period of one's life was secretly determined by God and known to him alone; any illness could presage death – thus Robert Yarrow called sickness 'the messenger of death'.[37] Robert Horne wrote 'I know not when I shall die, and therefore every day shall be as my dying day'.[38] Life had, therefore, to be a constant preparation for death. Puritans poured scorn on the Roman Catholic belief in death-bed repentances;[39] Horne wrote that they were a 'charm and a sorcery',[40] and that 'late repentance is seldom, or never true repentance'. Instead one needed to be in a constant state of repentance.[41]

Ariès has written that the move away from the death-bed scene to a constant preparation for death was a product of humanist writers and of the 'reformist elite of the Catholic and Protestant Churches',[42] with the consequence that 'death has become the pretext for a metaphysical

---

[36] Oliver Heywood, *Autobiography, Diaries* etc., ed. J. Horsfall Turner (4 vols., Brighouse and Bingley, 1882–5), vol. 1, p. 73 (hereinafter *Diaries*). See note 2 above on the literature on the history of death.

[37] Robert Yarrow, *Soveraigne Comforts for a Troubled Conscience* (London, 1634), p. 406 (hereinafter *Comforts*).

[38] Horne, *Life*, p. 116 and Stannard, *Death*, p. 77 quotes Cotton Mather, 'A prudent man will die daily'.

[39] On French death-bed repentance see McManners, *Death and the Enlightenment*, pp. 191–233. Although Catholics advised against too great a reliance on death-bed conversions, they nevertheless were seen to work, for 'a man's disposition in his dying moments decided his eternal destiny' (pp. 193–4).

[40] Horne, *Life*, p. 116.   [41] *Ibid.*, p. 69.

[42] Ariès, *The Hour of our Death*, p. 303.

meditation on the fragility of life that is intended to keep us from giving in to life's illusions. Death is no more than a means of living well'.[43] Ariès' view has to be modified in two respects. From the personal records of seventeenth century Puritans it is clear that there still remained an intensity around the death-bed. The formalised pattern of dying with its set speeches was a sign that Puritan society still retained death as one of the crises of life to be celebrated with ritualised behaviour learnt for the occasion. Moreover, in religious terms, the time of dying was that of most danger since this was when Satan's temptation was greatest.[44] Secondly, the life-long meditation upon death not only led one to pursue a better life, but also had another function: it integrated life with death and therefore enhanced the authority of the Church on the mundane level. Death, as religious writers had never tired of telling, was the gate-way to the world of the spirit and the destroyer of the social world and its hierarchy.[45] It was the leveller that struck down rich and poor alike:

Fearfull death, of all miseries the last and the most terrible... how quickly and suddenly stealest thou upon us? how secret are thy paths and ways? how universal is thy signiory and dominion? The mighty cannot escape thee, the strong lose their strength before thee, the rich with their money shall not corrupt thee. Thou art the hammer that always striketh: thou art the sword that never blunteth...[46]

[43] *Ibid.*, p. 301.
[44] Yarrow, *Comforts*, p. 393: 'He is not ignorant to take opportunity fittest for his purpose. And therefore now (above all other his desired times) he will devise and sound into the bottom of all his subtilties: to intrap, and so to make conquest of the Christian soules, knowing that this is the last combat that he is like to make with such a one... Assure thyself therefore that he will prepare the best he can stretch every limb in this final conflict.' Also Horne, *Life*, p. 71: 'there is business and work enough in the mind and external man of deaths condemned prisoner to resist and prepare against the extremity of that combat, which (because it is the last of the day) is like to be the sharpest'.
[45] Stannard, *Death*, pp. 16–17.
[46] Thomas Hastler, *An Antidote against the Plague* (London, 1625), pp. 35–6 (hereinafter *Antidote*). The theme of 'fearful' death seems to have been a Puritan one. Death was the 'king of Terrors', and Puritans combined their fear of death with the traditional view of death as a welcome release: Stannard, *Death*, pp. 78–99; Vovelle, *La mort et l'Occident*, p. 300. Jeremy Taylor's *Holy Living and Dying* shows many similarities with traditional and Puritan thought – 'that we should always look for death, every day knocking at the grave' (ch. 11, sect. 1) – but it differs from Puritan attitudes in not putting great emphasis on the death-bed scene itself, and on presenting a positive image of death: 'It is so harmless a thing, that no good man was ever thought the more miserable for dying, but much the happier' (ch. 3, sect. vii). Given the Puritans' belief in predestination such a view was logically impossible for them to hold, though in practice they sometimes did.

The constant meditation upon death diminished the reality of the secular world and allowed the Church's area of greatest expertise and legitimacy – knowledge of the world after death – to permeate the world of life. Puritans like Isaac Ambrose expressed the traditional merging of death into life:

We live and yet whilst we speak this word, perhaps we die. Is this a land of the living or a region of the dead? We that suck the air to kindle this little spark, where is our standing but at 'the gates of death'? Psalm 9.13. Where is our walk but 'in the shadow of death' Luke 1.19. 'What is our mansion-house but the body of death'? Romans 7.24.[47]

The systematic reminder of death found in advice books, sermons and books on the art of dying might well be interpreted (possibly cynically) as bolstering the indispensability (*qua* source of knowledge about death) and power of the Church in this world. It also served as the background for the Puritan writers' mingling together of religion and medicine which I discuss below.

The Church's emphasis on death gained plausibility because it reflected physical reality. Death and funerals were frequent experiences in seventeenth century society.[48] Moreover, seventeenth century England was a time of increasing mortality; the expectation of life fluctuated wildly because of epidemics, but declined overall through the century until by 1681 it had fallen by about ten years.[49] But whether people actually thought of death all the time is debatable. Although this was the baroque era with the skull as its remembrancer of death,[50] there were, not surprisingly, many people who show in their diaries and letters that they did not go around meditating on death

[47] Isaac Ambrose, *Ultima, The Last Things in Reference to the First and Middle Things* (London, 1650), p. 5 (hereinafter *Ultima*).

[48] Though the conclusion of some historians that other people's deaths were expected to occur at all ages and not just in old age has to be treated with some caution, see for such an instance: Stone, *The Family, Sex and Marriage in England 1500–1800*, pp. 54–66. Hervé LeBras shows, however, that in the France of the 1750s there was a high expectation that young children would have living parents and grandparents. Thus, the experience of death in the immediate family was not as high as a high mortality rate would suggest. H. LeBras, 'Living forbears in stable populations', in K. W. Wachter with E. A. Hammond and P. Laslett (eds.), *Statistical Studies of Historical Social Culture* (New York, 1978), pp. 163–88.

[49] E. A. Wrigley and R. S. Schofield, *The Population History of England 1541–1871*, pp. 413–14.

[50] Cotton Mather wrote 'Let us look upon everything as a sort of Death's Head set before us, with a *Memento mortis* written upon it'. Quoted in Stannard, *Death*, pp. 77–8.

all the time.[51] It is the exceptions, men like the mystic Francis Rous, who took to heart the injunction constantly to reflect on death.[52] Indeed, religious writers often complained that death, despite its experienced closeness, was far from the minds of people.[53] In other words, normative writings can affect the morality of a culture but not always thoughts and behaviour.

Turning now to religion and illness, it is clear that for both religious writers and laymen there was a close connection between religion and medicine. The links that produced this were various, and included the general intertwining of death and life. The union of those 'amorous twins',[54] the body and soul, had traditionally allowed the language of medicine to be applied to both. Richard Greenham wrote:

If a man troubled in conscience come to a minister it may be he will look all to the soul and nothing to the body: if he come to a physician, he only considereth of the body and neglecteth the soul. For my part, I would never have the physician's council severed, nor the minister's labour neglected: because the soul and body dwelling together, it is convenient, that as the soul should be cured by the word, by prayer, by fasting, by threatening or by comforting: so the body also should be brought into some temperature [health] by physic, by purging, by diet, by restoring, by music, and by such means; providing always that it be done so in fear of God.[55]

The use of medical language to describe the healing of the soul was widespread. Puritan theologians constantly used medical metaphors. Perkins wrote that a sinner was frequently compared in the Scriptures to a sick man: 'And therefore the curing of the disease fitly resembleth

[51] It is difficult to prove a negative, but see the diary of Adam Eyre, or even the more devout diaries of Henry Newcome and Roger Lowe. Oliver Heywood expressed his pleasure that his father started to think of God a few months before his death, and did not leave the preparation for death until the last moment: Heywood, *Diaries*, vol. 1, pp. 30 and 85.

[52] 'For myself, I have taken out many lessons of dying and I pray God I may so perfectly learn the art of it, that I may make good that heavenly sentence; that not only to live but to die choist is gain: and that by believing in Him, I may never die, which is his own promise.' Francis Rous, Bodleian Lib., Tanner MS. 62/2 fo. 530.

[53] McManners, *Death and the Enlightenment*, pp. 223–7 discusses the difficult problem of knowing who read books on dying, and whether they were acted upon. He concludes the literate minority did so only when absolutely necessary. The illiterate mass would have to rely on oral instruction by the curé.

[54] Hastler, *Antidote*, p. 36.

[55] Richard Greenham, *The Words of the Reverend and Faithful Servant of Jesus Christ*, 4th edn. (London, 1605), p. 159. On Greenham see Haller, *Rise of Puritanism*, pp. 26–8; Porter, *Reformation*, pp. 216–18.

the curing of sin', a sinner stands 'in need of Christ, the good physician of his soul'.[56] Dod wrote that the offences of God's children could be healed only by the medicine of the precious blood of the Lamb of God.[57] Religious writers used the medical metaphor as a way of moving from the more to the less familiar. Ambrose explicated Hebrews 1: 3, 'When he had by himself purged our sins', by using medical terminology:

See here the manner of the cure: there is a Physician he, (the patient *himself*) [i.e. Christ as physician and patient], the physic administered 'When he had purged' the ill humours evacuated, 'when he had purged our sins'.[58]

The figure of Christ the physician, the healer of the body as well as the soul also served to link this world with the next, medicine with religion. In 1665 during the plague the Anglican Richard Kingston wrote, in a vein common also to Puritans, that Christ by his death became not only 'physician of the dead',[59] but also of the living:

Other physicians, either out of hope of gain or to buoy up their credits and repute in this world, promise those cures which they can never perform: but here is one whose word is his deed, that archetypal verity, who having the issues of life and death in his hand, when he promises life cannot be guilty of a lie...[60]

Christ, of course, had healed the sick in body, and his example gave the church an entrée into the world of medicine. Kingston cited St Matthew's Gospel and Jesus curing the halt, the lame and the blind, and he declared:

the learned physicians are but shadows of this sun of righteousness, when he appears with healing on his wings. Have we the plague spots upon us? If God will be our physician their very redness shall serve for a blush to confess their impotency when he bids them vanish. Does a fever burn us, or a dropsy drown us? One word of his mouth will prove a julip to cool our veins, and a sluice to let out that lake of humours which would engulf us.[61]

The double face of physical and spiritual healing (cure of bodies, cure of souls) showed itself in the very words health and salvation. The Latin word *salus* was taken to mean not only health but also salvation, and health itself could mean salvation. The early English protestant

[56] Perkins, *Chain*, p. 365, citing Luke 4: 18 and Matthew 9: 11–12.
[57] Dod and Cleaver, *Seven Sermons*, p. 4.
[58] Ambrose, *Ultima*, p. 156.
[59] Richard Kingston, *Pillulae Pestilentiales: Or a Spiritual Receipt for Cure of the Plague* (London, 1665), p. 102.
[60] *Ibid.*, p. 103.   [61] *Ibid.*, pp. 105–6.

Thomas Becon had written:

God's word worketh marvellously unto the health of them that believe. And therefore in the word of God it is called the word of health, or salvation; as it is written: 'Ye men and brethren the children of the generation of Abraham...the word of this health was sent unto you.'[62]

The merging of the two worlds of life and death, of body and soul, and the dual and interchangeable senses of Christ the physician, medicine and health, probably helped the sick to move easily from medicine to religion and vice versa, and reflects the fact that there was more than one mode of healing available in the seventeenth century.

The utterances (or belief-system or ideology, as the reader's historical bent directs) of religious writers who indicate a duality or ambiguity between religion and medicine reflected the world of practice. Many ministers, such as Richard Baxter, acted as physicians; and even if they did not, they often quoted medical writers, as did Perkins and Ambrose; or like Ralph Josselin and Oliver Heywood had a developed knowledge of medical terms; or might be friendly with the town's medical men while their wives acted as sources of medical expertise especially at births, as was the case with Henry Newcome at Manchester.

Socially, clergymen and physicians belonged to the same stratum of society – at the lower end of the class of gentlemen, above 'the men which do not rule'.[63] In terms of career choice, medicine and religion could appear equal possibilities.[64] The general proximity of physician and clergyman was reflected by their personal contact at the sick-bed. Given the close intellectual, social and practical links between religion and medicine, it is not surprising that religious and medical explanations should come close together. In fact, as Charles Webster has noted, Puritan reformers argued that all clergymen should routinely act as doctors and provide a medical service;[65] clearly the close connections existing between religion and medicine already noted served as a background for such ideas.

Relations between the clergy and physicians were not always

---

[62] Thomas Becon, *Prayers and Other Pieces*, ed. J. Ayre for the Parker Society (Cambridge, 1844), p. 490.

[63] Laslett, *Lost World*, pp. 35–8.

[64] See *The Diary and Letter Book of the Rev. Thomas Brockbank 1671–1709*, ed. R. Trappes-Lomax (Chetham Soc., N.S., LXXXIX, 1930), p. 64 (hereinafter *Diary*), where Brockbank's father set out the choice of medicine or religion as equal possibilities.

[65] Webster, *Instauration*, pp. 259 and 289.

amicable, for proximity breeds rivalry: ministers objected to doctors dominating the sick-bed,[66] and the Puritan reformers put their schemes forward because they disliked the monopoly of the physicians.[67] On the other hand, physicians such as van Foreest, Cotta and Primerose attempted to establish a monopoly for orthodox, university-trained physicians and attacked ministers together with empirics and wise-women as dangerous to patients.[68] The attacks of the two groups upon each other is further evidence of their closeness.

To sum up: illness and death formed part of the teaching of the Church and were so emphasised that they were seen to permeate the whole of life. This moved people to be good throughout life rather than merely at their death-bed, and enhanced the authority of the Church in the world of life. At the same time, the extension of death into life,[69] and the parallel but more specific merging of religious and medical language were both signs of, and justifications for, the involvement of religion with the process of healing. This section of my essay should, therefore, help to explain why there were religious explanations of illness, and although it can be used as background for the well-known providential view of illness, it should also indicate that there was more to religion and illness than providence.

The individual and God's providence

One of the ways many Puritans spiritualised illness was to see it as God-given; it was a rod, and God was a father correcting (in the sense of guiding and admonishing as well as punishing) his children. The remedy for the Christian was to discover the reason for the correction. In Nehemiah Wallington's manuscript collection of Puritan letters, Paul Bayne's 'Letter of Comfort and Instruction in Affliction' advised:

---

[66] Perkins, *Chain*, p. 502.

[67] Webster, *Instauration*, pp. 250–64.

[68] Petrus Forestus, *De Incerto, Fallacii, Urinarum judicio...* (Leyden, 1589), trans. as *The Arraignement of Urines... Translated by James Hart* (London, 1623); John Cotta, *A Short Discoverie of the Unobserved Dangers of several sorts of Ignorant and Unconsiderate Practises of Physicke in England...* (London, 1623); James Primerose, *De Vulgi in Medicina Erroribus Libri Quatuor...* (London, 1638), trans. as *Popular Errors...* (London, 1651).

[69] John Carey, *John Donne: Life, Mind and Art* (London, 1981), p. 202 points to Donne's terror of death, yet impatience for, the Last Judgement. Donne's way of managing his fear of death is 'to treat death as a form of life, or to vivify it by giving it an active role in poems which are passionately concerned with living'. Although religious writers put death into life they also often saw events after death as a continuation of life.

First you must labour to apprehend God as a father correcting you by these infirmities. Secondly you must labour to find the cause why and to what purpose God doth follow you in such a kind.[70]

When in 1625 Wallington's wife was ill, his brother-in-law, Livewell Rampagne, wrote: 'I wrote doubtfully because I know not how it hath pleased God to dispose of my sister, who was then under his correcting hand.'[71] Rampagne made no reference to medicine, or to the natural course of the illness, but his attitude was not so much fatalistic as expectant of a higher power. Although Puritans stressed that the age of miracles was over, nevertheless in matters of providence, and illness was one such, God remained an active God, working amongst people. Although His purposes might be unknown, His presence was not.

As Keith Thomas and Alan Macfarlane have written,[72] illness was often seen in providential terms and it was included in the set of happenings or accidents such as fire, falling from horses and the occurrences of social life such as poverty which could be explained by God's providence. As illness, therefore, was one of the methods by which God showed 'his ways towards us', it was a subject to be noted by Puritan diarists along with the other happenings that indicated God's providence.

In this view of illness, guilt and a sense of sin (the natural allies and accompaniments of religion) were of course prominent. Health, a good night's sleep or recovery from illness were noted as a sign of God's favour, but the onset of illness stirred up anxiety, self-doubt and guilt. As Thomas has pointed out the illness of others could be perceived as a correction of oneself.[73] When Henry Newcome's child became ill, he blamed himself for having gone out the night before when, as he recorded at the time, at a private gathering for readings and prayers 'we had a pretty lively close of ye day'. So the next day he wrote:

Was sad this day. Could not sleep at night because of the child's illness. Surely my neglect of what I might have gotten last night, and needlessly going out as I did hath caused this sad affliction and withdrawment from my soul.[74]

---

[70] N. Wallington, *Letters on Religious Topics*, Brit. Lib., Sloane MS. 922, fo. 66r (hereinafter *Letters*).
[71] *Ibid.*, fo. 71r.
[72] Thomas, *Religion*, pp. 90–132; Macfarlane, *Josselin*, pp. 163–82.
[73] Thomas, *Religion*, p. 96.
[74] *The Diary of the Rev. Henry Newcome*, ed. Thomas Heywood (Chetham Soc., xviii, 1849), p. 107 (hereinafter *Diary*).

72

When his wife had a 'very sick night', Newcombe wrote 'I would humbly see the rod and him that hath appointed it and beg a good use of it'.[75]

Illness of others in a family could be perceived less as a punishment and more as a warning and a sign to alter one's life. The effect was the same: to change behaviour, and to act as a barometer to one's conscience. Newcome wrote at different times: 'Ye Lord awaken me to seriousness by my wife's illness'; 'My wife was ill this night, and so it occasioned me to be a little more serious. Such need have I of some load and ballast to keep my heart from carnality and security'; 'I have cause to be awakened and to draw nearer to God, my wife being so ill of a cold as she is.'[76]

The lack of institutional mediation between God and man helped to internalise this sense of guilt and anxiety, but its root cause was the ever-present doubt as to whether the individual was one of the elect. Newcome, describing a colleague's sermon on the spirit, wrote:

Despite of ye spirit is ye soule's apoplexy. Deprives of all life, motion, sense at once. Alas I doubt somet: I have a stroke of ye palsy on my soul taken all one side that I am defective in all I do and sadly partial: *But if I could be satisfied in this point that I am God's childe*, answer to all other objections would fall in of itself [my italics; note also use of medical metaphor].[77]

All his character faults, misfortunes, illnesses would be as nothing if Newcome could have known definitely that he was one of the elect.[78] But as he could not, the everyday occurrences of life took on significance and acted as indicators of God's decision. Illness, therefore, became one of the signs of what God had in store. Puritan theologians were aware of the possible dangers of such an approach, and cautioned that a life of illness and misfortune did not mean that one was not one of the elect.[79]

However, this was a period, like all others, when there existed a plurality of explanations for illness, and people moved easily between them. Thus belief in God's providence did not prevent Newcome from having recourse to medicine when someone was ill. Equally, when ill himself he went to the doctor. During April–May 1662

---

[75] *Ibid.*, p. 28.   [76] *Ibid.*, pp. 19, 137, 153.

[77] *Ibid.*, pp. 85–6.

[78] Certain signs might indicate if one was amongst the elect but there was no certainty: Miller, *The New England Mind*, pp. 50–3, also Stannard, *Death*, pp. 72–5, 83–5.

[79] Perkins, *Chain*, p. 492: 'And by the outward condition of any man, either in life or death, we are not to judge of his estate before God'.

Newcome became ill, he was bled and he took a rosemary posset to make him sweat; and after going to the apothecary, Thomas Minshull, he wrote: 'After supper I was a little at Mr Minshull's. I am it seems for ye jaundice.' The next day he wrote: 'Read my chapter and after duties, taking [blank] for ye jaundice, went a walking.'[80] The medical expert seems here in Newcome's mind to be deciding his bodily fate (of course the illness could be seen to originate from God) and Newcome immediately acted on the diagnosis by taking medicine. Having a religious view of illness did not exclude recourse to the physician and his remedies, and this was in keeping with the religious injunction to look after one's body; however, once in the hands of the doctors, the religious dimension to illness was forgotten for the time being.

It is clear that the providential view of illness, as well as stirring guilt, which Puritans probably welcomed as part of their spiritual life, also gave a rationale for why someone was ill. For instance, in Paul Bayne's letter 'against the passionate lamenting of the death of a brother', the images of God the punisher and God the healer came together – linked by the image of medicine as painful – and helped to make illness understandable:

God is wise who when he giveth us physic, doth put all the outward comforts we affect far from us. Lest his chastisements should work less kindly and with the purpose to us dear sister the physic must make us sick that doth us any good.[81]

The providential model of illness not only explained sickness, but also allowed recourse to a traditional practice: prayer. Prayer, a promise of repentance or some other religious activity, could be offered up to God in return for a cure. Wallington wrote of one such vow:

and I remember that in the year 1624 I was sick of a fever that I had little hope of life and then I turned my face to the wall (like Hezekiah) and prayed and promised unto God that if he would spare me a little longer O then I would frequent his house more than ever I have done and I would become a new man in the reformation of my life. And now God hath heard my prayers (as he did Hezekiah) in adding near fifteen years to my life.[82]

Richard Baxter wrote scathingly that 'sick-bed promises are usually soon forgotten',[83] but prayer and pleading to God to prevent and cure

---

[80] Newcome, *Diary*, p. 80.
[81] Wallington, *Letters*, fo. 62r.   [82] *Ibid.*, fo. 118v.
[83] Richard Baxter, *Reliquiae Baxterianae* (London, 1696), p. 90 (hereinafter *Reliquae*).

VI

illness was usual. Wallington wrote of others 'that were better than I who on their death-bed did so entreat the Lord to spare them and try them a little longer but the Lord would not hear to grant them their desire'.[84]

Prayers could be said in private but they were often part of communal healing. Puritan groups frequently had their own special days of humiliation, days set aside to assuage God's wrath where by prayer and fasting the community would plead with God that an individual's illness should be taken away or, in the case of an epidemic, that his people as a whole should be spared. Providence, therefore, although it affected individuals, could lead to a group response, and this should be borne in mind as a counter-balance to the picture of introversion and isolated individuality often painted of Puritans and their providential view of life.[85]

In the hands of Keith Thomas and others the providential view of illness has been paraded (and rightly so) as a historical wonder and curiosity. Some questions could now be put: What was the function of providence for religion? Did it retain the faithful by satisfying a need for explaining inexplicable events such as the onset of illness and by providing a method for recovery? The vengeance of God was seen to be inexorable, the case of plague often being taken to demonstrate the implacable efficacy of God's arrows of retribution,[86] but how much did this image of a powerful God depend on the failure of medicine, and to what extent was it used as a means of eliciting belief in God – the material success of the spiritual over the worldly, religion over

[84] Wallington, *Letters*, fo. 118v.
[85] Miller, *The New England Mind*, pp. 297–8; Haller, *Rise of Puritanism*, pp. 36–7, 90–1; Delany, *British Autobiography*, p. 56; Stannard, *Death*, p. 41 quotes Max Weber's 'unprecedented inner loneliness' of the Puritan.
[86] See William Gouge, *Gods Three Arrowes, Plague, Famine, Sword in Three Treatises* (London, 1631), p. 14 (hereinafter *Arrows*): '*Prepare to meet thy God O England*. This beginning of the plague is a real demonstration of a greater plague yet to come... The lion hath roared, who will not fear? The Lord God hath spoken, who can but prophecy?' Also pp. 65–6: 'Extraordinary it is, because the immediate hand of God in sending it, in increasing it, in lessening it, in taking it away, is more conspicuously discerned than in other judgements.' Hastler, *Antidote*, pp. 39–40: 'our sins have provoked *Bellatorum fortem*, the mighty warrior, the Lord of Hosts, the righteous judge, to whet his sword and bend his bow and made them ready to prepare the instruments of death, and arrows to destroy us: our customary sins have forced out the Lord's decree, and have brought forth three deadly weapons; his Sword and Famine hover over us...and we are already beset...with a conflict of many diseases; the Angel is darting the right aiming arrows of the Lord's wrath at every man's door: God's deadly tokens: the only marks of his displeasure'.

medicine? Such functional questions could be leavened by a psychological interpretation (always suspect in some historians' eyes). Apart from the well-worn approach that focusses on the figure of authority conjured up by God the chastiser and on the tremulous Puritan anxiously waiting for the next thunderbolt (Josselin's 'my dear angry Lord'),[87] another path could lead to the fear of illness and death and its channelling into a providential context. By focussing upon their putative sins rather than upon illness, Puritans could take away some of the anxiety that they felt about the latter — a form of conversion hysteria in reverse!

Finally, what of the duration and popularity of the providential view of illness? It was popular in the early to mid seventeenth century and amongst Puritans. Devout Anglicans such as John Evelyn and Lady Elizabeth Delaval also believed in providence and God's afflictions.[88] Many Anglicans, however, especially after the Restoration, tended not to refer to providence so much. Laud, who in his simultaneous belief in and denial of dreams, and in his astrological interests, was typical of the first half of the seventeenth century, nevertheless did not mention providence when noting his illnesses in his diary.[89] The attitude of the Anglican martyr was generally followed by later members of the Church in the more secular and less 'enthusiastic' Restoration period. For instance, the correspondents of the Hatton family, most of whom were conformists, writing in the later seventeenth century, used medical terminology when discussing illness and hardly mentioned God.[90] The early eighteenth century Yorkshire diaries of John Hobson

[87] Macfarlane, *Josselin*, p. 173; Delany, *British Autobiography*, p. 60 writes of 'the Calvinist image of man cowering before a wrathful God'.

[88] See, for example, Evelyn's account of the death of his son Richard where he commented 'The L. Jesus sanctify this and all other my afflictions: Amen', and when his youngest son died immediately after he wrote 'The afflicting hand of God being still upon us': *The Diary of John Evelyn*, ed. E. S. de Beer (6 vols., Oxford, 1955), vol. 3, pp. 210–11. Also *The Meditations of Lady Elizabeth Delaval*, ed. Douglas G. Greene (Surtees Soc., cxc, 1978 for 1975), p. 77: 'Pain seldom seizes us but physicians can tell what evil is the cause of it from whence our distempers proceed, and what are the most proper remedies (or at least they make us believe so), and by those remedies one may be cured, perhaps suddenly too; but if not me, who it may be God will punish longer making me smart under his rod, even till I humble kiss it, by suffering willingly, yet some other person in pain's might find ease by the physician's skill.'

[89] William Laud, *The Autobiography of Dr William Laud* (Oxford, 1839); this prints the diary.

[90] *Correspondence of the Family of Hatton, Being Chiefly Letters Addressed to Christopher First Viscount Hatton A.D. 1601–1704*, ed. E. Maunde Thompson (2 vols., Camden Soc., N.S., xxii, 1878).

and James Fretwell also described illness in medico-naturalistic terms.[91] The Reverend Giles Moore, rector of Horstead Keynes in Sussex from 1655 to 1679, was a strong supporter of the Restoration settlement. When in London he bought 'rolls on the burning of London, God's terrible voice in the City'. He noted that as his brother died 'he sent forth with great earnestness four or five most divine prayers'.[92] Yet these were mere echoes of Godliness. When he, or his maid, was ill, references to prescriptions and physicians predominate, and amongst the many details of his brother's illness the only reference to God was the one given above. God the healer seems to have receded into the background. A similar picture emerges from the diary of the Reverend Thomas Brockbank.[93] Of course, Anglicans did not ignore God, and thanks were often given to God for recovery after illness, for example by Pepys after his operation for the stone. However, after 1660 it was generally only Nonconformists – now an identifiable and limited part of the population – who seemed to view the occurrences of life in spiritualised and providential terms.

Even within Puritan ranks a providential view of illness was by no means universal. A Puritan might believe in providence but not see it working in illness. Richard Rogers, the Puritan lecturer and evangelist writing at the end of the sixteenth century, did not use the providential model in his diary when noting his illnesses.[94] However, clergymen *were* more likely to take a providential view of illness in their diaries. Oliver Heywood, Henry Newcome and Richard Baxter, who were by no means extreme Nonconformists and were close to Anglicanism in other respects, nevertheless contrast sharply with Anglican clergy in their constant recourse to providence. On the other hand, Puritan laymen less intensely devout than Roger Lowe or Joseph Lister were less constant in their reliance on providential explanations. It is almost as though the providential model of illness depended upon one's religious training and devotion. The young Simonds D'Ewes, when studying law in London between 1622 and 1624, showed himself in his diary to be a reasonably devout Puritan layman, but did not see illness as a punishment coming from God. Another layman, Thomas

[91] *Yorkshire Diaries and Autobiographies* (Surtees Soc. LXV, 1875) (hereinafter *Yorkshire Diaries*).

[92] 'Extracts from the Journal and Account Book of the Rev. Giles Moore', *Sussex Archaeological Collections*, 1, pp. 101, 109.

[93] Brockbank, *Diary*.

[94] M. M. Knappen (ed.), *Two Elizabethan Puritan Diaries* (Chicago and London, 1933) (hereinafter Rogers, *Diary*).

Dudley, the deputy governor of New England, could see God's hand in the diseases affecting his colony, yet he was able to distance himself from the providential view and, almost like a modern sociologist, see behind the systems of medical and religious explanations. On the causes of the widespread deaths in the colony in 1630–1 Dudley wrote in a Hippocratic vein:

The natural causes seem to be in the want of warm lodging and good diet to which Englishmen are habituated at home, and in the sudden increase of heat which they endure that are landed here in summer, the salt meats at sea having prepared their bodies thereto...

He also mentioned

the poorer sort, whose houses and bedding kept them not sufficiently warm, nor their diet sufficiently in heart. Other causes God may have, as our faithful minister Mr Wilsonne (lately handling that point) showed unto us, which I forbear to mention, leaving this matter to the further dispute of physicians and divines.[95]

It is difficult to tell whether being a layman, having a cosmopolitan range of experience (Dudley had been page to the Earl of Northampton, clerk to a judge and steward to the Earl of Lincoln) or living in the metropolis (as did D'Ewes) produced a greater detachment from a providential way of thinking. Detailed research linking place in society, domicile and personal experience to religious attitudes may elucidate the issue, but I suspect that, as in all periods, there will be frequent contradictory findings, especially as the period up to 1660 was a time of great confusion as regards the religious identity of the gentry (for instance, Dudley's superior was the wealthier John Winthrop who was a consistent believer in providence).

Moreover, much of the evidence has an inherent bias. As one of the purposes of writing a diary was to express the communion between the individual and God, it is almost inevitable that a diarist would favour a providential view. The fact that a Puritan diarist like the parliamentary Captain Adam Eyre[96] did not constantly look for the hand of God in daily life, or like D'Ewes hardly mentioned it, shows that not all Puritan diaries were written as a reckoning of God's ways to man and vice versa. No doubt the rising consciousness of the 'middling' sort of people expressed in politics, commerce and religion found an outlet in diary writing. But, for those imbued with the

95 Everett Emerson (ed.), *Letters from New England* (Amherst, 1976), p. 76 (hereinafter *New England*).   96 See *Yorkshire Diaries*.

providential view of things, namely clergymen and devout laymen, the perception of illness as God's correction was habitual. However, together with or underlying the providential view of illness are found more widespread ideas about illness, which are discussed later in the essay.

The plurality of models of illness

Religion held no monopoly in explaining illness. Even thorough-going Puritans often used medical or physically based explanations. This is not surprising given the intellectual and social proximity of religion and medicine discussed earlier. However, from mediaeval times there had been a third way of understanding illness. Magic and folk-wisdom still permeated the English countryside in the seventeenth century.[97] This was oral knowledge and so generally hidden from us, often only surfacing in some disapproving mention in court record, letter or diary. In other words, we know of popular magic only through literary sources, and they almost always disapprove, unless they take an explicitly magical or Paracelsian approach. The magical tradition, however, lies outside the scope of this essay. My focus rests upon religious and naturalistic (medical) explanations, for these were the ones employed both by religious writers and by Puritan diarists.

Although, as we shall see, medical and religious explanations could at times be used by Puritans without relation to each other, there was a standard perceived relationship between the two. In the minds of Puritans, medicine, like other aspects of life, was integrated with religion. For instance, medical remedies were seen as a gift of God, put on earth for men's use. Perkins wrote:

In the preserving of life, two things must be considered: the means, and the right use of means. The means is good and wholesome physic, which, though it be despised of many as a thing unprofitable and needless, yet must it be esteemed as an ordinance and blessing of God.[98]

Perkins added that the medicines had to be authorised 'by the word of God and prayer'.[99] They had to be 'lawful and good' and 'by prayer we must entreat the Lord for a blessing upon them, in restoring of health, if it be the good will of God. 1 Tim. 4.3'. In this way Puritans (and Anglicans like Robert Burton)[100] placed medicine within the

97 See Thomas, *Religion*.   98 Perkins, *Chain*, p. 505.
99 *Ibid.*, p. 506.
100 Robert Burton, *The Anatomy of Melancholy*, ed. Floyd Dell and Paul Jordan-Smith (New York, 1938), pp. 384–6, 389–91 (part 2, sect. 1, member 2 and 4).

bounds of religion, for the word of God (the Bible) defined what was acceptable medicine, and a remedy worked on a specific occasion only because of prayer (which thus gave religion priority over medicine) and God's blessing.

In Perkins' eyes what was allowed by God's word was essentially the medicine of orthodox Galenic physicians. He condemned uroscopy, astrology and enchanters who, he wrote, were in fact witches and wizards though they might be called cunning men and women. Perkins' advice on the choice of physician could be found in many Galenic text-books (in a scholium he cited the attack on uroscopists by Lange and Foreest who were both Galenists). Moreover, the physician should be of 'good conscience and good religion', a sentiment echoed by John Sym who likewise attacked empirics and required physicians to be 'conscionable for religion and piety that God may bless their labours the better'.[101] The requirements that the medicine used should be lawful was understandable given the existence of magical remedies – Perkins condemned the use of spells and charms which 'are all vain and superstitious: because neither by creation, nor by any ordinance of God's word have they any power to cure a bodily disease'.[102]

The attack on empirics shows how moderate Puritan clergymen were closely in tune with their fellow professionals, the Galenic physicians, and had a similar interest in attacking competitors, especially of the oral or 'little' tradition. (It would be an interesting test of Charles Webster's link between Puritanism and Paracelsianism[103] to examine the attitude of moderate Puritan theologians and diarists to Paracelsian medicine.)

The definition of medicine as God-given 'means' not only placed religion on top of medicine, but also had implications for the sick person. The need to gain God's blessings upon 'means' by prayer was an expression of obedience to God. By praying and showing his willingness to accept God's control over medicine the individual avoided the possibility that God might take the use of means as an expression of rebellion, as a method of escaping punishment. In this way the possible conflict between religion and medicine could be avoided, and Puritan diarists and autobiographers – men like Ralph

---

[101] Sym, *Self-killing*, p. 15.
[102] Perkins, *Chain*, p. 506. Burton, *Anatomy of Melancholy*, p. 382 also condemned magic ('sorcerers are too common: cunning men, wizards, and white-witches as they call them, in every village'), but unlike Perkins he accepted astrology (p. 390).   [103] Webster, *Instauration*, pp. 273–82.

Josselin, Henry Newcome, Joseph Lister and Richard Baxter – took special care to note that the success of a remedy was due to God's blessing.[104] The Puritan Lady Brilliana Harley wrote to her son in 1640:

Edward Pinner hath been very sick. I sent to Doctor Wright to him, who hath been here the most part of this week, and hath given him physic which hath done him (by the blessing of God) upon that means, much good.[105]

Was there any conflict between providential, God-controlled means of medicine, and a naturalistic medicine in which a remedy would work whether God's blessing was given or not? Certainly, Puritan writers were aware of the possibility that people could rely too much upon means and not enough upon God, and that they could sin by thinking that medicine worked without God's blessing – that is, that it worked naturalistically. John Sym wrote:

In taking of physic we are always to observe these subsequent cautions. First, that we *dote not* upon, nor *trust*, or *ascribe too much* to physical means; but that we carefully look and pray to *God* for a blessing by the warrantable *use* of them. For, it is *God* that both directs the *physicians* judgement and conscionable practise about a *patient*, and also puts virtue into, and gives healthful operation to the medicines.[106]

Sym also argued that a man might indirectly kill himself when he 'doth not depend upon God, for a blessing upon means, who by his over-riding providence directs the course and blesses the means'. The possibilities were that men would 'slavishly enthrall' themselves to means and so exclude God or 'perplex themselves if they cannot have them [means], or that the success answers not their expectation: because the Lord disposes things so, as he also may effect his work and will, often by crossing ours'.[107] The God of the early seventeenth century was not yet the giver of immutable laws to be discovered by reason and by the scientist, as was thought in the late seventeenth and eighteenth centuries. For Puritans who believed in providence, all things were subject to the secret will of God, and reason could not discover his plan, though a minister, as in the case of plague, might interpret his actions.[108] However, there was some uniformity in the working of

---

[104] Miller, *The New England Mind*, p. 234 writes that the idea of means 'prevented believers from being lured into the heresy of natural autonomy'.

[105] *Letters of the Lady Brilliana Harley*, ed. Thomas Taylor Lewis (Camden Soc. LVIII, 1853), p. 91.

[106] Sym, *Self-killing*, pp. 14–15.   [107] *Ibid.*, p. 92.

[108] Gouge, *Three Arrows*, p. 13 gave ministers a privileged position as interpreters of God's word (the Scriptures) who could discern what particular sins had brought on the plague.

nature. God, after all, could achieve his ends through natural means, in other words he used the natural (God-given) tendency of a remedy to behave in a particular way. Perkins, for instance, wrote of how a life-span was measured by a predetermined amount of 'radical moisture' in the body.[109] God's determination of a person's existence was thus achieved by natural means. The acceptance of the workings of nature and, more especially, the exhortation not to depend too much on means show that Puritan writers implicitly recognised the existence of naturalistic explanations which might be divorced from providence. And their teaching can be seen as an attempt to exclude the latter possibility from people's minds.

Ralph Josselin, who is discussed in detail elsewhere in this volume by Lucinda McCray Beier, illustrates in his diary how providential and naturalistic explanations of illness could be interchanged – sometimes connected in his mind, sometimes not. The two do not seem to come into overt conflict; after all, even today recourse both to prayer and to doctors often takes place without any inner stress.

Josselin had a sore and suppurating navel between 1648 and 1650. His attitude was that God could heal it directly or could do so indirectly by blessing 'the remedies applied'.[110] When the remedies did not work he 'applied nothing to it hoping in god it will do well'.[111] Here God worked directly rather than through means. Sometimes, providential and naturalistic explanations were placed side by side. At one time Josselin saw his sore navel as God's way of minding him of his folly, but at the same time he wrote that his going outside and taking cold may have been a precipitating factor, and he also added: 'And I observe that I swett very much too or three nights before it was sorish.'[112] Josselin's attempt to make sense on a natural level of his illness by looking for precipitating causes is independent of his ideas of what caused God to make him ill (though Josselin, being a good Puritan minister, would have probably used the standard link between divine ends and means and replied that God worked by indirect means, by cold, to achieve his correction). However, it is clear that Josselin's anxiety was not limited to the divine level, for he was anxious about the natural possibilities threatened by his sore navel, writing: 'heard of one that after 2 years illness was killed with a rawness in his navel, but god shall heal me of this infirmity, and I shall praise him'.[113] Here,

109 Perkins, *Chain*, p. 506.
110 *The Diary of Ralph Josselin*, ed. Alan Macfarlane (Oxford, 1976), p. 141 (hereinafter *Diary*).   111 *Ibid.*, p. 147.
112 *Ibid.*, p. 157.   113 *Ibid.*, p. 159.

Josselin was setting the divine against the natural. Again, when noting cases of smallpox he wrote that God's providential will could allay the natural, contagious nature of smallpox: 'he can preserve my family or me when others ill';[114] and he prayed 'the lord stand betwixt the whole and sick, and suffer his rod to proceed no farther if it be his will'.[115]

There were times for Josselin, however, when naturalistic and providential explanations of illness coincided. He employed medical metaphors for religious purposes and carried them through their origins in physical illness:

This day I had a little pose and roughness of rheume in my throat, my god will ordain all for my good...my desires are with David that god would purge and wash me thoroughly from my sin, oh let not the humour have no settling stay behind if it be thy pleasure.[116]

Here Josselin slid from the medical to the religious and perhaps back again. He moved from a description of his body to wish God to purge and wash him of sin, then he asked that the humour (of sin? of phlegm?) have 'no settling stay behind': the language could apply just as well to his chest or throat as to his soul. In a sense we are seeing the homely medical metaphor of Dod and Cleaver, Perkins and Ambrose put powerfully into practice; for it draws religion into medicine by borrowing medicine's language, but also appropriates medicine for religion by showing that there is a supreme, providential physician who cures both body and soul. Perhaps it was such language and such metaphors which allowed the possible tensions between religious and naturalistic (medical) explanations of disease to remain hidden from view. Certainly if God was a physician and worked like one then the potential conflict could be evaded, and Josselin did at times picture God like this: 'the lord is pleased to give me some mixtures and rubs in my condicions that my heart may upon every thing look up to him'.[117]

Turning to naturalistic ideas of illness, it is clear that Puritans often thought of the natural causes of illness in two ways. There was knowledge, possibly derived from professional medicine but certainly current in society, involving humoral ideas and specific disease conditions such as 'ague', 'rheum', 'gout', 'fit', 'palsy', etc. Secondly, and more generally, there was an ability to make sense of an illness

---

[114] Ibid., p. 154. [115] Ibid., p. 158.
[116] Ibid., p. 204. [117] Ibid., p. 206.

by referring to some precipitating event, often described in terms of wet, cold, dry and warm. This latter type of knowledge seems to have been widespread and to have transcended differences of domicile, religion and status. D'Ewes, for instance, wrote 'being somewhat thin clothed I got there a most fierce and bitter cold';[118] Josselin, as we have seen, felt that going outside and taking cold might have produced his sore navel; whilst the poor Puritan servant Roger Lowe wrote 'I went to Leigh and was ill wet'.[119] Thomas Dudley reported 'there died Mrs Shelton, the wife of the other minister there, who, about eighteen or twenty days before, handling cold things in a sharp morning, put herself into a most violent fit of the wind colic and vomiting, she at length fell into a fever and so died'.[120] Pepys also tried to make sense of his illnesses in this way: 'this day under great apprehensions of getting an ague from my putting on a suit that hath lain without ayring a great while, and I pray to God it do not do me hurt'.[121]

This way of thinking, relying upon a qualitative (hot, cold, dry, wet) view of things, had analogies with the more complex and technical system of orthodox medicine, which in its practice was also qualitative despite the advent of Paracelsian and then mechanical ideas which tended to change its theoretical structure. It may be that an anthropological analysis, as MacDonald has suggested,[122] instead of, or as well as, a social history approach will give insight into what seems to have been a common resource in literate society (and most probably in non-literate ones as well). Anthropologists have studied hot–cold/dry–wet systems of ideas in various societies. The need of sick people to find for themselves a precipitating cause for an illness is something that we find today,[123] and a psychological as well as an anthropological perspective may be helpful in understanding it. For this type of explanation, depending as it does on the sick person's actual

---

[118] *The Diary of Sir Simonds D'Ewes (1622–1624)*, ed. Elizabeth Bourcier (Paris, 1974), p. 124 (hereinafter *Diary*).
[119] William L. Sachse (ed.), *The Diary of Roger Lowe of Ashton-in-Makerfield, Lancashire 1663–74* (London, 1938).
[120] Emerson, *New England*, p. 82.
[121] Pepys, *Diary*, vol. 6, p. 32.
[122] Michael MacDonald, 'Anthropological perspectives on the history of science and medicine', in P. Corsi and P. Weindling (eds.), *Information Sources in the History of Science and Medicine* (London, 1983), pp. 61–80.
[123] As I write, newspapers report the death of a girl whose parents believed that the piercing of her ears was responsible, despite doctors' statements to the contrary.

experience and his own verbalisation of it, which is usually different from the complex and probably alienating reasoning of the medical profession, has the function of giving personal understanding of, and hence a measure of personal control over, illness.

The vocabulary of illness

The vocabulary used to express knowledge of illness varied greatly. Richard Rogers gave few descriptions of his own illnesses and hardly any of other people's. When visiting the sick he recorded no details of the illnesses that they suffered from; what we have is the laconic: 'One of these days I visited a goodly sick woman with comfort.'[124] Apart from mentioning a cough and cold,[125] Rogers did not have a developed vocabulary for illnesses (at least in his diary), though as one of the early 'physicians of the soul' he did for his psyche and its troubles, for his great interest was 'seeing myself':

And I had this med[itation] one morn[ing] that, comparing this course in which I view my life continually with the former wherein I did it by fits and thus was oft unsettled, out of order, and then either not seeing myself, though I had been less unwatchfull [sic] walked in great danger by every occasion or, seeing it, could not easily recover myself, and so went unfit, many hours and sometimes days, for my calling, sometimes dumpish and too heavy, sometimes loose and many fruits following, as no study but unprof[itableness].[126]

Clearly Rogers' emphasis was on his mind not on his body, and the adjectives 'unsettled' and 'out of order', 'unfit', 'dumpish', 'too heavy', 'loose' all testify to the fact that he had developed a rich and variegated vocabulary of fine distinctions to describe the state of his mind. Napier's patients also seemed to have the same wealth of vocabulary for their mental states,[127] so this fullness of language may not have been limited to Puritans; certainly as Haller points out it is found in the literature of the time.[128] Whether Rogers had the same full vocabulary for physical illness but did not put it in his diary is impossible to tell.

In the diary of Roger Lowe the vocabulary both for his mental and for his physical states was very limited. As his is almost a unique diary,

[124] Rogers, Diary, p. 70. On Rogers see his editor's introduction and Haller, Rise of Puritanism, pp. 35–45.
[125] Ibid., p. 83.   [126] Ibid., p. 70.
[127] On the vocabulary of psychological states see MacDonald, Mystical Bedlam, p. 243.
[128] Haller, Rise of Puritanism, pp. 31–3.

from a poor but literate servant, it is worth looking at it in a little detail. 'Sad' was one of Lowe's major descriptive terms for mental trouble and 'sick' for physical. He often put the two together, expressing the typical union of body and mind: 'Tuesday, I was sadly sick and had a very sick night, but the Lord restored me in the other morning.'[129]

Lowe, however, gave a little detail of his own and others' physical illnesses. Obvious, visible ailments were noted, Lowe at different times recording that 'A tedious stitch took in my back, so I was unable to stay shop, and held me very sore till noon, and then the Lord helped me'; 'I was in an afflicted state in my body by reasons of cold'; 'and so we parted and were ill wet'.[130] However, more serious complaints were vague, in a sense unknowable, for affliction and recovery belonged to God. From March to May 1666 Lowe suffered from some illness which was probably serious but which he did not identify, apart from his references to God's affliction and mercy; the physical descriptive terms used were 'ill', 'pains', 'well'.[131]

When describing the illnesses of others Lowe noted some obvious ailments and well-known conditions. He mentioned toothache (often specifically noted by diarists), accidental poisoning by arsenic, 'a hurt by a fall off a horse', 'neck broken in riding', 'dropsy', 'falling sickness', 'troubled with sores'. However, he was usually less specific when describing illness.

At first sight this is surprising, for his acquaintance with illness and death was far greater than that of a modern lay person. Although not a minister, he visited the sick regularly (as Puritans were enjoined to do); he was present at death-beds and he attended many funerals. Judging from other diaries such as William Bulkeley's[132] and Adam Eyre's, this was not unusual for a lay person in the seventeenth century. Lowe certainly gained some knowledge of illness and death from his exposure to the sick. (Accounts of death-bed scenes not only portrayed the piety of the dying, but also described their symptoms and thus expressed medical knowledge, and being read became sources of knowledge.) Lowe thought that he knew the signs of approaching death:

This evening old Izibell and John Hasleden and I went to Gawther's and were merry when we parted. We went all together into old John Jenkins', we

[129] Lowe, *Diary*, p. 56.   [130] *Ibid.*, pp. 22, 75, 86.   [131] *Ibid.*, pp. 99–101.
[132] *The Diary of Bulkeley of Dronwy, Anglesey 1630–1636*, ed. H. Owen (Anglesey Antiquarian Society, 1937), pp. 27–172.

thought he would have died this night. When I was with him he shook me by the hand and I conferred with him. After a while I parted. [In fact he did not die that night.][133]

On another occasion Lowe wrote: 'I went into old William Hasleden's in Ashton, his wife was sick and I read in the *Practice of Pietie*, and as I was reading she gave up the ghost.'[134] However, despite his familiarity with the sick, Lowe had little vocabulary to describe different diseases or perhaps had no interest in having one. He went to a large number of funerals, but gave no cause of death, and on his visits to the sick, with few exceptions he seemed uninterested in recording what particular illness was involved. Lowe was interested in medicine only in so far as it related to religion. So he recorded a religious rhyme for staunching blood;[135] and a visit to 'one George Clare, who lay sick' provided a religious motif: 'I went into church yard to look at graves, as is my common custom, and there stayed a while admiring the common frailty of mankind: how silently now they were lying in dust.'[136]

For Lowe the sick were sick, and no explanation or diagnosis of their condition was required; but the sick, even if strangers, could act as the focus of social activity and be the recipients of religious comfort. We should thus remember that the sick were not only perceived in 'medical' terms but also in religious and social terms.

It may also be the case that Lowe's knowledge of medical terminology was slight. Certainly men like Newcome, Josselin, Heywood who were ministers and in daily contact with sickness, and who sometimes read medical authors, used a wider vocabulary. And Richard Baxter, who had a consuming interest in his own illness as well as being a minister and a medical practitioner, came close in his autobiography to emulating the language found in medical text-books (whether contact with physicians produced an acquaintance with medical terminology, or whether it was a shared resource of a particular section of society needs further research). However, it is possible that these men were the exceptions and that many people were specific only about accidents (broken legs etc.), obvious ailments (toothaches, colds, joint pains) and a few well-known illnesses (dropsy, ague, etc.), with the large majority of cases being labelled 'sick'. In other words, for some people knowledge of illness as shown by a differentiated terminology may have been slight. Or, it may be the

---

[133] Lowe, *Diary*, pp. 42–3.
[135] *Ibid.*, pp. 76–7.
[134] *Ibid.*, p. 109.
[136] *Ibid.*, p. 57.

case that there was a difference between the first and second half of the century. The diaries of Robert Bulkeley, Adam Eyre and the reports of the early American colonists tend to support the view that in the earlier part of the century less medical terminology was used, while the diaries after 1660 are richer in the vocabulary of illness. A comparison of the diary of Laud and the autobiography of Baxter, the former written in the first half of the century and the latter in the second half, also shows this difference. However, generalisations are dangerous; Baxter was *so* interested in his health that his knowledge would probably have been as great had he been living at the beginning of the century.

To conclude the more general part of this essay: it should now be apparent that physical illness was only partly 'spiritualised', that there was a guarded note of acceptance by Puritan writers of physical medicine and that, given the wide diversity of knowledge and vocabulary amongst different people, generalisations are most difficult.

So far I have discussed problems and approaches; the people involved have not really shown their faces. The English historian in taking the thematic approach has tended to use snippets of evidence to support a particular point; this means that a person's overall 'life trajectory' or experience as shown in a diary or autobiography is lost in the attempt to describe particular problems and to produce generalisations. This is especially unfortunate in such a personal matter as attitudes to illness. By looking in some detail at the autobiographies of Joseph Lister and Richard Baxter I hope to remedy the defect.

The autobiographies of Joseph Lister and Richard Baxter

A Puritan autobiography, as opposed to a diary, highlighted significant events and episodes in the author's life.[137] Rather than a day by day account of illness we are presented in the autobiographies of Lister and Baxter with a selection of significant illnesses; and health and illness are treated in a more considered if distanced fashion, being remembered after a period of years.

Joseph Lister (1627–1709) was an apprentice, and a servant, who finally became reasonably well off after the death of his wife's uncle who left land worth £20 a year. Although not a minister himself, Lister sent his sons into the ministry. His autobiography is full of examples of God's providence, whether it was saving him from accidents or

---

[137] On Puritan autobiographies see Delany, *British Autobiography*, and Watkins, *Puritan Experience*.

illness; however, the autobiography is not a mere recital of pious paradigms but, like Lowe's diary, also a lively and almost innocent account of social life (his reasons for not marrying his master's daughter spring to mind).

Lister's first brush with divine providence came when he fell off a horse and 'I was taken up for dead...O how near was I to death at this time! and had I died then, surely I had gone down to the pit'.[138]

Another example of God's providence occurred when, as an adult, he was at Hartlepool and he was caught by the tide. Lister put his trust in God:

Then I cried unto the Lord, who can do everything; and I thought, though I be in the sea, I am not in the whale's belly; and if I was, yet God could demand deliverance for me; so I depended upon his ability to save me...yet God enabled the horse to grapple with the flood.[139]

Here Lister's horse as well as God could help him, but in most accidents it was God alone who could be a protector. In illness, however, medicine and doctors could be of use as well as God. This brings us back to the problem of the perception of illness as naturalistic and/or divine. After his ordeal, Lister came home wet and fell ill (he saw illness in functional terms: he could not rise, food was disagreeable and appetite and sleep departed from him). His reaction was to send his urine to a physician who, without knowing of the episode with the tide, could form no judgement except that 'the person had been under some sad overpowering fear'. Rather than wait upon providence Lister acted. He was dissatisfied with his physician:

I fell into a violent fever, in which, after I had laid some weeks in great extremity and the doctor ordering me nothing but some easy cordial things, I desired him to give me a bill, for I purposed employing another man; for though I was not against cordials for relieving and strengthening nature, yet I thought it very proper to have some working physic that might be likely to weaken and remove the distemper, which he was not willing to give me.[140]

There are some points to note here. Lister was a free agent, who like Josselin and anyone else who could afford it, could decide on his own treatment. We in the age of the National Health Service have forgotten how easy it is to change a doctor if the patient is paying. However, Lister like Josselin had his own opinion of medical matters, and the

[138] Joseph Lister, The Autobiography of J. L...., ed. T. Wright (London, 1842), p. 4.
[139] Ibid., p. 42.   [140] Ibid., p. 43.

plastic, qualitative language of seventeenth century medicine – ' working physic ... weaken and remove the distemper' – was far easier for lay people to use than that of modern medicine. Lister could not only sack his doctor, but he was also much more able to make a decision on the rationale of his treatment and could do so whilst using the language of the physicians. One might also say that by helping himself, Lister was not waiting upon God's providence, for, as Perkins wrote, the Christian had the duty actively to look after the health of his body. Lister got a new doctor:

a good man, I believe, and they said a young convert ... He first let me blood, and then gave me what he thought proper, and *God so blessed his prescriptions*, that I did soon recover. [my italics][141]

Even if it appears illogical to us that God should work through one doctor and not the other, it was not to a Nonconformist, for every moment was subject to God's providence. Providence worked not uniformly but at each moment of time, and in the face of providence consistency was a meaningless concept – and the doctor being a convert may have helped.

Yet the difference between blind acceptance of providence as in the case of accidents and an ability to act to evade illness was still there. Although Lister recovered, he fell ill again, not because of providence but because he walked into the garden and was 'much worse than before'. In this case Lister's actions did not bring healing but disease. Nevertheless, his explanation was a naturalistic rather than a providential one. The point, however, is that Lister was able to use both explanations without feeling any tension between them. Providence in a sense encompassed the natural, for it could work through natural means. Certainly, after being close to death both from drowning and illness, Lister saw providence behind all his recent experiences. He got back to Bradford among his Christian friends who:

assisted me in returning a thanks-offering to the Lord for his past mercies, for I had been under a series of gracious and merciful providences for a long time past.[142]

Lister's attitude to death was not one of anxiety. Like Josselin he was sure that he would go to heaven. He wrote of his relapse: 'I now lay long in a languishing condition, expecting nothing but death; and being easy, and well satisfied about my future state, was borne

[141] *Ibid.*, p. 43.   [142] *Ibid.*, p. 45.

comfortably.'[143] This serenity may have been unusual, for the Puritan's belief in his predestination ensured that no worldly event such as a death-bed confession or repentance could change God's unknown decision as to his fate after death. Hence, anxiety should in theory have continued up to the moment of death. But the older tradition of dying well to which Puritans still subscribed emphasised that the dying person should achieve a state of peace and reconciliation with God.[144]

For both Catholics and Puritans the approach of death was usually something that was known to the ill person. The religious preparation for death would be enough to ensure this.[145] Lister perceived the intimation of death in terms of execution (a recurring image in diaries). After his wife's death, he was attacked by a 'violent fever' so that:

> for a week or ten days I was, in the judgement of almost all spectators, a gone man; and I had received the sentence of death in my own apprehension, and yet, at last, even to a wonder, God was pleased to rebuke the distemper, and raise me up again. Bless the Lord, O my soul and all that is within me praise his holy name![146]

Illness and death were spectacles in which the spectators and the patient could make their own judgement; the medical expert did not have a monopoly on prognostication. At the same time, God was the ultimate judge, giving his sentence of death through bodily intimation to the patient. Whatever the theologians might have said and a Puritan expected after death, loss of life was still a punishment (an execution).

Richard Baxter (1615–91), the Puritan divine, also discussed his health and illnesses in his autobiography.[147] Baxter left the materials for an autobiography which were published after his death as *Reliquiae Baxterianae* (1696). In it are accounts of his involvement in religion and politics as well as intimate details of his personal life. Health and illness were given places of great importance. Baxter saw himself as suffering pain and illness continually through his life. He perceived these illnesses as being sent by God, but his interest in providence was, on this subject, at times only nominal in relation to the large amount of detail about

---

[143] *Ibid.*, p. 44.
[144] Stannard, *Death*, pp. 69, 78–9, 88, describes the conflicts of the two views.
[145] Puritan theologians stressed that physicians should tell the patient if the prognosis was bad and call a minister. In France a physician was required by law to advise the patient to call in a confessor on the second day of a serious illness: McManners, *Death and the Enlightenment*, p. 244.
[146] Lister, *Autobiography*, p. 57.
[147] On Baxter see G. F. Nuttall, *Richard Baxter* (London, 1965); Delany, *British Autobiography*, pp. 72–6; Watkins, *Puritan Experience*, pp. 121–43.

his ailments. It was his illnesses *per se* that interested Baxter, their symptoms, causes, treatments and his sufferings under them. In short, Baxter was morbidly obsessed with his ailments, but as I do not want to label Baxter with what his doctors tagged him with, this will be my last pejorative comment about Baxter's interest in his own health.

The reasons that Baxter gave for writing about his health varied. At the beginning of the book Baxter stressed the importance of his body for understanding his soul:

And because the case of my body had a great operation upon my soul, and the history of it is somewhat necessary to the right understanding of the rest, and yet it is not a matter worthy to be oft mentioned, I shall here give you a brief account of the most of my afflictions of that kind, reserving the mention of some particular *deliverances* to the proper place. [my italics: Baxter was indicating the formal structure of a Puritan autobiography][148]

The same note of apology is present later when Baxter gave another reason for talking about his health. Students and physicians might learn something and other men's health might benefit, so 'I must here digress, to mention the state of my vile body, not otherwise worthy the notice of the world'.[149] Whatever the ostensible reasons for writing about his health, its place in his autobiography is clearly justified for he must have spent many hours both suffering from, and thinking about, his illnesses. Not only did he treat himself (which was quite usual) but, like other ministers, he became a medical practitioner.

Baxter opened his case history by describing his general constitution ('sound...but very thin and lean and weak and especially of a great debility of the nerves').[150] The structure of his narration was totally secular and 'medical'. He listed his childhood illnesses and how he had caught a chronic catarrh and cold which he was afraid had turned into a consumption. From this point on we have a catalogue of treatments, and Baxter's explanations of why they failed. His account would have provided Molière with good material for his satire on medicine, but for Baxter the treatments did not fail because they were *useless*, but because they were not *appropriate* – the physicians had neither properly diagnosed the illness and its causes, nor correctly assessed what treatment would supply the required qualities to counteract the illness. At first, Baxter ate garlic, 'but this put an acrimony into my blood, which naturally was acrimonious'. Baxter then sought advice:

---

[148] Baxter, *Reliquiae*, p. 9.
[149] *Ibid.*, part III, p. 173.   [150] *Ibid.*, part 1, p. 9.

After this the spitting of blood increased my fears. After that Sir Henry Herbert advised me to take the flower of brimstone, which I continued till I had taken seven ounces; which took off most of the remainder of my cough; but increased the acrimony of my blood.[151]

Then Baxter consulted an 'unskilful physician' who persuaded him that he had a hectic fever:

and to cure that I took much milk from the cow, and other pituitous cooling things, and constantly anointed my stomach and reins [kidneys] with refrigerating oils of violets and roses; and was utterly restrained from my usual exercise! By this time I had an extream chilliness without, and yet a strange scurf on my tongue, with a constant desire of stretching, that I thought I would almost have endured the rack; and an incredible flatulency at the stomach, and a bleeding at the nose.[152]

Clearly Baxter did not agree with his doctors. It would be tedious to recount the diagnoses, the treatments, and the reasons for their failure. Baxter wrote he had 'at several times the advice of no less than six and thirty physicians, by whose order I us'd drugs without number almost, which God thought not fit to make successful for a cure'[153] (who was to blame – God or the doctors?). A number of epistemological and social issues are involved here.

Baxter felt that his knowledge was equal to the physicians'. It was not of a different kind from theirs, but Baxter thought that he could apply it better than the doctors. He believed that his illnesses stemmed 'from latent stones in my reins, occasioned by unsuitable diet in my youth'.[154] He had observed that his catarrh and cough had come on after eating raw apples, pears and plums (note the search for a precipitating cause), and he was confirmed in his opinion that diet was at the root of his troubles when Sir Theodore Mayerne (physician to James I) advised him to eat apples 'which of all things in the world had ever been my most deadly enemies', with the result that:

Having taken cold with riding thin clothed in the snow, and having but two days eaten apples before meat, as he persuaded me, I fell into such a bleeding as continued six days, with some fits of intermission; so that about a gallon of blood that we noted was lost, and what more I know not.[155]

In the end, perhaps because he felt he knew better, Baxter 'at last forsook the doctors for the most part except when the urgency of a symptom or pain constrained me to seek some present ease'.[156]

[151] *Ibid.*, part 1, p. 9.
[152] *Ibid.*, part 1, p. 9.
[153] *Ibid.*, part 1, p. 10.
[154] *Ibid.*, part 1, p. 10.
[155] *Ibid.*, part 1, pp. 9–10.
[156] *Ibid.*, part 1, p. 10.

It was not epistemological freedom that was the crucial issue; Baxter never really successfully exercised such freedom. He never escaped from doctors; he was always asking their opinion despite his rejection of them. The reasons for this attraction are difficult to grasp (perhaps Baxter partly accepted physicians' claims that only they should make humoral interpretations of illness). Moreover freedom to diagnose and treat his illness was not the crucial factor in making him reject the physicians; it was a particular action of the doctors that mattered.

Baxter was variously diagnosed as suffering from a hectic fever, from scurvy and then came the blow: 'divers eminent physicians agreed that my disease was the hypochondriack melancholy'.[157] This was a diagnosis that Baxter did not want (it was one that was to recur), for it labelled him as mad, or possessed, or at least highly fanciful. Robert Burton wrote of windy or hypochondriack melancholy that physicians found it very difficult to locate the part affected. Signs of the illness included the tendency of the patient to exaggerate symptoms and to change physicians very often.[158] This particular category of melancholy was less associated with the extreme forms of madness, but it did fit Baxter and the label deprived him of the reality of his symptoms. He denied the diagnosis:

And yet two wonderful mercies I have had from God that I was never overwhelm'd with real melancholy. My distemper never went to so far as to possess me with any inordinate fancies, or damp me with sinking sadness, although the physicians call'd it the hypochondriack melancholy.[159]

Baxter had been willing to suffer for two years debilitating treatments for scurvy, but 'hypochondriack melancholy' was too much for him; although he was attracted to doctors and sought their expertise, their rejection of his symptoms and pains made him withdraw from them for a while. Interestingly, Baxter's denial of the doctors' diagnosis was based upon God's providence – 'mercies'. The strategy of using God's authority to counter that of the physicians was to recur.

Baxter came back to the question of 'hypochondriack melancholy' when he described how later on in life his kidneys started to trouble him. He first discussed his general state of health:

---

[157] *Ibid.*, part 1, p. 10.
[158] Burton, *Anatomy of Melancholy*, pp. 350–2, 392–3 (part 1, sect. 3, memb. 2, subsect. 2, and part 2, sect. 1, memb. 4, subsect. 2).
[159] Baxter, *Reliquie*, part 1, p. 10.

94

I have lain in above forty years constant weaknesses, and almost constant pains: My chief troubles were incredible inflations of stomach, bowels, back, sides, head, thighs as if I had been daily fill'd with wind...Thirty physicians (at least) all call'd it nothing but hypochondriack flatulency, and somewhat of a scorbutical malady: great bleeding at the nose also did emaciate me, and keep me in a scorbutickal atrophy.[160]

Baxter was fighting the doctors through the pages of the autobiography. This shows how much power they had in his eyes and how necessary a diagnostic label was for Baxter to legitimate his disease (unless the label was melancholy). Baxter wrote that 'I thought myself, that my disease was almost all from debility of the stomach, and extream acrimony of blood by some fault of the liver'.[161] Then in 1658 he suspected renal stones and

thought that one of my extream leanness might possibly feel it: I felt both my kidnies plainly indurate like stone: But never having had a nephritick fit, nor stone came from me in my life and knowing that if that which I felt was stone, the greatness prohibited all medicine that tended to a cure: I thought therefore that it was best for me to be ignorant what it was.[162]

Rather than thinking that he did not have kidney stones because he did not have colic Baxter took the gloomier view – the stones were so big that they could not be dislodged. After fifteen years his pains redoubled:

1673 it turned to terrible suffocations of my brain and lungs. So that if I slept I was suddenly and painfully awakened: The abatement of urine, and constant pain, which nature almost yielded to as victorious, renewed my suspicion of the stone, And my old exploration: and feeling my lean back, both the kidneys were greatlier indurate than before, that the membrane is sore to touch, as if nothing but stone were within them.[163]

The physicians replied that 'the stone cannot be felt with the hand!' Baxter asked for them to feel his back and they had to agree that the kidneys felt hard but with what 'they could not tell'. The reaction of the physicians was to tell Baxter that if both kidneys had such big stones then he would have been 'much worse, by vomiting and torment, and not able to preach, and go about'.[164] This argument between doctors and patient went on with Baxter relying on the

---

[160] *Ibid.*, part 3, p. 173.   [161] *Ibid.*, part 3, p. 173.
[162] *Ibid.*, part 3, p. 173.   [163] *Ibid.*, part 3, p. 173.
[164] *Ibid.*, part 3, p. 173.

authority of 'Skenkius[165] and many observators' that kidney stones could lie unsuspected. The debate had its spectators and the label of 'hypochondriack melancholy' could be hurtful when disseminated at large, and this indicates again the legitimating powers of the doctors:

I became the common talk of the city, especially the women; as if I had been a melancholy humourist, that conceited my reins were petrified, when it was no such matter, but mere conceit. And so while I lay night and day in pain, my supposed melancholy (which I thank God, all my life hath been extraordinary free from) became, for a year, the pity or derision of the town.[166]

Baxter had the last word, stating that 'all physicians had been deceived', and as he perceived 'that all flatulency and pains came from the reins by stagnation, regurgitation and acrimony I cast off all of their medicine and diet'.[167] He decided to clean out his intestines twice a week with a mixture whose ingredients he gave. The result was that God eased his pains. The structure of the argument is important. Baxter gives his own diagnosis and aetiology, and applies an appropriate remedy (cleaning out the guts should get rid of stagnation and acrimony). Cause and remedy now make sense, and it is the success of the latter that justifies his belief that the doctors were deceived and his diagnosis was correct. Yet Baxter could not hide his anxiety, and his arguments were not totally convincing to himself; he gave a whole barrage of reasons why he was right, but could not shake off in his mind the authority of the doctors. He had to justify his illness. One of his arguments was that God had been merciful to him, despite his constant sufferings, for he had 'not one nephritick torment nor acrimony of urine (save one day of bloody urine) nor intolerable kind of pain. What greater bodily mercy can I have had?'[168] Baxter tried here to turn the doctors' arguments by recourse to God's providence. Again, as with Josselin, but in a different form, we have the divine being set up against the naturalistic and secular. Baxter also attacked the concept of hypochondria itself. Humoral medicine was enormously elastic and could explain most symptoms, and would *prima facie* not

---

[165] Skenkius may have been Johannes Schenck (1530–1598) who published a book of medical observations reprinted in the seventeenth century, or more probably his son Johann Georg Schenck who wrote on calculi.

[166] Baxter, *Reliquiae*, part 3, p. 173.

[167] *Ibid.*, part 3, p. 173. [168] *Ibid.*, part 3, p. 174.

need to have recourse, if recourse it was, to hypochondria to hide ignorance. But this is what Baxter thought was involved:

I have written this to mind physicians, to search deeper, when they use to take up with the general hiding names of *hypochondriacks* and scorbuticks, and to caution students.[169]

Baxter was willing to accept the framework of orthodox medicine if not his place within it. Whether he was seen as 'deviant' by society is difficult to judge, for Baxter's appeal to God's providence as determining the nature of his illness – even if that providence produced the topsy-turvy result of kidney stones without symptoms – was sanctioned by Nonconformist tradition, though its force was being challenged as Anglican rationalism came to the fore.

The extent of Baxter's 'deviancy' is also difficult to assess, for men like Josselin were willing to treat themselves, the number of recipe books of drugs was large, and despite the pretensions of the Royal College of Physicians there was no set pharmacopoeia. So that when Baxter made up his own drugs he was not, in the wider context, being 'deviant'. His actions would not have been interpreted in the way that a rejection of orthodox medicine for herbalism would be today. Yet, in his own mind, Baxter was being 'deviant': the doctors could not be ignorant; they were in principle powerful and knowledgeable; he had to justify his reaction against them. Part of his strategy was to place his own alternative remedies within the framework of orthodox medical theory, but then give them further validation by referring their powers to God. When Baxter had a constantly running eye, his doctor prescribed chalk to counteract the acidity of his stomach, but Baxter wanted to try something of his own:

At last I had a conceit of my own that two plants which I had never made trial of, would prove accommodate to my infirmity, *heath* and *sage*, as being very drying and astringent without any acrimony: I boiled much of them in my beer instead of hops, and drank no other: When I had used it a month my eyes were cured, and all my tormenting tooth-aches and such other maladies.[170]

Baxter found that it was the sage that was most effective and he described its effect on different types of people. His choice of sage was based on the same reasoning that his doctor had used, but God was responsible for its nature and power – God the Physician ('This I thought myself obliged to mention to the praise of my heavenly

[169] *Ibid.*, part 3, p. 174.   [170] *Ibid.*, part 1, p. 82.

physician, in thankfulness for these ten years ease; and to give some hint to others in my case').[171] Baxter used the idea of God the Physician and the belief that God blessed medicines to put God against the physicians: 'In a word, God hath made this herb do more for me (not for *cure* but for *ease*) than all the medicines that ever I used from all physicians in my life.'[172] Preferring his own medicine, Baxter appealed to another system – that of divine medicine. His separation of the divine and the naturalistic view of illness was more explicit than Josselin's, perhaps because of his love/hate relationship with orthodox medicine. The paradox with Baxter is that he did not believe exclusively and consistently in providential medicine. Far from it: although at times he used the divine physician against the human and also referred to instances of divine providence in relation to his illnesses, the tenor of Baxter's views on illness was frequently naturalistic. Immediately after his thanks to the 'heavenly Physician' Baxter added that the sage was diminishing in effectiveness because of constant use:

Though now, through age and constant use, this herb doth less with me than at the first; yet am I necessitated still to use it...After sixteen or seventeen years benefit it now faileth me, and I forsake it.[173]

Baxter moved from the providential to the naturalistic; he did not mention the possibility that sage no longer worked because God had withdrawn his blessing from it. In a sense, both medical theories and God's providence were bodies of knowledge (resources) that Baxter used when appropriate. He was not aware of it, but we are. Whether one should concentrate on Baxter's consciousness, or on a more distanced 'social', 'objective' view is a moot point.

Although Baxter made much use of orthodox medical categories, at times he also perceived illness in a predominantly religious sense. Like Lister, Baxter saw God as a judge handing out sentence and punishment. That Puritan relationship to God, more personal even than that of human beings with each other, was fully present in Baxter. On occasion he viewed his pain and illnesses not as medical entities but as the language that God used. After detailing his persecution for refusing to conform Baxter wrote:

But God was pleased quickly to put me past all fear of man...by laying on me more himself than man can do...day and night I groan and languish under God's just afflicting hand...As waves follow waves in the tempestuous seas,

[171] *Ibid.*, part 1, p. 83.
[172] *Ibid.*, part 1, pp. 82–3.   [173] *Ibid.*, part 1, p. 83.

so one pain and danger followed another, in this sinful miserable flesh: I die daily, yet remain alive: God in his great mercy, knowing my dulness in health and ease, doth make it much easier to repent and hate my sin and loath myself, and contemn the world, and submit to the sentence of death with willingness than otherwise it was ever like to have been. O how little is it that wrathful enemies can do against us, in comparison to what our sin, and the justice of God can do? And O how little is it that the best and kindest of friends can do, for a pained body, or a guilty sinful soul, in comparison of one gracious look or word from God. Woe be to him that hath no better help than man! And blessed is he whose help and hope is in the Lord.[174]

Here illness was put into a framework where the secular is excluded in favour of the divine. Illness is merely one of the providential instruments or signs of God, used as part of a communication with his own, which was far more intimate and effective than any human relationship. The afflictions of Lowe, Josselin and Newcombe were all part of this communion between God and man.

Yet, the language was notoriously ambiguous. Baxter himself pointed this out. At the time of the Great Plague, God's providence upon the whole community was variously interpreted according to particular interests:

Yet under all these Desolations the *wicked* are *hardened*, and cast all on the fanaticks: and the true dividing fanaticks and sectaries are not yet humbled for former miscarriages, but cast all on the *prelates* and imposers: And the ignorant vulgar are stupid, and know not what use to make of anything they feel: But thousands of the sober, faithful servants of the lord, are mourning in secret...From *London* it is spread through many counties, especially next London. Where few places, especially corporations are free: which makes me oft groan and wish, LONDON AND ALL THE CORPORATIONS OF *ENGLAND* WOULD REVIEW THE CORPORATION ACT AND THEIR OWN ACTS AND SPEEDILY REPENT.[175]

If it was easy to interpret the cause of plague to suit one's own prejudices, it was also convenient to have a nosebleed at a particular time. Much of Baxter's autobiography was a justification for his Nonconformist stance, though he was at pains to stress that he was against Charles I's execution and in favour of a monarchy. Baxter had been chaplain to the Parliamentary Army and when it seemed that it would move decisively against the King he tried to stop it. But providential nosebleed came in the way and excused him from taking any further action:

[174] *Ibid.*, part 3, p. 192.　　　　[175] *Ibid.*, part 2, p. 448.

I came to our Major Swallow's quarters at Sir John Cook's house...in a cold and snowy season, and the cold, together with other things coincident, set my nose on bleeding. When I had bled about a quart or two, I opened four veins, but, it did not good. I used divers of other remedies for several days to little purpose; at last I gave myself a purge which stopt it. This so much weakened me and altered my complexion, that my acquaintance who came to visit me scarce knew me. Coming after so long weakness, and frequent loss of blood before, it made the physicians conclude me deplorate after it was stopped; supposing I would never escape a dropsy.

And thus God unavoidably prevented all the effect of my purposes in my last and chiefest opposition to the Army; and took me off the very time when my attempt should have begun...But the determination of God against it was most observable: For the very time I was bleeding the Council of War sate at Nottingham, where (as I have credibly heard) they first began to open their purposes and act their part...And as I perceived it was the will of God to permit them to go on, so I afterward found this great affliction was a mercy on my self; likely to have had small success in the attempt, but to have lost my life among them in my fury. And thus I was finally separated from the Army.[176]

Thus high politics, providence, physicians and a nosebleed all came to be mixed together.

There is much else in Baxter's autobiography to interest the historian: his view that God made use of sickness to acquire converts, his observation that the 'Religiouser sort' were protected from the plague until they boasted of it, and his use of a Gold Bullet for 'a case like mine' would all provide evidence of the multifaceted face of illness in this period.[177]

P.S. In 1766 and up until 1830 the stone from Baxter's bladder was in the British Museum at Montague House.[178]

This essay is part of a larger study of health and illness in seventeenth century England. I would like to thank Roy Porter and George Yule for their advice and help.

[176] *Ibid.*, part 1, pp. 58–9.
[177] *Ibid.*, part 1, p. 90; part 3, p. 1; part 1, p. 81.
[178] G. F. Nuttall, *Richard Baxter*, p. 42.

VII

Medical Ethics in
Early Modern England

Early modern England had no codified medical ethics, there was no *Handbook of Medical Ethics* of the type that the British Medical Association publishes nowadays. Instead, there was available a body of Hippocratic writings, for instance the *Oath, Decorum,* the *Law,* which described how a doctor should behave both with the patient and with other doctors (the two bases of much of modern medical ethics) and which was often cited in the early modern period. Other more general ethical value systems also influenced medicine.

Christianity was a major influence, as was Aristotelian ethics which formed a general context for the Hippocratic texts familiar to early modern physicians. In a sense, what we have here is ethics in medicine, whilst medical ethics can be found in the Hippocratic and Galenic texts which refer to specific norms of conduct as they relate to the details of medical practice. The distinction is, however, one that would not have been recognized in the sixteenth or seventeenth centuries.

Ethics were used in early modern medicine by competing groups of practitioners to argue for the rightness of their practice and the wrongness of that of their opponents. Ethics formed part of the epistemological, economic, political and legal weapons that were employed by the competing factions in English medicine at this time. The context for medical ethics was, therefore, assertive rather than deliberative. The polemical writings of the learned, university-educated physicians and those of their competitors indicate how ethics were put to work in the struggles of a medical market-place largely unregulated by law, and this is the focus of the chapter. However, the fact that ethics were put to such use should not lead to the inference that they were not strongly believed in. It is too often the case that historians diminish the force of people's beliefs whilst placing such beliefs into larger economic and social frameworks, and I do not wish to do so. The two opposing sets of ethics, one based on the classical tradition, the other on Christianity, which I will be discussing in this chapter represent two strands of thought and of belief which were central to the culture of the sixteenth and seventeenth centuries. It is difficult to overestimate their force and reality.

Tradition and the Good and Learned Physician

The learned physicians, who had invested time and money being taught the medicine of Hippocrates, Galen and other classical writers in Latin, if not in Greek, naturally based their medical ethics on classical sources. There were not many of them in sixteenth century England and they often give the impression in their writings of feeling beleaguered and surrounded by competitors. The founding of the College of Physicians of London in 1518 gave them an institutional home and also some authority, for the college regulated the practice of physic (internal medicine) in London and seven miles round it by issuing licenses to practise, by prosecuting unlicensed practitioners and by punishing instances of dangerous practice. The College could also supervise the activities of apothecaries and surgeons. At a formal level, therefore, the learned physicians were at the top of the medical ladder in status and authority. However, in practical terms all this was precarious. The College was limited geographically (it was founded on the model of the college of physicians in Italian cities), its powers of supervising and prosecuting irregular practice in London were never very effective and over time these became more and more diluted till by the beginning of the eighteenth century they had become practically non-existent.[1] In reality, the learned physician was faced with effective competition from a wide variety of sources. Illness was often treated by other members of the family: mothers and wives undertook to cure and care for the most serious of illnesses. Informal medical care was available from neighbours, clergymen and their wives and the charitable ladies who treated the sick poor. Wise men and women, empirics, uroscopists, astrologers, herbalists and others provided cheaper medical treatments than did the learned physicians.[2] In such a context of a largely unregulated medical market-place and with different views of what constitutes medical knowledge it is not surprising to find ethics being used to justify one group or another.

The learned physicians were mostly concentrated in London,

Medical Ethics in Early Modern England

their clientele was relatively prosperous, yet they still felt threatened by competition. Their attacks on their competitors were fuelled by the knowledge that the rich (and even royalty), as well as the poor, patronized empirics. They were united by a shared medical education based on Hippocratic and Galenic writings which defined the good physician and in which, especially in the latter, there was a constant criticism of empirics and empirical medicine. Not surprisingly, therefore, the classical traditions, until at least the later seventeenth century, were used by the learned physicians to define the ethical behaviour of a physician at the bedside and to characterize the bad practitioner. John Securis' *A Detection and Querisome of the Daily Enormities and Abuses Committed in Physic* (1566) provides a typical example. A close examination of its contents illustrates how, in a very rennaisance manner, ancient opinions and injunctions were made relevant to contemporary concerns and provided an ethical value system.

Securis was an orthodox physician concerned with upholding the position of learned medicine. He practised in Salisbury and had been a pupil in Paris of Sylvius, the ultra-conservative physician and anatomist. Securis began his book by describing the good ethical, physician, he repeated the *Oath*, and enumerated the evils of unlearned medicine. His aim was a reformation of medicine, and he appealed in support of this to the Hippocratic principle of doing no harm to the sick and to the related one of achieving monopoly in the profession (i.e. only the doctors who do no harm should be allowed to practise). Securis asked:

> What doth it prevaile for us that be lerned to procede (as I saide) in any degree of maister, of bacheler, or doctor, and so to be allowed and have authoritie to use our science? When every man, woman, and chyld that lyst, may practice and use phisicke *(idque impune)* as well as we? And so, many tymes not only hinder and defraud us of our lawfull stipende and gaynes: but (which is worst of all and to much to be lamented) shall put many in hasarde of their lyfe, yea and it be the destruction of many. Is this tolerable? Will the magistrates alwayes wynke at this? Shall there never be no reformation for suche abuses? God of his great mercy graunt that ones they may be reformed. For if they be not, verily it wyll greatly discourage men of learnying hereafter to apply them selves to the studye of Physyke, whereby the healpe, succour and safegard of many of sick man, woman, and chylde shall be hyndered and secluded....'

A way of highlighting abuses in medicine was to present as a contrast a composite picture of the good physician and his good practice. Securis wrote 'before I speake of ye abuses and enormities of phisike, I wil shew and declare first, what is the part office and condition of a good Phisition.'[4] Securis gave in Latin and English the central part of the *Oath* which directed and confined the actions of the physician to a virtuous path. He then went on to cite the *Law*, which, in a fashion to be echoed by Aristotle and Galen, had emphasized that a long period of study in medicine constituted an ethical requirement for the proper practice of medicine.

> Who soever saith, he wyl truly get him the knowledge of phisicke, he must satisfie his mynd, and as it were be accompanied with these guides, with nature, science, a place mete and convenient for study and learning, an institution from childhood, a labor and peinful diligence with a long time.[5]

A look at the beginning of the text of the *Law* shows why it was still relevant. Securis, who saw all around him empirics, mountebanks and quacks making money, and who deplored the government's weak and limited laws against them, must have identified with the situation described in the *Law*:

> Although the art of healing is the most noble of all the arts, because of the ignorance both of its professors and of their rash critics, it has at this time fallen into the least repute of them all. The chief cause of this seems to me to be that it is the only science of which states have laid down no penalties for malpractice. Ill repute is the only punishment and this does little harm to the quacks who are compounded of nothing else. For a man to be truly suited to the practice of medicine, he must be possessed of a natural disposition for it, the necessary instruction, favourable circumstances, education, industry and time. The first requisite is a natural disposition, for a reluctant student renders every effort in vain. But instruction in the science is easy when the student follows a natural bent, so long as care is taken from childhood to keep him in circumstances favourable to learning and his early education has been suitable. Prolonged industry on the part of the student is necessary ...[6]

Securis cited other Hippocratic works which defined the body and the character of the doctor, from *The Physician* he learned that 'the physician must be of a good coloure and comely countenance and of a good disposition of the body: he muste also be had in estimation among the common people, by commonly apparell and by swete savours [smells] (so that he be not suspected of to much excesse) for by suche meanes the pacientes are wont to be delited.'[7]

This was no antiquarian copying of ancient texts. The charter of Charles I to the Barber-Surgeons stated that 'no such apprentice

Medical Ethics in Early Modern England

[wanting to enter into apprenticeship] be decrepid, deformed' as well as 'or have any corrupt or pestilential disease.'[8] Many of the classical qualities required of the physician had force in Securis' time, and perhaps they still do.

What Securis did was to bring together into one place many different passages from Hippocrates and Galen which originally dealt with different aspects of medical ethics. As well as purity in mind and acts (the *Oath*), study and learning (the *Law*) Securis adds the character of a doctor. He must have 'a modest and sobre mynde', be not only modest in his talk 'but also in other things concerning his behaviour, he must be wel disposed: for there is nothyng that getteth a man better estimation and authoritie than to bee endued with an honest lyfe and good manners.' The need for reputation, *doxa*, for getting trade, in the end joined both physicians and empirics, and medical ethics could be useful in achieving it. Securis added that the physician's 'countenance must be lyke one that is given to studye and sadde'[9] (cf. the Act of 1522: 'That no person ... be suffered to exercise and practise physic, but only these persons that be profound, sad and discreet, groundedly learned and deeply studied in physic'[10] – note the coupling of moral character with deep knowledge, which had Platonic and Aristotelian origins, and served to place classical learning in the renaissance in an ethical framework.) But the physician should not over-do this, for he could 'be taken to be stubborn and scornful', yet he should not always be laughing for then he 'is taken for a lewde person'.[11] Reputation was all. Securis repeated the advice of *On Decorum* on how the doctor should be gentle and courteous, brightly consoling yet firm with the patient at the bedside,[12] (advice to be repeated by John Gregory two centuries later, and indicating not only a long-lasting and common appreciation of how a scholar and a gentleman should behave, but also that the conjunction of manners with medical ethics was not present in the eighteenth century alone).[13]

Ethical injunctions also helped to convey some of the tricks of the trade. The physician should not 'minishe his gravitie, for unlesse the paciente have in reverence and estimation his phisicion as a god, he shall never follow and obey his councell'.[14] The monopolistic aspirations of orthodox learned medicine were put at risk by internal competition and advertising, and Securis advised fellow physicians not to do down fellow physicians:

> They be so covetous that they would have all, and do al them selfe, and they, have envy many tymes at other honest men having cures, when they have none. Thys doinge verelye they bringe them selves

Medical Ethics in Early Modern England

in greate contempte, and dothe as it were abate and blemishe the
honorable science of phisicke, which requireth rather to be sought,
earnestly with great sute, with humilitie, reverence and prayinge,
then to be offered, and as it were objected undiscretely to every
man, and in every place, lyke a blinde harpers songe or a Pedlars
packe. The common proverbe saith, that offered service stynketh.[15]

Securis easily mixed traditional medical ethics with contemporary
concerns, the classical past was still relevant to the present. The
Northampton physician John Cotta also believed this. A
conservative Galenist physician, perhaps a Puritan, Cotta relied
largely on learning and study in the universities, as Harold Cook has
pointed out, to distinguish a physician from an empiric,[16] though
when describing 'The True Artist' [the good physician] Cotta also
stressed the need for the physician to gain experience and to know
nature for 'Without the knowledge of nature our life is death, our
sight blind, our light darknese, and all our waies uncertaine'.[17] In his
*A Short Discoverie of the Unobserved Dangers of Severall Sorts of
Ignorant and Unconsiderate Practisers of Physicke in England* (1612),
Cotta stated that he would not describe 'vertue' as it was 'beside my
promised performance'.[18] Rather, he stressed the need for learning,
industry and past authority ('precept'),[19] and from Galen he took his
model of the best physician, the man who was rational, who
combined reason with experience over a long period of study. In this,
Cotta, in effect, does come near to 'vertue' for, as Aristotle wrote at
the beginning of the second book of the *Nicomachean Ethics,* virtue is
acquired by habit over time by a process of learning and is not innate
– at this most general level there is a shared process for becoming
virtuous and for becoming a good doctor hence Galen's equation of
the two.[20] For my purposes Cotta's book is significant not only for its
reiteration of the traditional values that identified the learned
physicians and the empiric with regard to medical knowledge, but
for its stress on the dangers in medical practice. It is this thread that I
want to follow, and I shall consider what kind of ethical issues
relating to practice troubled medical writers. Tradition provided a
framework with which to categorize empirics, and given Galen's
analysis of the poverty of experience in medical practice, it supplied
the dialectical ammunition with which to shoot them down. It also
provided a picture of the ideal physician that was suited to the world
of the virtuous, scholarly, middling and respectable physician. But
there was more to medical ethics than a restoration of tradition.

Medical Ethics in Early Modern England

Danger, Choosing a Doctor and Reputation

At the end of the seventeenth century a call for medical reform, that echoed some of the earlier sentiments of the learned physicians, came from Hugh Chamberlen, the royal accoucher, the empiric fined by the College of Physicians, the member of the family famous for its use of the forceps and the projector of such schemes as a land bank – a typical larger than life entrepreneur of the long eighteenth century. In his *A Few Queries Relating to the Practice of Physick* (1694) before setting out his scheme for a rate-supported medical service, he asked:

> Whether the Practice of Physick doth not very much want a just and due Regulation, and is not capable of great improvements for the benefit of Mankind? And whether it doth not well deserve such Reformation, since it concerns Life and Health, the dearest earthly injoyments?

More specifically Chamberlen asked:

> Whether there can be contrived (if the Government please) any just and proper Test or Standard whereby to try the several Abilities of Physicians much more truly and certainly than any we have at present?

He replied:

> This were at least to be wisht, if there were no hopes to reduce it to practice, for not to know how to distinguish the skilful Physicians from the ignorant is next to having none.[21]

Here is one of the main reasons why ethics became involved in the very definition of good medical practice and runs so strongly, though sometimes hidden away, in the writings of opposing medical practitioners. Without a system of medical licensing that applied to the whole country or which had general public support and recognition, the qualities that made a good physician became a matter for debate and analysis. The definition might for some groups include elements which today we can easily recognize as ethical such as the charitable physician which I discuss later.

Other aspects of what made a good doctor are less easily fitted into our ideas of what constitutes ethics in medicine or medical ethics. For instance, the actual procedures used by doctors could indicate if one was a good doctor who cured, or a bad one that harmed the patient. This mix of the moral and the technical, of character and skill, was characteristic in early modern medicine and

VII

Medical Ethics in Early Modern England

is one that, except for extreme cases, we find difficult today to recognize as subject matter for medical ethics. Obviously total ignorance or gross negligence come within malpractice and modern medical ethics. But in early modern England normal medical practice (which today is a defence in English malpractice suits) could be labelled bad, dangerous and hence unethical. The good doctor, therefore, was defined by the type as well as the extent of his technical knowledge together with his moral behaviour, as indeed Galen had written centuries before. This occured in a context in which there was no general consensus amongst the different groups in the medical market-place on what was normal medical knowledge and practice. The imputation of danger and harm could be placed on any medical practice, so that potentially all medical actions might be problematical and fall within the ambit of medical ethics. The issue was how to defend one's own practice, how to convince patients that it was safe and how to prove that the practices of one's opponents were dangerous. Rhetoric, advertising, and denigration became mixed with medical ethics.

The learned physician advertised his superior skill by stressing the lengthy and individualized treatment (and preventive care by means of regimen) he offered: how he judged the individual's constitution, how he recognized the cause of the illness, how he achieved a fine fit between the patient, the disease and the remedies and how he took into account the day-to-day progress of the patient. Eleazar Dunk in 1606 wrote of this personalised treatment:

First the learned Physician is to search out the proper signes of this disease, and by them to distinguish it from others that hath some affinity with it: then he looketh into the cause of it ... he examineth the naturall constitution of the patient, his present state of body, his former course of life, his age, his strength, the time of the disease, the season of the yeere etc he considereth the qualities and quantity of the humors; from whence the matter of the disease floweth ... by what passages it moveth, whether swiftly, or slowly ... Out of an advised consideration of all these, first a diet is to be appointed: this cannot be the same in every one that laboureth of this sicknesse, but it requireth great variety and alteration agreeable to the foresaid circumstances. Then followeth the consultation of the meanes of the cure: what kinde of evacuation is fittest, whether opening a veine ...

Without the method and the judgement of the physician danger lurked:

In the great variety of these doubts, difficulties and distinctions

105

Medical Ethics in Early Modern England

there is a necessary use of sound judgement, confirmed by long study and profound knowledge both in philosophy and Physicke. It is therefore cleere that the practise of Empiriks, being destitute of these helps, must needs be unfit and full of perill.[22]

The practitioners of this type of medicine, men like John Cotta, James Hart, James Primrose,[23] considered it, like Galen before them, the best and safest type of medicine (hence ethically the best). Yet the population did not always agree. As I have argued elsewhere there was a great deal of similarity between learned physicians and empirics, for instance, both in the end gave medicines and applied procedures.[24] The learned physicians realized that some members of the public believed that the empirics were more successful. One might be sure of the virtue of one's own particular form of medical knowledge and practice, but was the outside world so convinced? Reputation was all. In their analysis of why the world was not always convinced, the learned physicians used ethical arguements to attack the behaviour of patients, and the way they were influenced by the people around the bedside.

Cotta deplored how people chose their doctors:

It is strange to observe how few in these dayes know, and how none almost labour to know with election and according to reason, or reasonable likelihood, to bestow in cases of their lives the trust and care of their crazed healths, but for the most part wanting a right notice of a iudicious choice, take counsel of common report which is a common lier or of private commendations which are ever partiall. The unmindfulnesse hereof, and the more minde of mindlesse things, do steale from men the minds of men.[25]

The arrogant, yet whining, complaint that the patients did not automatically realize that rational, learned, medicine was best permeates the writings of the rational physicians. If medicine needed to be reformed of its unethical practitioners, the empirics, there was also a need to reform the patient (the two were frequently seen as conspiring together). The ethical righteousness of the physician can only be real in a practical sense if recognized to be so by the patient. Yet the moral and intellectual superiority assumed by the learned physicians made a denigrating attitude to the public almost inevitable. Richard Whitlock in his *Zωotomia. Or Observations on the Present Manners of the English* (1654) took the part of the learned physicians and wrote 'the people love to be cheated'. He listed their sins: being influenced by the novelties and boasts of their practitioners, trusting the judgement of incompetents

Medical Ethics in Early Modern England

when choosing a practitioner, being impressed by a pseudo-skill in diagnosis, not realizing that the accidental success of an empiric is no guarantee that it will happen again – it is 'no more a rule for curing the same againe ... then one Swallow bringeth a Summer', and the physician 'is the last or late sent for' and unjustly gets blamed for failure. Whitlock also blamed patients for refusing to take the physician's treatment and substituting their own, or that of their neighbours' 'kitchen Physick'[26]. Without the patient's obedience the physician's honourable success could not come about:

Sicknesse posteth to us, but crawleth from us: happy it were for Patients, honourable for physitians successe of their labours, if men would but truly deserve the name of Patients, when sicknesse is on them, if they would take counsell timely, and obey it patiently.[27]

If patients did not choose rightly, if they did not obey, then much of the failure of learned medical practice was explained: 'To conclude, through the default of Physitians, the Theory of Physick is for the most part Conjecture, or Controversie, through the default of Patients, the practise is but Lottery.'[28]

The bedside was a place which could make or break a physician's reputation. Here women were especially blamed, for as well as having no authority to practise medicine themselves, they also threw doubt on the physician's practice. Cotta wrote:

Here therefore are men warned of advising with women counsellors. We cannot but acknowledge and with honor mention the graces of womanhood, wherein by their destined property, they are right and true soveraignes of affection; but yet, seeing their authority in learned knowledge cannot be authenticall, neither hath God and nature made them commissioners in the sessions of learned reason and understanding (without which in cases of life and death, there ought to be no daring or attempt at all).... We may justly here taxe their dangerous whisperings about the sicke, wherein their prevalence oft being too great, they abuse the weake sense of the diseased, while they are not themselves; and make just and wise proceedings suspected, and with danger suspended. For it is not sufficient for the Physition to do his office, except both the sicke himselfe, and also all that are about him be prudently and advisedly carefull unto good reason: without which love it selfe may be dangerously officious, the error of friendship a deed unto death....[29]

Both patients and onlookers in early modern England acted at times as practitioners and were, in a sense, like the empirics, rivals of learned practitioners and could be accused like them, of doing harm. There is clearly an ethical dimension in Cotta's diatribe against women. He details acts made morally suspect: 'they abuse the weake sense of the diseased', the contrast with 'just and wise proceedings' and the result of 'danger', and 'death' (though the honour of the physician and of his office lies just below the surface in all this). The breaking of moral and technical norms leading to harm to the patient epitomizes medical ethics. Moreover, the sense of this being medical ethics is reinforced when we remember that what is going on here is an attempt at exclusivity in medical practice.

In defence of a doctor's reputation very general ethical norms or prejudices were also brought into play. The assumed superiority of men over women in matters of medicine was supplemented by references to the bad practices of the common people. Cotta warned in a tone reminiscent of that to be found in Elizabethan and Jacobean government references to the dangerous mass of the poor:

> Oft and much babbling inculcation in the weake braines of the sicke may easily prevaile with them, to forget both that which their owne good hath taught them, and also by a borrowed opinion from others indiscrete words, to corrupt their owne sense. It is the common custome of most common people thus ordinarily to molest and trouble the sicke. Their presense therefore is dangerous and carefully to be either prohibited or better governed. Common and vulgar mouthes easily incline scandalously to prejudice the things they know not.[30]

The mixture of superiority and underlying defensiveness lay at the heart of the defence of learned medicine. The art was not to be blamed, others were:

> Hence it is in thes daies a customary worke to disswade physicke, while men not making right choice of their Physition, or perverting good counsell by their owne peevish frowardnes, and thereby multiplying unto themselves continuall occasion of complaint, unjustly therefore accuse art, which they never duly sought, nor found, nor used, and therefore never know. The offences that men justly take, are the faults, the blots, the staines of unperfect workemen, not of art; whereof art is as guiltlesse as they are void of art.[31]

Wrong judgement, lack of reason and restraint, imperfect know-ledge, all these accusations expressed in the emotive terms of social superiority of the early seventeenth century, bear some analogy with classical Aristotelian ethics that was part of the university education shared by the physicians. The choice of actions define the just man, so also in the case of medicine. The emphasis is on the individual rather than on the out-reaching relationship of the individual to society as in Christianity or on the parts of society as in utilitarianism. As Aristotle wrote in Book five of the *Nicomachean Ethics:* 'but how actions must be done and distributions effected in order to be just, to know this is a greater achievement than knowing what is good for the health; though even there, while it is easy to know that honey, wine, hellebore, cautery and the use of the knife are so, to know how, to whom, is no less an achievement than that of being a physician.'[32] In constrast to the more social values of Christianity as applied to medicine (discussed below), the learned physicians were, I feel, most at home with the Aristotelian ethical position that focused on the right actions of the individual qua individual as judged against 'justice' or in the case of the learned physicians 'the art'.

At a time when patients could easily dismiss their physicians, and when they had a wide choice of different types of practioner, the learned physicians were not in a position to persuade patients to accept painful or uncomfortable treatments through the authority conferred by a monopoly or quasi monopoly of practice, backed up by legislation. The patient's personal preferences and dislike of unpleasant procedures could be translated into dismissal of the learned physicians. The right actions in relation to the art might be subverted by the promise of more pleasant treatments than those offered by the physicians. Cotta wrote of how 'many ignorants may speake faire and pleasing and commend things that look smooth and smiling upon the liking of the sicke' and how it is usual for 'many unskilfull busie-bodies under colour and pretext of gentle and safe dealing, to make familiar and ordinary the use of perileous medicines.'[33] Clearly medicine could appear harmful and painful, and this view was held throughout the seventeenth century. Chamberlen referred to it when he asked whether "tis better for a Physician to be a knave and increase his Practice by humouring the Fools and letting them die their own way; or to be honest and lessen his practice in saving them with methods displeasing, because really there are no other can help them.'[34]

Again he asked:

> Whether 'tis not safer for a Doctor to let his Patients die their own way with a gentle wrong Method, than to endeavour to help them with a rough right one, and to miss?

He replied:

> 'tis very probable it is, for the gentle method displeaseth none, and

the Doctor, though he never endeavoured to save the Patient, still continues his Interest and Credit in the Family, because the Patient and Friends believe he did, not being able to judge; but on the other hand the Doctor, that endeavours to save, and misses, shall be esteemed a murtherer, because of the seeming violent medicines used and be discarded and hated, though he used the best skill then known to save the Patient.[35]

Normal clinical practice today is largely out of the net of medical ethics. One reason is that clinical trials and statistical analysis decide in the end on whether and to what extent a remedy or technique is safe or effective (though there may be a wider ethical dimension, for instance, in the case of embryo implantation, or in the allocation of resources that goes beyond the mere question of safety). Moreover, there are legal procedures such as inquests or civil cases for malpractice which can decide how far a medical practitioner has gone beyond the normal and the accepted. In the early modern period such legal methods of discovery were largely ineffective or not used.[36] In his time as Cotta put it, the medical errors of the ignorant (and, one could add, of the learned) were 'for want of knowledge unespied, or by the privacy smothered. For if they kill, a dead man telleth no tales: or if by chance they save one life, that shall be a perpetuall flag to call more fooles to the same adventure.' Instead of being able to use the modern advertising power of science other means such as word of mouth recommendation had to be employed for gaining credit in one's practice. Living almost a century later Chamberlen was able to look forward in a Baconian fashion to 'a true History of Cures' which would register the outcome of cures.[37] Failing such a method (and even that is neither 'objective' *per se*, nor avoids all debate), a practitioner's reputation was at the mercy of the public, and ethical values were employed in attacking or defending it.

Christian Charity and Dangerous Remedies

Christianity provided medicine with a different set of ethical values. The ethics of the classical world had largely been individualistic rather than social and were often devoid of charity and of altruism in relation to the care of the sick (though as Vivian Nutton points out in this volume Galen did encourage the physician to be philanthropic). However, the care of the sick was one of the six works of charity of the early Church, and Christianity, which had ever before it the example of Christ healing the sick, the lame and the blind, emphasized the value of giving care both at an institutional level (in monasteries, and then in church-run hospitals) and at the personal level of providing for the poor and needy sick. Although the Protestant Reformation cast doubt on the efficacy of good works for getting to Heaven, charity and the duty of neighbours to look after each other was still emphasized by radical Protestants. The opponents of the learned physicians used such Christian values to attack the ethical basis of their practice.

Their attacks had added point, because Christian ethics were largely absent from the writings of the learned physicians and, at least until 1660, this was a time when Christian belief was extremely important for society at large. The sources for the ethics of the learned physicians were largely classical and founded on the need for both learning and exclusive practice and on the rectitude of a person's actions in relation to the art. If God was mentioned it was often in terms of natural theology and the study of God's workmanship rather than the social ethic of charity.[38]

Christian ethics were also used to support new medical doctrines and practices, and to attack those of the learned physicians. In 1585 Richard Bostocke published one of the earliest English Paracelsian works. In the title of his book he emphasized the heathen and unchristian origins of classical learned medicine: *The Difference Between the Auncient Phisicke, First Taught by the Godly Forefathers, Consisting in Unitie, Peace and Concord; and the Latter Phisicke Proceeding from Idolaters, Ethnickes and Heathens; As Galen, and Such Other Consisting in Dualitie, Discorde and Contrarite. And Wherein the Naturall Philosophie of Aristotle Doth Differ from the Trueth of Gods Worde, and is Iniurious to Christianitie and Sound Doctrine.* Bostocke pointed out that not only was Greek medicine and philosophy unchristian in doctrine, it was also unchristian ethically in that it lacked charity. He wrote that if the Galenists would no longer be under the 'Wings and protection of Princes, Privilidges and Charters', then 'the Chymicall doctrine agreeing with Gods worde, experience, and nature may come into the Scholes and Cities in stede of Aristotle, Gallen, and other heathen' and people could decide if 'Galen and other heathen or the Chimests were most to be followed and allowed. And whose writings and travailes were more available for mans health, either conserving or restoring, and who seeketh more paynefully, faythfully, sincerely, charitably and Christianlike for the certein helpe of his neighbour, and not for lucre or veine glory and pompe, the auncient Chemical Phisition or Gallen and his followers.'[39]

The Christian ethical values of helping one's neighbour and

Medical Ethics in Early Modern England

giving charitable care were powerful. Despite the Reformation and the consequent breakdown in England of church-organized charitable care for the poor and sick poor, the feeling that one ought to help one's neighbour in adversity remained. Alan Macfarlane has shown that many witchcraft accusations were made because the accused felt guilty that he or she had not provided charitable help to the person subsequently accused of witchcraft (their reasoning was that the person who had asked for charity then bewitched them out of a sense of revenge or spite). Bequests to the poor, and donations to the parish poor box continued despite the creation of the secular poor law system based on the parish rates.[40] At the time of the Civil War, the importance of Christian charity as a major social value was emphasized even more. As Charles Webster has pointed out, various reformers of medicine of the 1640s and 1650s wished to have a medical care service that would encompass all the country or at least would provide medical treatment for the poor[41] (though parishes were already paying for the medical treatment of the sick poor).[42] A sense of charity underlay such proposals and this is reflected in the choice by Gabriel Plattes, in his utopian *Macaria* (1641), of ministers as providers of such care – for they would be embued with charity rather than profit.

At various levels, then, Christianity, the most potent belief system of the early modern period, whose influence extended from politics down to the details of the household economy, was used to attack orthodox medicine for being based on pagan learning and values (though, of course, for many Christians the medieval assimilation of classical knowledge into Christianity had got rid of the contradictions that were being pointed out). Greed was seen as especially unchristian and, as Luis García-Ballester has shown in an earlier chapter, it was a quality associated from the Middle Ages with the learned physician. The learned surgeon, William Clowes, advised in 1579 the young surgeon not to be greedy: 'not too covetous for mony, but a reasonable demaunder/Being good unto the poore, let the rich pay therefore.'

Nicholas Culpeper, in the mid-seventeenth century complained that physicians would not come 'to a poor mans house who is not able to give them their fee ... and the poor Creature for whom Christ died must forfeit his life for want of money'.[43] Culpeper, who was one of the most prolific writers of popular medical books, had fought on Parliament's side in the Civil War and he integrated his religion into his medicine. It supplied the ethics for his medicine. Culpeper also contrasted the cheapness of his native God-given remedies, appropriate to the means of the poor, with the expensive and often exotic remedies of the Galenic physicians.⁴⁴ Charity, alternative medicines and care for the poor were opposed to expensive, fleecing, physicians. Securis had revealingly quoted the saying 'that phisicke unles it be earnestly sought and well payde for, it will never prosper nor worke well with the pacientes.' He quickly added that he did not mean that physicians should not 'be alwayes liberall and mercifull to the poore, on whom his living dependeth not but on the rich'.⁴⁵ The many books on remedies for the poor, with their references to charitable physicians and their self-help approach carried the implied accusation against orthodox physicians of avarice and of a lack of charity. 'J.E.' wrote in support of Robert Pemel's ΠΤΩΧΟΦΑΡΜΑΚΟΝ or *Help for the Poor* (1653):

> What Herbs, Flowers, Min'rals,
> Trees the earth doth bear
> For men his use and help, prepared are:
> Intended them unto poor peoples good;
> As well as of rich Lords, and Ladies, Gent.
> Poor people in pain meet help and ease do want;
> But oh the love of gold and sordid gain,
> That doth the Lords rich bounty much restrain!
> Let a rich man lie sick, or pained be,
> Upon his least request, to him doth flee
> The Physick Doctor, or the Surgeon
> Their Soveraigne Medicines them to try upon;
> And him to cure, the love of rich reward,
> Which there he hopes, makes him the rich regard:
> But let the poor, sick or diseased lie,
> Let him send for them, let him call and cry,
> They are as deaf as Baal to his Priests;
> He hath no gold to grease them in their fists
> Loe here a pitiful Samaritan,
> That taking care for the poor needy man,
> Doth him provide of easie medicines
> Which nor are costly, nor are hard to finde;
> So his own Doctor in need he may be,
> Without the care of any Doctors fee....⁴⁶

The learned physicians did not directly reply to the age-old accusation of greed and of a lack of charity but Cotta and others like him did realize that religion threatened their attempts at monopoly: God had given the gift of healing to the apostles, and this posed the possibility that it could be acquired without learning and application, especially by clergymen (as descendents of the apostles) or by wise-women and others as a 'natural' talent (on the latter see below). The learned physicians reiterated Calvin's claim that the age of miracles was past and that God's ministers could not heal miraculously any more. Cotta also cited Calvin's doctrine on keeping to one's calling as forbidding 'pastor physicians' and he pointed to the dangers to patients of ministers being called away from caring for them by the duties of their other calling.[47] The Calvinist concern with public order was congenial to the physicians. Cotta opposed charity with the imperative of one's calling, and contrasted private acts of charity with the public policy of the commonwealth (a very conservative and typically Calvinist position).

> It is indeed a deed of mercie to save and helpe the sicke, and a worke of charitie to advise them for their health and ease: but the common good and public weale and the law for both inhibit the doing of every good by every man, and both doth limit and refraine it unto some speciall and select sort of men, for necessary causes, and respects unto good government and policie, and for avoiding confusion which is the ruine of publicke weales. Shal then Divinitie teach and allow for private deeds, ends and respects of charitie and mercie, to break publicke edicts, to trangress lawes, to condemme magistracie, to confound and disturbe good order?[48]

Richard Whitlock also wrote in support of learned medicine and opposed the Christian ideal of charity and of helping the poor that motivated 'Shee-Doctors' with the effectiveness of orthodox medicine:

> The Physick of Almes I allow them, but am out of charity with their Almes of Physick (by their owne hands:) with the former they may feed Christians, but with the latter they too often with Christians feed the Wormes; Or if they would be charitable in this way, let them pay for the Physick of the poor, the noblest way of giving Physick, and will have its Fee from Heaven.[49]

However, in the later seventeenth century the feeling that the regular physicians lacked Christian charity did touch a nerve and the College of Physicians set up charitable dispensaries. When the apothecaries in the Rose case (1704) accused the physicians of wanting to create a monopoly so that poor people who could not afford a physician's fees would be unable to go to the cheaper apothecary, the physicians replied by pointing to their dispensaries for the poor.

The Christian picture of the 'compassionate physition' not only included charity but also humane, kind medical practice that did not involve dangerous, cruel and painful treatments The

Medical Ethics in Early Modern England

radical Noah Biggs asked Parliament to reform medicine and wrote in his *Mataeotechnia Medicinae Praxeus. The Vanity of the Craft of Physick* (1651):

> ... till the body of Physick [i.e. orthodox Galenic medicine] be changed and reformed there's little hopes that a better sanation of Diseases or a Melioration of the languid condition of men and women will follow then what has been hitherto, and what that has been let the clamours of the Sick, and standers by, the cries of Widows and Orphans and the ocular unsuccessfulness of Physicians in their own practice, decide whether the things that I now move for ... do not groan for a Reformation.[50]

Perhaps the 'unsuccessfulness of Physicians' does not fall within medical ethics, after all we all die. Yet as one reads Biggs' convoluted work it is clear that he was condemning orthodox medicine for malpractice. The nature of medicine, its theories, beliefs and remedies produced illness, diseases could be iatrogenic.

> Oftentimes a man is chain'd to his bed by small disease ... and [the Galenists] only make them rage more by their remedies, when they undertake to expell them.[51]

As well as being disease-making, medicine created death, it experimented recklessly and was tainted with cruelty:

> Speculation, the alone Patron of idleness, and lazinesse, which weakly understood, and violently put in practise, hath made a shambles, rather than a Sanctuary, to butcher men violently and devour and destroy them insensibly, then give ease or succour. For there is nothing more hard, more inhumane and full of Cruelty, among all humane Arts, through so many ages undertaken and usurp'd, then that art, which by a concentrick subscription doth make new experiments by the deaths of men, where the Earth covers the vices, the errors and fraud of its professors.[52]

Biggs used religion as part of his condemnation of the cruelty of learned medicine. He stressed that the erroneous opinions were those of 'Pagans and Infidels' and wrote of the 'ruines, the dangers and dreadful effects, the ignorence, errors, abueses, impieties and cruelties of Physitians.'[53]

The ethical rhetoric of dangerous and tormenting remedies was common currency in the medical market-place and amongst learned physicians. Cotta had also written of:

> Quacsalvers, banckrupt-apothecaries, and fugitive Surgeons every where over-travelling the face of this kingdome ... do sell ... these

Medical Ethics in Early Modern England

generose and noble secrets carrying on the outside the titles of
famous medicines, and being within infamous poysons. And by this
means quicke and desperate experiments, with such as thus like to
gaine them grow vulgar medicaments.[54]

Cotta also mentioned how medicines in the wrong hands could
cause disease. Yet the force of the argument was not equal.
Unorthodox practitioners, often using Christian values, developed
further the view that their remedies were milder and less dangerous
than those of the faculty. William Walwyn, the Leveller, advertised
in his *Physick for Families* (1669) his medicines and their cures. He
presented them as 'Kindly and Powerful' rather than being
'hazardous, painful and dangerous'[55] (he went into detail to show
the danger and pain involved in Galenic practice).[56] Significantly, he
justified his whole enterprise by the Biblical injunction 'to love our
Neighbour as ourselves'[57] and more specifically he argued:

> The Scripture saith, a merry heart doth good like a medicine: And
> if so, in true consequence, ought not the Operations and Effects of
> kindly and real Medicines to resemble those of a merry heart;
> certainly it can be no absurdity to expect it.[58]

Walwyn also stressed that Christianity was above philosophy, it
provided both a moral pattern for the physican and knowledge
hidden from philosophy.

> So I conceive my charitable intentions, sufficiently justified by the
> Text: The truly Christian Vertu of Compassion, being as essentially
> needful in a physitian, as in the most tender hearted Samaritan....
>
> Nor did I decline the common Road of Physick, for any other cause
> Imaginable, but for its manifest uncertainty in Principles,
> Roughness, Harshness, and Cruelty in Methods, Impropriety,
> Impotency, and danger in Medicines. Nor found out any way to
> relieve my understanding, when at first at so great a loss, but by
> withdrawing my thoughts from out the wilderness of all the
> uncertain Notions and Guesses of Philosophy and giving them free
> liberty in the walks of Scripture; where the true Original of men the
> sole subject of Physick (hid from Phylosophy) being apparent....[59]

Christianity was a way for the unorthodox to reject philosophy, the
classical tradition, and it could supply not only the ethical values of
compassion and neighbourliness but also give insight into medicine.
Morality and knowledge were very close together, something which
is also clearly apparent in classical medical ethics. Christianity,
moreover, provided the characteristics for the 'Conscionable

Medical Ethics in Early Modern England

Compassionate Physitians'[60] who Walwyn had in mind as the model of what was best in medicine, and Christianity was used to make orthodox medicine appear unfeeling, that is cruel and barbarous in its remedies, avaricious and uncharitable in its human relations.

Thomas O'Dowde, one of the instigators of a society of chemical physicians which it was hoped would be set up in opposition to the College of Physicians, though in politics O'Dowde was not a political radical having followed the royalist cause, presented himself as a charitable physician in his *The Poor Man's Physitian or the True Art of Medicine* (1665). He used the Christian model of the good physician: '... and rather than not do good for Gods sake, I will traverse all the Streets, Lanes and Alleys of this great and glorious city, to find out the Poor and Necessitous, wanting help and Medicine; and leave the Rich to them'[61] [the Galenists]. The title of his book shows, again, how morality, 'poor man's physician', was related to a particular position on medical knowledge: in this case 'the true art of medicine' lay in O'Dowde's belief in chemical remedies. The morality helps to give credence to the knowledge, in turn the knowledge has ethical value (is not dangerous etc.). It is worth taking a closer look at O'Dowde's work for it exemplifies the way in which morality and medical knowledge and skill came within an ethical framework, though some might feel that his use of Christian ethics arose more from motives of gain than from conviction, and that he used them in order to attract patients.

The title page of his book cited the passage from Mark 5:26 which criticizes medicine for its pain, rapacity and lack of success, rather than the more usual one from Ecclesiasticus 38:1, 'Honour a physician with the honour due unto him, ... for the Lord hath created him'. The passage from Mark reads: 'And had suffered many things of many Physicians, and had spent all that she had, and was nothing bettered, but rather grew worse.'

The Biblical context, the assertion that physicians could make the patient worse, plus the allusion to their rapacity encapsulates the ethical framework that O'Dowde used to justify his own practice. The same combination had occurred when the law at one time opened the door for empirics. The statute of 1542/3, which allowed unlearned practitioners to practise in a limited way, has not been seen as containing ethical statements, but it did:

> the company and fellowship of surgeons of London, minding only
> their lucres, and nothing the profit or ease of the diseased patient,
> have sued, troubled, and vexed divers honest persons, well men as
> women, whom God hath embued with the knowledge of the

Medical Ethics in Early Modern England

nature, kind and operation of certain herbs, roots and waters, and
the using and ministering of them to such as been pained with
customable disease ... the said persons have not taken anything for
their pains or cunning [skill] but have ministered the same to poor
people only for neighbourhood and God's sake, and of pity and
charity. For although the most part of the persons of the said craft
of surgeons have small cunning, yet they will take great sums of
money, and do little therefore, and by reason thereof they do
oftentimes impair and hurt their patients, rather than do them
good; in consideration whereof, and for the ease, comfort, succour,
help, relief, and health of the king's poor subjects inhabitants of
this realm, now pained or diseased, or that hereafter shall be pained
or diseased.

Be it ordained....[62]

From the statute (often dismissed as the 'Quack's Charter') a
picture was drawn of the ethical, good practitioner practising
charitably with God's means and more effectively than the unethical, bad, money-grubbing, monopolistic and harmful surgeons who
would not cure someone unless they were sure to get more than the
cure was worth and 'many rot and perish to death for lack of help
of surgery.'[63] By being labelled harmful the practice of the surgeons
was put into the sphere of ethics, and this was made doubly so by its
association with greed and lack of charity.

To return briefly to O'Dowde. What characterizes the description
of his cases is that they are, like the language of the statute, assertions
of fact and opinion. There is no argument for or against a position;
we are dealing, as in the prescriptions of the *Oath* (and in advertisements), with absolute values and judgements, often expressed in
graphic and violent language. The context was not appropriate for the
deliberative debating of issues of a Warnock Report. The cases did not
give rise to ethical problems but to ethical condemnations.

O'Dowde, like Biggs, referred to the cruelty and barbarism of
the physicians, their experimenting with people's lives and leaving
them for dead when they could be cured. Here are some examples:

Mr Savage, at the Queens Head ... afflicted with violent Convulsive
Fits, and extraordinary Dropsie and Scurvy and past all hopes of
either life or recover, was perfectly cured by me in four days of
Medicine, to his great admiration, after being long the Experiment
of the Galenick Artists.

Mr Garret ... under so prodigious a Dropsie and Scurvy, as after the
Experiment of some able Artists, left as a dying man, not able to

eat, drink, sleep, walk, lie, sit or stand; and thus weary of life and the most dejected of all men, was perfectly cured by me in four days of Medicine, when before assigned a peremptory day to dye in.[64]

Mr Rowley, a Baker ... under a five years Dropsie Lask and Bloody Flux, a Patient, whose story is so remarkable, as to call Angels and men to witness against the barbarous inhumanity of those persons that stile themselves Doctors.

There follows the gruesome story of twin incisions into the scrotum and the division of the foreskin 'to the end', but though left in agony O'Dowde cured him.[65]

O'Dowde continued:

A merchant of good account, (this last Patients Neighbour) and under the like Distemper, method and Doctor, was cured by being sent to his Grave, according to Art and Method [keywords identifying an orthodox Galenist], Cum Privilegis, good Mr Doctor.

In all this, I appeal to all the fair Ladies and good Wives of this Nation, whether the Galenist or the Chymist, is the true Artist and Friend to Nature and Health, that thus restores languishing Nature, and makes it erect, and servicable as ever, or those than thus inhumanely butcher a principal part.[66]

It is not enough to refer only to Christian values of charity (the language of the last quotation is perhaps nearer to advertising than to Christianity) to explain what lies behind these cases. O'Dowde was saying 'my treatments are better, safer, more efficacious than the treatments of my opponents which are deadly, cruel and unsuccessful.' The actual treatment used became an ethical issue. Both the Christian and the Hippocratic doctor agreed that the patient should not be harmed, the disagreement, however, lay in what was good for the patient, and what constituted harm. This was expressed through a mixture of technical medical language and ethical values, the boundaries between the two being, because of the nature of the disagreements, imprecise.

The Law

The involvement of the law in medicine often puts ethical norms onto a formal footing and signifies the presence of the State. Discussion of this and of the law in general provides a further context that helps us to understand the state of play in the relationship between ethics and medicine in early modern Europe.

In post-Reformation England outside legal authority or agencies

Medical Ethics in Early Modern England

did not exist that would decide whether one type of medical practice was ethical or not (they hardly exist today). In a society where the study of canon law had been abolished by Henry VIII, where explicit statute law covered few civil or criminal contingencies, and where the apprehension of criminals was left to the victims of the crime and to lay officials such as the amateur constables and justices of the peace,[67] it was not likely that the law would be involved in any major way with the enforcement of ethical medical practice.

Medical ethics were not codified in law, and the development of English law in the early modern period goes against such a development. Common law, with its piecemeal, precedent approach and its hostility to the codifying tendencies of the continental Roman law tradition, was not the instrument with which to forge a legal-ethical framework for medicine. The ways in which trials were conducted also argued against the creation of such a framework. There was a general lack of expert evidence, (and when it was presented it was not given special status), the jury was still 'of the country' with special knowledge of the local situation, if it was no longer, as in the Middle Ages, composed of neighbours who acted as evidential testators as to the accused, still it had not yet been transformed into the nineteenth-century jury having no prior knowledge of the victim and of the accused and concerned with assessing the objective truth of the evidence.[68] English law at this time was on the whole neither investigative, nor inquisitorial, nor concerned with a scientific approach where juries put aside local knowledge and decided solely in terms of the court room evidence, nor did the law attempt to set down in writing every possible contingency (the latter is still not yet with us in England, but no doubt the influence of European legal-systems as expressed through the Common Market will achieve this). Another way of putting the same point is that it was only in the nineteenth century that the State began to legislate in detail on the activities of its citizens. In the early modern period the English State kept to a hands off policy except on particular areas where its interests were involved as in religion, or where devastating crises such as plague or famine occurred or where it perceived danger to itself as with vagrancy and the poor. The implementation of the law was left to local lay officials or to assize judges travelling on the different circuits around the country. The legal system was simple and largely amateur, and it was usually the judges rather than Parliament who decided how the law was to be developed. It is only in the nineteenth century with, for example, the influence of utilitarianism in penal and welfare matters, that the role

Medical Ethics in Early Modern England

of the Parliamentary legislator becomes dominant. It is, of course, no accident that it was around this time that codified medical ethics were developed, though in England the *laissez-faire* approach was strong enough to keep such ethics on a voluntary basis.

Given this context it is not surprising that we do not find codified medical ethics let alone a code with legal force. What we do have are statutes, sometimes contradictory, which were limited to a local area, London, which gave power of enforcement and of judgement, not to judges and juries at large, but to corporations. Where the common law was involved its tendency was to limit the power of the corporations and also to leave the law on malpractice undeveloped.

In the statutes and charters setting up the College of Physicians, Company of Barber-Surgeons and Society of Apothecaries there was an acceptance of the superiority of the learned physician, a recognition of grades amongst medical practitioners, with the physicians having a supervisory role over the apothecaries, and being able to do surgery. Safeguarding the public was a constant theme. Guarding people from being deceived by empirics and from the dangers of their unskilful practices was often the expressed purpose of the law-makers. The language could have come straight from Securis and Cotta. Nevertheless, as we have seen there was an alternative in law. The Act of 1542/3 expressed a different set of values, emphasizing charity and alternative, non-elite knowledge. That such a body of ethics in medicine, separate from the official, College classical tradition, was recognized by sections of government is confirmed when one looks at the way patrons of empirics sought to prevent the College taking action against them. In 1581 Sir Francis Walsingham, Secretary of State to Elizabeth, interceded 'in favour of one Margaret Kennix an outlandish, ignorant, sorry woman', as Charles Goodall apologist for the College put it. Walsingham wrote:

> Whereas heretofore by her Majesties commandment upon the pityfull complaint of Margaret Kennix I wrote unto Dr Symmondes [the former President of the College] ... signifying how that it was her Highness pleasure that the poore wooman shoold be permitted by you quietly to practise and mynister to the curing of diseases and woundes, by the meanes of certain Simples, in the applieing whereof it seemeth God hath given her an especiall knowledge, to the benefit of the poorer sort, and cheefly for the better maintenance of her impotent husband, and charge of Family, who wholy depend of the exercise of her skill; forasmuch as now I am enformed, she is restrained either by you, or some other of your

Medical Ethics in Early Modern England

> College, contrary to her Majesties pleasure, to practise any longer
> her said manner of ministring of Simples, as she hath done, wherby
> her undoing is like to ensue, unles she maie be permitted to
> continue the use of her knowlege in that behalfe. I shall therefore
> desire you forthwith to take order amongst your selves for the
> readmitting of her into the quiet exercise of her small Talent, least
> by the renewing of her complaint to her Majesty thorough your
> hard dealing towards her, you procure further inconvenience
> thereby to your selfe.[69]

Given such *ad hoc* pleading, it is clear that this was not a time for a
legal framework of medical ethics. What we have here are two sets
of ideals being used by two different centres of power. The ethical
values used by Walsingham implicitly opposed those of the College,
and appealed to God, to helping the poor and to natural knowledge
or talent (royalty and its courts, despite Bostocke's comment above,
often favoured empirics). The College in its reply referred to the
danger to her Majesty's subjects, the weakness and insufficiency of
Kennix, and it tried to incorporate Walsingham to its ranks and to
its point of view 'most humbly beseeching your Honor, that as
most excellent Virtues and Learning hath made you famous to the
World and posterity, so it might please you to be a favourable
patron to such as have been trained and brought up therein.'[70]

It is a trite but often true point that the law reflects the views of
the public, and mostly of those in power. The College found
opposition to its policing of medicine from powerful figures – the
Queen on various occasions, Walsingham, Howard, Essex and
others. The monopolistic values of the College were not held by
everyone in power. The judgement of Coke in Bonham's case
(1608/9) is indicative of this as, crucially for medical ethics, Coke
broke the link between licensing and skill: 'but he who practises
physic in London, in a good manner, although he doth it without a
licence, yet it is not any prejudice to the body of man'.[71] The
College could not, according to Coke, convict someone of
malpractice merely because they were not licensed. (Coke felt that
the learning of a university graduate was sufficient – so his ideal was
still that of learning). The effect of the judgement was not long-
lived,[72] what is significant about it is that it was one of the few cases
in which the courts became involved in the area of medical ethics.

The law on malpractice was largely underdeveloped. The specific
offence of malpractice was recognized by the public courts (the
College believed its right to convict for malpractice was a private one).
In Groenvelt's case (1697) the Court of King's Bench decided that:

Medical Ethics in Early Modern England

mala praxis is a great misdemeanor and offence at common law,
whether it be for curiosity or experiment, or by neglect, because it
breaks the trust which the party has placed in the physician,
tending directly to his destruction.[73]

However, the criminal courts do not seem to have elaborated further
on this. The detailed judgement of whether malpractice had occurred
was left in the sixteenth and seventeenth centuries for the physicians
to decide. As Chief Justice Holt held, in Groenvelt's action for false
imprisonment against the College, there was no appeal from matters
that fell to the College members to judge as experts:

> Though the pills and medicines were really 'salubres pillulae et
> bona medicamenta' no action lies against the censors, because it is
> a wrong judgement in a matter within the limits of their
> jurisdiction; and a judge is not answerable, either to the king or
> the party, for the mistakes or errors of his judgement in a matter of
> which he has jurisdiction.[74]

The College doctors did get some support from the law. And it is
clear from the cases of malpractice tried by the College in the
sixteenth and seventeenth centuries that its finding of malpractice
depended on whether the practitioner had any education i.e. was he
or she an outsider, whether wrong or poisonous sort of medicines
had been used (in the sixteenth century these would often be
chemical which Galenists opposed) and whether harm had
occurred,[75] the threads of classical medical ethics came together
when they were enforced by a body steeped in the classics.

The law on malpractice as developed by the common law was
not all on the side of learned medicine. The balance of opinion by
the beginning of the eighteenth century held that if a patient died
and the practitioner was unlicensed this was not of itself sufficient to
constitute a criminal offence. The supposed legal immunity of
physicians could provoke bitterness. In Volpone there is:

> *MOSCA:* No, sir, nor [physician's] fees
> He cannot brook; he says they flay a man
> Before they kill him.
> *CORBACCIO:* Right, I do conceive you.
> *MOSCA:* And then, they do it by experiment,
> For which the law not only doth absolve 'em,
> But gives them great reward; and he is loath
> To hire his death so.
> *CORBACCIO:*It is true, they kill with as much licence
> as a judge.[76]

Medical Ethics in Early Modern England

However, it is not enough to assess whether and how far the ethical standpoints of the College physicians were policed or received full support. What should be recognized as well is that although the law contributed little to ethics in medicine or in a more narrow sense to medical ethics, even here two ethical approaches can be discerned – that of learning and that of Christian charity. Allied to the latter, but not always, there was an anti-monopolistic sentiment (as seen in the Lords' judgement in the Rose case).[77]

Conclusion

Reference to continental Europe provides a confirmation and a contrast to England, and can serve as a conclusion. On the continent there were the same diatribes about the unethical nature of empirical practice, the same complaints about disobedient patients, about the undue influence of onlookers, and about the doctor being brought in too late to the harm of his reputation when the patient died. Laurent Joubert's *Erreurs Populaires au Fait de la Medecine* (1578) dealt with many of these issues in quite a systematic and focused fashion. As the previous chapter has shown, in Italy the same defences of learned medicine can be found, as indeed they can also in Germany, for instance, in the writings of Johannes Langius.

However, it often seems that more learning was employed than by English physicians, for instance, by writers such as Ioannes Siccus, *De Optimo Medico* (1551), Baptista Condrochius, *De Christiana, ac Tuta Medendi Ratione* (1591) and Rodericus a Castro, *Medicus Politicus* (1614). Perhaps the poverty of the classical tradition in medicine in England has something to do with the sense of a lack of developed argument. England, despite Linacre, Caius and Harvey was a relative backwater in terms of the European renaissance of classical medicine. The richness and elegance of Siccus' depiction of the best doctor contrasts with the crudity of Securis' paraphrases of classical texts, and Cotta's even balder use of the sources. Yet in terms of substance there was little difference between the Continental and English ethical defences of learned medicine. What was different was the Catholic and Canon Law context of much of the European writing. Paulus Zacchias, who was personal physician to Innocent X and Alexander VII and Protomedicus to the Papal State, in his *Quaestiones Medico-Legales* (1621–35) dealt with many issues that concerned Canon Law and lay on the border between medicine and Canon Law. Zacchias was concerned with topics such the viability of the foetus, the causes of

Medical Ethics in Early Modern England

foetal death, types of madness, poisoning, impotence, malingering, torture, witchcraft, miracles, virginity, types of wounds and so on. The medical-forensic nature of many of these subjects stemmed from the canon lawyers' need to produce answers to a wide variety of contingencies having both moral and physical components. This gave a sharper but also more dialectical character to Zacchias' work. He asked questions related to specific aspects of medical practice. For instance, could necessary and urgent amputation of limbs be carried out with a safe conscience when there was a risk of gangrene. Zacchias replied that it was better to leave the patient in the hands of God than attempt such a treatment, which promised no ultimate safety and whose horror and pain was obviously most troubling.[78]

Again, in England the lack of detailed codes of law such as the *Constitutio Criminalis Carolina* (1532) which Charles V wished to apply to all the territories of the Empire meant that there was missing the sense of legislative authority which was present in some Continental medical writing.[79] It was this sense of a relationship between the law and medicine that led Johannes Bohn to write his *De Officio Medici Duplici Clinici nimirum ac Forensis* (1704). For instance, he wrote that a patient's secrets should not be divulged to any busybody, but only to those with a legitimate interest such as magistrates and to those who would be less safe by coming into contact with the patient by reason of contagion, or when the unfit, the impotent, the mad, the epileptic etc. attempt to marry.[80] Medical ethics, clearly, sometimes develop in response to the presence (or the needs) of the law and the State. In England medicine was largely oblivious to both.

Notes

1. On the College of Physicians see G. Clark, *A History of the Royal College of Physicians*, 2 vols (Oxford: Oxford University Press 1964–6); on the College in the Seventeenth century see H. J. Cook, *The Decline of the Old Medical Regime in Stuart London* (Ithaca and London: Cornell University Press, 1986).

2. On the medical market-place and on recent social history of early modern England: Lucinda McCray Beier, *Sufferers and Healers. The Experience of Illness in Seventeenth Century England* (London: Routledge, 1987); Roy Porter (ed.) *Patients and Practitioners. Lay Perceptions of Medicine in Pre-industrial Society* (Cambridge: Cambridge University Press, 1985); Roy Porter and Dorothy Porter *In Sickness and in Health. The British Experience 1650–1850*, (London, 1988); Roy Porter, *Health for Sale, Quackery in England 1660–1850* (Manchester: Manchester University Press, 1989);

VII

Medical Ethics in Early Modern England

Doreen G. Nagy, *Popular Medicine in Seventeenth Century England* (Bowling Green, Ohio: Bowling Breen State University Popular Press, 1988).

3. John Securis, *A Detection and Querisome of the Daily Enormities and Abuses Committed in Physic* (London, 1566), sig B3 r–v.
4. *Ibid.*, sig A2r.
5. Gent., sig A3v.
6. G. E. R. Lloyd (ed.) *The Hippocratic Writings* (Harmondsworth: Penguin Books, 1978), 68. I have kept to the traditional title, *The Law*, rather than *The Canon* of Lloyd's edition.
7. Securis, *A Detection*, sig A3v – A4r.
8. In J. W. Willock, *The Laws Relating to the Medical Profession* (London, 1830), clxxxiii.
9. Securis, *A Detection*, sig A4r.
10. Willcock, *The Laws*, xi.
11. Securis, *A Detection*, sig A4r–v.
12. *Ibid.*, sig A4v–A5r.
13. John Gregory, 'Lectures on the Duties and Qualifications of a Physician' in *The Works of the Late John Gregory M.D.*, 4 vols (Edinburgh, 1788) vol 3, 21: the bad behaviour of patients can 'cloud his [a physician's] judgement and make him forget propriety and decency of behaviour' in this situation appears the advantage of a physician 'possessing presence of mind, composure, steadiness, and an appearence of resolution.' Gregory's lectures have been unjustly overshadowed by the emphasis placed on the work of Percival.
14. Securis, *A Detection*, sig., A5v.
15. *Ibid.*, sig., C6v.
16. Harold Cook, unpublished paper 'Intellectual Property and Propriety: Professional "Monopolies" and the Physicians of Early Modern London'.
17. John Cotta, *A Short Discoverie of the Unobserved Dangers of Several Sorts of Ignorant and Unconsiderate Practisers of Physike in England* (London, 1612), 116.
18. *Ibid.*, 132.
19. *Ibid.*, 125–8.
20. On Galen see Vivian Nutton's chapter in this volume and Galen, *Quod Optimus Medicus sit quoque Philosophus*, in C. G. Kuhn, *Claudii Galeni Opera Omnia* (Leipzig, 1821) vol I, 61.
21. Hugh Chamberlen, *A Few Queries relating to the Practice of Physick* (London, 1694), 68–70.
22. E. D. [Eleazar Dunk or Duncan], *The Copy of a Letter Written by E. D. Doctour of Physicke to a Gentleman* (London, 1606).
23. Like Cotta, Hart and Primrose wrote defences of Galenic medicine: James Hart *KAINIKH, or the Diet of the Diseased* (London, 1633); James Primrose *De Vulgi in Medicine Erroribus* (London 1638) translated by Robert Wittie into English as *Popular Errors* (London, 1651).

Medical Ethics in Early Modern England

24. Andrew Wear 'Medical Practice in late Seventeenth and early Eighteenth-Century England: Continuity and Union' in Roger French and Andrew Wear (eds), *The Medical Revolution of the Seventeenth Century* (Cambridge: Cambridge University Press, 1989), 294–320.
25. Cotta, *A Short Discovevie*, 9.
26. Richard Whitlock, *Zwotomia. Or Obsevations on the Present Manners of the English* (London, 1654), 86 and 110–22.
27. *Ibid.*, 124.
28. *Ibid.*, 133.
29. Cotta, *A Short Discoverie*, 25.
30. *Ibid.*, 28.
31. *Ibid.*, 28.
32. Aristotle, *Nicomachean Ethics*, Book v, ch 9 [1137a11–18] in the translation of J. L. Ackrill, *Aristotle's Ethics* (London: Faber and Faber, 1973), 110.
33. Cotta, *A Short Discoverie*, 31.
34. Chamberlen, *A Few Queries*, 67–8.
35. *Ibid.*, 93–4.
36. Catherine Crawford in a recent study has pointed out that there were very few malpractice suits in the early modern period.
37. Chamberlen, *A Few Queries*, 76–7.
38. It is significant that when Cotta does mention God in his description of the true artist or physician it is in the context of knowledge and not charity. The physician's calling to study God's workmanship, nature, is an added reason for gaining knowledge, and one can use God as a guide: 'Not to speake of his excellent subiect (which is the life and health of mankind), his divine direction in his calling (led by the unchanged order and wisdome of God himselfe, manifested and set forth unto him in the structure and frame of heaven and earth) doth exact and require in him all possible perfection to sound and fadome the depth and height thereof. For as it is manifoldly and unmeasurably infolded and wrapped up in the intricate wisdome of his universal workmanship, so must long dayes and time carefully spent, indefatigable studie, paines and meditation, restlesse vigilance, a cleare eye of understanding, and sincere affection worke and labour it out .... And this must the true Physition ever behold God as his guide, and be governed and directed by his hand. For God is nature above nature, and nature is his hand and subordinate power, he is the giver of health and life in nature....' *A Short Discoverie*, 120.
39. Richard Bostocke, *The Difference Between the Auncient Phisicke ... and the Latter Phisicke....* (London, 1585), sig., Fiiir–v.
40. Alan Macfarlane, *Witchcraft in Tudor and Stuart England* (London, 1970); Paul Slack, *Poverty and Policy in Tudor and Stuart England* (London, 1988).
41. Charles Webster, *The Great Instauration. Science, Medicine and*

VII

Medical Ethics in Early Modern England

Reform 1626–1660 (London: Duckworth, 1975) 246–64

42. On the parish care of the sick poor see Margaret Pelling, 'Healing the Sick Poor: Social Policy and Disability in Norwich 1550–1645', *Medical History*, 29 1985, 115–37 and Andrew Wear, 'Caring for the Sick Poor in St. Bartholomew Exchange' in W. F. Bynum and Roy Porter (eds), *Living and Dying in London, Medical History Supplement* II, (London, 1991).

43. William Clowes, *A Briefe and Necessarie Treatise touching the Cure of the Disease called Morbus Gallicus* (my ed, London, 1585), 42r. Nicholas Culpeper, *A Physical Directory or a Translation of the London Dispensary Made by the College of Physicians of London* (London, 1649) sig. A1V.

44. Nicholas Culpeper, *The School of Physick* (London 1659) 7–40; Culpeper was following, often verbatim, Timothie Bright's, *A Treatise wherein is Declared the Sufficiencie of English Medicine* (London, 1580).

45. Securis, *A Detection*, sig., C6v–C7r.

46. Robert Pemel, *Help for the Poor*, (London, 1653), sig., A1r–v.

47. Calvin, *Institutes of the Christian Religion*, Book iv, ch XIX, sections 18–21; also see Calvin's comments on the healing miracles in his commentaries on the Gospels. The denial of miraculous healing was related to the Protestant denial of the efficacy of the Catholic sacraments and the anointing of the sick 'the greasy sacrament of the Papists' as William Perkins, the outstanding Puritan divine, put it: William Perkins, *A Golden Chaine* (London, 1612), 501.

48. Cotta, *A Short Discoverie* 88.

49. Whitlock, *Zφotomia*, 55.

50. Noah Biggs, *Mataeotechnia Medicinae Praxews. The Vanity of the Art of Physick* (London, 1651) sig., b3v.

51. *Ibid.*, 8.

52. *Ibid.*, 14.

53. *Ibid.*, sig. b3v and 17.

54. Cotta, *A Short Discoverie*, 33.

55. William Walwyn, *Physick for Families* (London, 1669), 2.

56. Walwyn wrote that his medicines if taken by those in health should nourish and not harm them (*ibid.*, 21) whilst for instance: 'The next sore troubler of the sick are Vescicatories, or Raisers of small and great Blisters, by irksome fretting, if not venomous Pleisters, sometimes flaying off all the skin from the backs, otherwhiles the shoulders, leggs ... to extream torments, expecially when those new places are rubb'd and irritated for diversion of venomous inflammations, hidious Curses and Excrations having been noted the impatient Effects of such cruelties; of which Nature also are the use of cupping Glasses, drawing of Silk through the Neck-skin, Leeches, and Issues, all full of pain, hazard and dangers (*ibid.*, 18). Note the religious distaste of 'Curses' the result of cruel medical practices.

Medical Ethics in Early Modern England

57. *Ibid.*, sig., A2r.
58. *Ibid.*, sig., A2v.
59. *Ibid.*, 3.
60. *Ibid.*, 6.
61. On O'Dowde see Harold J. Cook, *The Decline of the Old Medical Regime in Stuart London*, 148–50. Thomas O'Dowde, *The Poor Man's Physician, Or the True Art of Medicine* (London, 1665) 3rd edition, Preface, unpaginated.
62. Willcock, *The Laws*, clxxvii–clxxviii
63. *Ibid.*, clxxviii.
64. O'Dowde, *The Poor Man's Physician*, 15–6.
65. *Ibid.*, 20–1.
66. *Ibid.*, 21–2.
67. Ronald A. Marchant, *The Church under the Law*, (Cambridge: Cambridge University Press, 1969); R. H. Helmholz, *Roman Canon Law in Reformation England* (Cambridge: Cambridge University Press, 1990), Helmholz makes the point that although the faculties of canon law at Oxford and Cambridge were closed down manuscript sources indicate that some canon law was taught within a civilian context 152–4; good accounts of the investigative and judicial processes in England are in J. S. Cockburn, *A History of English Assizes 1558–1714* (Cambridge: Cambridge University Press, 1972); Cynthia B. Herrup, *The Common Peace. Participation and the Criminal Law in Seventeenth Century England* (Cambridge: Cambridge University Press, 1987); J. H. Gleason, *The Justices of the Peace in England 1558 to 1640* (Oxford: Oxford University Press, 1969); Norma Landau, *The Justices of the Peace 1679–1760* (Berkeley: University of California Press, 1984).
68. J. H. Baker, *An Introduction to English Legal History* (3rd ed. London: Butterworths, 1990); S. F. C. Milsom, *Historical Foundations of the Common Law* (2nd ed. London, 1981); T. A. Green, *Verdict According to Conscience* (Chicago: Chicago University Press, 1985). O. F. Robinson, T. D. Fergus, W. M. Gordon, *An Introduction to European Legal History*, (Abingdon: Professional Books, 1985).
69. Charles Goodall, *The Royal College of Physicians of London* (London, 1684), 316–7.
70. *Ibid.*, 317–9.
71. Willock, *The Laws*, lxxxvi (8. Coke's *Reports* 107–21).
72. Harold J. Cook has given an excellent account of Bonham's case 'Against Common Right and Reason: The College of Physicians versus Dr. Thomas Bonham' (American Journal of Legal History, 29, 1985, 301–22.
73. Willcock, *The Laws*, cxxxvi.
74. *Ibid.*, cxlix–xl.
75. Some of the cases appear very serious, for instance, that of the surgeon John Lamkin. He admitted practising medicine, but he was

also tried by the College for malpractice: 'He was afterwards charged
for Mala praxis upon several Patients (as his dropping of Oil of
Sulphur into a Patient's eyes, from whence an inflammation ensued
.... which endangered a total blindness; His prescribing Stupefactive
Pills to a Citizen troubled with an Iscury, by which he fell into a total
suppression of Urine, and made not one drop of water for ten days,
but died most miserably on the 11th) which being proved before the
President and the Censors, he was forwith commited to prison
propter malam praxin et immodestos mores, and fined 20l.' A year
later Lamkin was again brought before the College and imprisoned
for further illegal practice, the Archbishop of Canterbury interceded
for him then withdrew, and then someone else interceded with the
result that he was released on a bond of £40 that he would not
practice in the future. Goodall, *The Royal College of Physicians*,
331–2. From this case and others it is clear (as in Bonham's case)
that the College mixed together its attempts to have control or
monopoly of medical practice with protecting the public from
malpractice, self-interest with altruistic concern at patients being
harmed. The lack of State involvement limited the College's
effectiveness as a judicial body. This is clearly seen in the decision of
the College in 1635 to remit John Hope, an apothecary's apprentice
to the higher courts, when they found that he had given an infusion
of Coloquintida from which the patient died. The Censors certified
that 'it was evil practice [malpractice] in the highest degree, and
transcending the Censure of our College; and therefore we remit it in
all humility to the higher Courts of Justice.' Goodall, *The Royal
College of Physicians*, 442.
76. Ben Jonson, *Volpone* 1.iv.26–33. I am grateful to Dr Gordon
Campbell for this passage.
77. Willcock, *The Laws*, xciv–xcvi. See also Harold J. Cook, 'The Rose
Case Reconsidered: Physicians, Apothecaries, and the Law in
Augustan England' *J. of the History of Medicine*, 45, 1990, 527–55.
78. Pauli Zacchiae, *Quaestiones Medico-Legales* (3rd ed. Amsterdam,
1651), 635.
79. See Esther Fischer-Homberger, *Medizin vor Gericht. Gerichtsmedizin
von der Renaisance bis zur Aufklärung* (Berne: Hans Huber Verlag,
1983).
80. D. Johannis Bohnii, *De Officio Medici Duplici Clinici nimirum ac
Forensis* (Leipzig, 1704) 95.

VIII

CARING FOR THE SICK POOR IN
ST BARTHOLOMEW'S EXCHANGE: 1580–1676

The first part of this essay looks at the care of the sick poor in one small London parish, St Bartholomew's Exchange (see map, figure 1), between the 1580s and the 1670s. The second part puts some question-marks around the interpretation that I give to the parish material. The care of the sick poor appears to have analogies with the later care of the sick poor in hospitals, but in the second part I argue on structural, if not on socio-historical, grounds that a case can be made for seeing elements common to both the care of the poor, dependent sick and that of the well-to-do, independent sick.

St Bartholomew-the-Little, or St Bartholomew's Exchange as it came to be known, was a wealthy London parish traversed by Throgmorton Street and Threadneedle Street. It was 4·1 acres in area, which was on the low side for London.[1] Figure 2 shows that in 1579, 86 houses were rated to pay for the clerk's wages. In the seventeenth century the number of houses rated gradually rose, but then fell disastrously to three after the Great Fire. Rebuilding quickly made up the numbers.[2]

The affairs of the parish were reported in the Vestry Minute Books and the Account Books.[3] They disclose a world centred around the church, its upkeep, the selection and payment of its officials, and the care of the investments and property that originally had come to it in the form of charitable gifts and bequests. The books were written by the churchwardens, who also noted the other business of the parish, the

---

[1] Roger Finlay, *Population and metropolis*, Cambridge University Press, 1981, 168. St Bartholomew's was quite respectable for size, if one excludes London's outlying districts.

[2] The figures are taken from Edwin Freshfield (ed.), *The Vestry Minute Books of the parish of St Bartholomew Exchange in the City of London 1567–1676*, 2 vols, London, privately printed, Rixon & Arnold, 1890; vol. 1: pp. 7–8, 18–19, 36–7, 48–9, 59–60, 74–5, 86–7, 103–4,131; vol. 2: pp. 3, 35, 53–4, 76–7, 96–7, 102, 110–11 (hereafter cited as *Vestry Minute Books*). Shops have been excluded, as have houses with no named inhabitants. The figure for 1732 comes from Freshfield's 'Introduction', p.vi. Apart from 1732, the figures are for houses rated for purposes such as payment for the sexton's, raker/scavenger's wages, for which all the parish including the poor were likely to be rated. Figures taken from the rates for the poor naturally do not include the poor and are less than the other figures. For instance, in 1579, 86 houses were rated for the clerk's wages and 55 for the poor; in 1630, 91 were rated for the sexton's wages and 74 for the poor.

[3] Ibid.; and Edwin Freshfield (ed.), *The Account Books of the parish of St Bartholomew Exchange in the City of London 1596–1698*, London, privately printed, Rixon & Arnold, 1895. (Hereafter cited as *Account Books*.) Many similar books survive for the other London parishes.

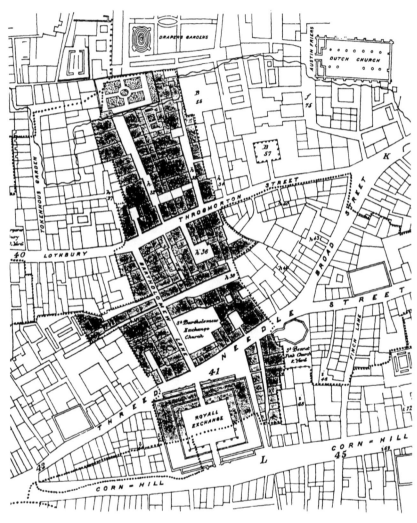

PLAN OF THE PARISH OF S⸱ᵗ BARTHOLOMEW BY THE EXCHANGE.
From Ogilby's Map of London, 1677.

References to Courts and Alleys.

h 32. Angel Court	h 37 Bartholomew Court	h 46; Horse Shoe Alley
h 33. Copt Hall Court	h 38 Noggs Head Court	h 27 Whalebone Court
h 35 New Court	h 39 Ship Court or Caple Court The inheritance of	h 31 Warnford Court
h 36 Shorters Court	Sir Robert Clayton Knt & Alderman M⸱ʳ John Harris	i 53. Castle Alley

Figure 1. Parish of St Bartholomew by the Exchange. Reproduced from Edwin Freshfield (ed.), *The Vestry Minute Books of the parish of St Bartholomew Exchange . . . 1567–1676*, London, 1890.

The sick poor in St Bartholomew's Exchange

ordering and care of vagrants and the poor. Even though poor relief had been partly secularized, as the State attempted to produce at the beginning of the seventeenth century a uniform system of poor relief by means of legislation, the care of the poor remained a church matter as in the days of voluntary relief.[4] The Vestry and Account Books detail the assessment of parishioners for poor relief and give the names of those parishioners who received pensions and relief in money or in kind and the amounts involved. There are also brief minutes of the discussions amongst congregation and officials concerning particular cases. Money spent on emergencies, for instance the medical expenses of parish pensioners, was noted down. The books also detail decisions and expenses concerning the disposal of vagrants, the care of out-of-parish women who gave birth, and the care and education of foundlings. In all, they give us an insight into the little world of the parish, a world that in terms of its organization, finance, and control over people was far more significant than its counterpart today.

The parish had a regular income from legacies, though most of the costs of poor relief were drawn from rates on householders. In terms of other London parishes, St Bartholomew's must have been well-off, as by the middle of the seventeenth century it was contributing money, on the Lord Mayor's orders, towards poor relief in other parishes such as Aldgate and Bishopsgate Without.[5]

The parish supported (that is, gave a weekly sum to) a maximum of around twelve pensioners, whilst there was a fluctuating group of poor numbering about twenty or less that included pensioners, which received bread, cheese, sea-coal, and money at different times, usually as the result of an annual disbursement of a legacy or as a one-off gift. The parish also had to look after foundlings, who were often "nursed" (the term includes the care of older children) outside in places such as Ware and Walthamstow. The numbers again were very small, below ten, but the foundlings constituted a heavy burden when seen as a proportion of the poor account. In 1634–35 the amount expended on the poor came to £73.4s.10d., of which £39.0s.10d. was spent on foundlings and £34.4s.0d. in various ways on the poor. In detail, the parish gave nine parishioners pensions totalling £12.18s.4d. for the year; £5.15s.8d. worth of sea-coal, £5.4s.0d. of cheese (partly given in money), and £6.10s.0d. of bread were distributed to the poor; expenses concerning the Beadle and the Overseers of the Poor and to do with the poor-rate came to 8 shillings. Other sums spent on the poor were £1.8s. for releasing the parish pensioner Widow Empson from prison, and £2 for the lodging of another pensioner, Peter Hartly, whose father had left money to the

---

[4] On poor relief see E. M. Leonard, *The early history of English poor relief*, Cambridge University Press, 1900; E. M. Hampson, *The treatment of poverty in Cambridgeshire 1597–1834*, Cambridge University Press, 1934; Geoffrey W. Oxley, *Poor relief in England and Wales 1601–1834*, Newton Abbot, David & Charles, 1974. Long after this paper was written, the standard work on the subject was published: Paul Slack, *Poverty and policy in Tudor and Stuart England*, London, Longman, 1988. For a European perspective, see Brian Pullan, *Rich and poor in Renaissance Venice*, Oxford, Basil Blackwell, 1971. For detailed micro-studies that focus on the poor themselves, see Paul Slack, 'Poverty and politics in Salisbury 1597–1666', in Peter Clark and Paul Slack (eds), *Crisis and order in English towns 1500–1700*, London, Routledge & Kegan Paul, 1972, 164–203; the essays by Tim Wales, 'Poverty, poor relief and the life-cycle: some evidence from seventeenth-century Norfolk', and W. Newman Smith, 'The receipt of poor relief and family situation: Aldenham, Hertfordshire 1630–90', both in Richard M. Smith (ed.), *Land, kinship and life-cycle*, Cambridge University Press, 1984, pp. 351–404 and 405–20 respectively.

[5] *Account Books*, 141, 173.

VIII

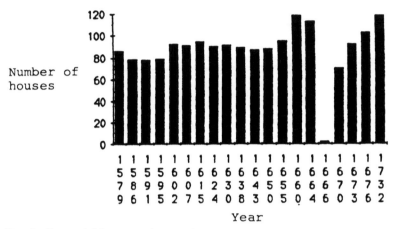

| 120 |
| 100 |
| 80 |

Number of
houses

| 60 |
| 40 |
| 20 |
| 0 |

1 1 1 1 1 1 1 1 1 1 1 1 1 1 1 1 1 1 1 1 1
5 5 5 5 6 6 6 6 6 6 6 6 6 6 6 6 6 6 6 6 7
7 8 9 9 0 0 1 2 3 3 4 5 5 6 6 6 7 7 7 3
9 6 1 5 2 7 5 4 0 8 3 0 5 0 4 6 0 3 6 2

Year

Figure 2.   Houses rated for scavenger's wages, etc.

parish for his care. When the newborn foundling Mary Throgmorton was discovered, the parish laid out a total of £3.15*s*.2*d*. for her nursing for twenty-eight weeks until her death, christening, clothing, and the search for her mother; Goody Hasard, one of the parish pensioners, was given £6.4*s*. for nursing and clothing Sara Potts for a year; and £26.11*s*.8*d*. was spent on the care, clothing, travel, and schooling of five other foundlings nursed outside the parish. Foundlings were often apprenticed, and in 1634–35 the parish paid out £2.10*s*. for the apprenticing of Mercie Bartholomewlane.[6]

These figures are reasonably typical, if on the low side. In the Cromwellian period the amount spent on the poor in St Bartholomew's increased. In 1657–58, when the parish was receiving more money from a generous legacy and from property rents, £139.19*s*.11*d*. was spent on the poor account.[7] The numbers of the poor are small and it is not worth spending too long putting them into any statistical form. The advantage, however, of having the record of a small number of poor in one place over a long period of time is that one can go down to the level of individuals and study their interactions and careers.

Help to the individual was governed by the system of parish provision for the poor set up by the 1597–98 and 1601 Poor Law Acts. The two churchwardens and the two to four overseers of the poor drawn from "substantial householders" of the parish,[8] together with the system of assessing a rate for poor relief from the parish

[6] Ibid., 98–9. See also Valerie Fildes, 'The infant wet-nurse and her role in infant care, 1538–1800', *Med. Hist.*, 1988, **32**: 142–73.

[7] *Account Books*, 160–1. This excludes the sum of £100 lent to the Grocers' Company and included in the accounts under money paid on the poor account.

[8] John Pound, *Poverty and vagrancy in Tudor England*, Harlow, Longman, 1971, 106; who prints an excerpt from the Poor Law of 1601 (*Statutes of the Realm*, vol. 4, pt. 2, pp. 962–5).

The sick poor in St Bartholomew's Exchange

householders, ensured that in a small parish there continued to be the same intimate connection between donor and recipient as when contributions were voluntary.[9] This connection was given visible expression when the poor were forced to give public thanks for the parish's charity. At a Vestry meeting in 1582:

> The most of the parishioners being assembled it was ordered and agreed that for all such bread as is given and distributed to the poor every Sunday in this parish Church, that the said poor immediately after the epistle and gospel every Sunday shall come up into the chauncell and there give the Lord thanks for his blessings bestowed upon them and for such of the said poor as will not come in form afore said it shall be at the liberty and discretion of the church warden for the time being to give and bestow their bread to the poor present.[10]

In 1627–28, the parish paid 5s.10d. for "9 Tickets [or labels] of pewter with the letter P, and the name of the Pensioners to wear".[11]

The public labelling of the pensioners gives us a clue to their relationship to the parish. They belonged, quite literally, to the parish, and when they died their possessions became parish property. Their pensions were granted "with this caution that they and everyone of them behave themselves well and orderly and be always ready to perform their best service to every inhabitant of this parish".[12] However, the relationship between parish and pensioner was not simply coercive or degrading. After all, it was concerned with charity and there was apparently a good deal of benevolence. It is on this mixture of benevolence and coercion and its various forms that I shall concentrate.

THE SICK POOR

The general position of the poor outlined above helps us to understand how the sick poor in St Bartholomew's were looked after.[13] Sickness was one of the characteristics that helped to define the status of a poor person in the eyes of the parish authorities and to determine their response. Many of the poor receiving pensions from the parish were likely to be, or to fall, sick.

In 1600. the twelve pensioners were described as "being past labour and very poor, allowed pensions". Most were widows, or men with many children, and in the demographic terms of the time all were very, very, old:

---

[9] Ordinances and laws that made contributions to the poor compulsory came in fits and starts. London levied a compulsory poor rate in 1547; Norwich, more successfully, in 1570; and the government in 1572.

[10] *Vestry Minute Books*, vol. 1: 14.

[11] *Account Books*, 75. Beggars and vagrants had been "badged" by the authorities from 1514 in London: Leonard, op. cit., note 4 above, 25–6. In 1600, recipients of pensions in London were ordered that they "shall every day openly wear a badge upon their left sleeve"—refusal merited suspension of relief: A. L. Beier, *Masterless men: the vagrancy problem in England 1560–1640*, London, Methuen, 1985, 155.

[12] *Vestry Minute Books*, vol. 1: 56 (1607).

[13] On the sick poor see, as well as the works cited in note 4, Margaret Pelling 'Healing the sick poor: social policy and disability in Norwich 1550–1640', *Med. Hist.*, 1985, **29**: 115–37; Thomas R. Forbes, *Chronicle from Aldgate: life and death in Shakespeare's London*, New Haven, Conn., Yale University Press, 1971.

	Weekly pension
Phillip Williamson and his wife, aged either of them 80 years and very poor	2/–
Widow Atkinson, bedrid, extreme poor	6d
Widow Hall, aged 70 years, very poor	7d
Widow Preston, aged 70 years and very poor	7d
Widow Sherbrooke, aged 70 years and very poor	7d
John Rankyn, aged 85 years, with wife and many children, very poor	2/–
Widow Boothe, aged 70 years, past labour, and very poor	8d
Widow Wood aged 80 years and very poor	8d
Widow Cuttings, aged 80 years and very poor	8d
John Saunders, aged 66, poor and many children	8d[14]

Clearly people of this age group would more often fall ill and need help. For instance, Goodwife Hall (listed above) was given a total of twenty-five shillings "in her sickness" between 15 July and 23 November 1599, over five different occasions.[15] As the parish became accustomed to the new poor law, the pensioners may have been chosen at an earlier age, as many of them were pensioners for quite long periods. However, they remained mainly widows, men incapable of supporting families, or people totally incapable of working.

There was a two-fold system of health care for the parish poor. One was run by the pensioners themselves; the other had recourse to "official" medicine in the form of seeking out and paying for the advice and remedies of surgeons, physicians or apothecaries. The parish gave special sums in addition to the pensions and hand-outs, to give access to both systems. In the parish's health system there were appointed, from the ranks of the pensioners and the poor, "keepers of the sick" as well as "searchers" who would certify cause of death and "searchers of the sick suspected" (that is, of having plague).[16] The system was in existence early on. In 1577 (a plague year),"It was ordered that these women . . . receiving the alms of the parish . . . being able upon request shall keep any sick person that shall happen within the parish of what desease soever it be, upon pain to lose the alms to them refusing given."[17]

This threat was not an empty one, for in 1582 the Vestry meeting agreed that those "nominated to be keepers of sick folks and such as be visited with the plague" should get more than the ordinary poor: "in all distributions not only so much as any other in the parish but also shall have each of them as much more, as well in bread every Sunday as in coals and money given out of the church box." Those serving the parish got "4d for a day and 4d for a night and meat and drink, to be paid by them that shall have need of them". However, the carrot was not enough and the minutes list five widows who refused to keep sick persons with the result that "they shall have no relief by the said parish neither in bread, coales nor in money as they were wont, but the same to be distributed where more need is".[18] In the end, most of the women agreed to be searchers or keepers of the sick.

[14] *Account Books*, 8.
[15] Ibid.
[16] *Vestry Minute Books*, vol. 1: 5, 13, 27.
[17] Ibid., 5.
[18] Ibid., 13.

The sick poor in St Bartholomew's Exchange

This was the only example in the St Bartholomew's records of relief being refused to those who did not agree to look after the sick or to be searchers.[19] In fact, it paid the poor to help the parish authorities. Sometimes they would be given money to look after foundlings before they were put to nurse, or a widow might nurse one on a long-term basis herself. Although a pension might be lowered to take account of the extra income, in general it seems that it was profitable for a pensioner to help the parish. (One difficulty in calculating how much a poor person was earning is that any income from such outside sources as tailoring or laundry-work is unknown: parishes often seem to have supplemented earned income and, as the person grew less able to work, the amount given by the parish increased.)[20] Widow Hasard, one of the two searchers in the 1630s (the official posts of keepers of the sick seem to have lapsed), made £5.4s. in 1635, in addition to a yearly pension of £1.6s., for looking after Sarah Potts.[21] A shilling a week early in the seventeenth century and a bit over a shilling in the second half of the century might have been just sufficient to live on, though some contemporaries thought not.[22] Between 1633 and 1648, Widow Hasard got a regular income for looking after Sarah. For instance, in 1643–44 the parish "paid widow Hasard for clothing Sarah Potts 20/-, for her boarding and schooling £4.19s.8d. at 23d. per week, £5.19s.8d.".[23] (The pensioners also helped at the christening of foundlings, and for this, significantly, they were also paid—an early example of good deeds being put on a commercial, contract basis.)

The system of parish welfare was of mutual benefit to the parish and the parish poor. It is in this context that the sick were cared for. Widow Hasard was paid a total of one pound "at several times from the 17 of August to the 2 of October 1640 for Peter Hartly when his leg was broke".[24] Evidence of the poor looking after their own for a price is present for the whole of the period. In 1602, Goodwife Wharleton, who was poor but not in absolute poverty, was paid 2s.6d. a week to look after

> Ann Smith a poor maid born in this parish of age 27 years the daughter of John Smith sometime Sexton of this parish deseased which poor maid [is] alleged to be lame and sickly praying to be releaved by the parish which was yielded unto. Viz, that the Church wardens should provide her of her apparell, diet and lodging, till she recovered health and strength to get her living by her own service and labour at the charge of the parish.[25]

This may have been a special case, for the poor were usually enlisted in caring for the sick in cases of old age, often in the days before death, and of chronic ill health.

[19] In 1581, the Lord Mayor ordered that, if the viewers gave the wrong certificate or refused to serve, they should be imprisoned. Thomas R. Forbes, 'The searchers', in Saul Jarcho (ed.), *Essays on the history of medicine*, New York, Science History Publications, 1976, 148–9.

[20] On this, see Wales, op. cit., note 4 above.

[21] *Vestry Minute Books*, vol. 1: 124.

[22] Keith Wrightson and David Levine, *Poverty and piety in an English village: Terling, 1525–1700*, London, Academic Press, 1979, 40–2. Gregory King calculated the income of a pauper family as £6.10s. per annum: Peter Laslett, *The world we have lost—further explored*, London, Methuen, 1983, 32–3; Wales, op. cit., note 4 above, 356–7; Keith Wrightson, *English society 1580–1680*, London, Hutchinson, 1982, 32–4.

[23] *Account Books*, 123.

[24] Ibid., 116.

[25] Ibid., 20; *Vestry Minute Books*, vol. 1: 47.

VIII

The Vestry and the overseers of the poor seem to have been flexible in their response to the needs of the poor, and sickness was the most frequent reason for temporary increases in pensions or for extra payments to cover the expenses of illness. The accounts for 1602 note, "paid to goodwife Garladye for a benevolence in time of her childrens sickness, which was taken out the poor's money in the chest . . . £1–00–00".[26] Frequently, help was slow in coming, the parishioner being made absolutely penniless first, as when "old John Griffin's daughter" got some allowance "towards the reclaiming of her apparell which she was constrained to pawn in the time of her sickness".[27]

The example of Widow Bulling and her daughter-in-law, Mary Bulling, illustrates the relationship between the patient, the carer, and the paymaster. Widow Bulling had been a searcher and pensioner, together with Widow Hasard. Mary Bulling was not a pensioner, but one of the poor who received bread and coal. In 1659, Widow Bulling got an additional five shillings a week on top of her pension of two shillings a month: "upon consideration of the great age and decrepitude of the widow Bulling then bedrid". Mary Bulling "desired 3/– per week to look to her" but the Vestry decided "she should have but two shillings six pence per week".[28] Mary looked after her for twenty-seven weeks. When her mother-in-law died, Mary "desired the parish would give her those few old things her mother left behind her. Twas agreed. In regard of the readiness of Mary Bulling to serve the parish upon occasions, that she should have them."[29]

And Mary Bulling did serve the parish, as, for instance, in 1661, when "Elizabeth Southern, a woman having no habitation" gave birth: the parish provided food, fire, straw, and "the nurse", who was Mary Bulling, "to tend her till she was able to go away". Mary got nine shillings for "tending her and cleaning the house", with the rest of the poor also joining in "the bread and beer", which cost seven shillings, for "the pensioners and company" at the child's funeral.[30] Mary's career repeated that of her mother-in-law. She became a searcher and, like Widow Bulling, got extra money from the parish just before she died.

Two points can be made from the example of the Bullings. First, the parish did pay proportionately much larger sums to people who were so ill and aged that death was probable, and who certainly stood no chance of being made well enough to work (as in the case of Ann Smith). This is rather different from the practice in Norwich, where relief to the sick poor appears to have been tied to the aim of getting people back to work.[31] Second, the payment to Mary Bulling and to other poor people for looking after each other says something about the ideology of neighbourly and family help which was so prevalent in early modern England. Even a relative[32] could expect, and received, payment for looking after someone who was ill. If the seventeenth century

---

[26] *Account Books*, 19.
[27] *Vestry Minute Books*, vol. 1: 89.
[28] Ibid., vol. 2: 71.
[29] Ibid., 72.
[30] Ibid., 84; *Account Books*, 173.
[31] See Pelling, op. cit., note 13 above. Pelling also points out that Norwich transferred responsibility for the sick poor to lazar-keepers and medical practitioners by contracting out their care and cure to the latter.
[32] Mary Bulling may have been more than a relative by marriage, for most references have "Widow Bulling" as her mother, and only one as her mother-in-law.

The sick poor in St Bartholomew's Exchange

saw the rise of capitalism, then here is perhaps a small example of the process: the ideals of voluntary mutual care being transformed into a financial arrangement—a transformation not yet complete, as is shown by the present debate as to whether the State should pay women to care for their mothers.

It may be that the system that I have briefly illustrated—of the poor being paid to help each other—was one that was cheaper than other alternatives, such as bringing in help from medical experts. However, the parish did pay for medicines and for the cost of surgeons and apothecaries. We may be on safer ground to talk of the poor providing nursing care rather than medical help, as the records do not say precisely what kind of help was given (though the boundary between nursing and medical care must have been very blurred, and the seventeenth-century practices of lay and family medical care amongst the middling classes[33] would lead one to the conclusion that medical care as well as nursing was given).

The moral ideal of family and neighbourly care found in books of practical divinity[34] and in practice in actual examples (seen especially in childbirth)[35] does not appear to have been invoked by the parish authorities in an attempt to get health care on the cheap. This may be partly due to the types of poor involved, who were often aged and without family. Yet the parish, after it was bequeathed some houses in 1643, housed its poor in one small area, many of them in one house;[36] and with its coercive powers it could have forced them to look after one another without payment (as the Geffrye almshouses did at the beginning of the eighteenth century)[37]— perhaps using the ideal of neighbourly love to justify its doing so—but it did not take that option. The frequency of the examples of the poor being paid to look after the poor means that care of the sick and dying even outside the regular medical context—for instance, when Widow Hasard was dying, her "daughter" Sarah was paid two shillings for washing her linen[38]—was viewed as a commercial matter.

---

[33] On this, see the essays in Roy Porter (ed.), *Patients and practitioners*, Cambridge University Press, 1985.

[34] The works of the early seventeenth-century theologian, William Perkins, are full of practical divinity, as is William Gouge's *Of domesticall duties*, London, 1622. For discussions of practical divinity, see William Haller, *The rise of Puritanism*, New York, Harper Torchbooks, 1957, 22–6; C. Hill, *Society and Puritanism in pre-revolutionary England*, London, Secker & Warburg, 1964, 443–81; John Morgan, *Godly learning: Puritan attitudes towards reason, learning and education 1560–1640*, Cambridge University Press, 1986, 142–71.

[35] See Adrian Wilson, 'Participant or patient? Seventeenth-century childbirth from the mother's point of view', in Porter (ed.), op. cit., note 33 above.

[36] In 1652, the vestry minutes note: "ordered that the poor people that are pentioners to the parish shall go to the general rooms following in Dibles Alley. Margaret Racy and Ann Wheeler in the first room, widow Hasard in the second room upward, goody Tedder in the 3 room upward. At the same vestry agreed with Mrs. Fox to give her £5–10–00 a year for one year . . . for a little house in Dibles Alley. At the same vestry agreed and ordered that Mrs. Chandler shall have the upper chamber and the garret of that house, Goody Shory to have the lower chamber and the use of the kitchen in common between her and Mrs. Chandler". *Vestry Minute Books*, vol. 2: 20.

[37] Rule 25 of the almhouses stated: "That none of the almspeople shall refuse to be aiding and assisting one another; and in case of sickness, 'tis expected they shall, by turns attend, assist and be helpful to each other, and live in peace and unity with each other: and which of them shall refuse their good offices to another in sickness, shall, upon good proof be expelled the house". Neil Burton, *The Geffrye almshouses*, London, Geffrye Museum, 1979. I am grateful to Mr H. J. M. Symons of the Wellcome Institute Library for the reference. The analogy between parish and almshouse care of the sick may well be worth exploring.

[38] *Account Books*, 184

49

VIII

The second type of health care system to which the poor and the parish had recourse was the familiar one provided by apothecaries, surgeons, and physicians. The foundlings often needed medicines and expert attention. In 1638, Widow Hasard was given ten shillings "to pay Mrs. Tedman for the Cure of Sarah Potts and for a powder", Hercules Wilson got 2s.6d. "that he laid out for physic for the child Mary Bartholomewlane when she was sick", and in 1639 the orphan Thomas Baldwin had seven shillings laid out for the "healing of [his] . . . head".[39] The pensioners often petitioned for their medical bills to be paid. In 1631, Bridget Harris's daughter was "under the surgeon's hand", and it was certified to the Vestry "that the widow Harris had one of her daughters that hath a lame hand in danger to loose it which had cost her much money above her ability and was thereby come into debt towards whose relief it was ordered [the churchwarden] should pay her four pounds."[40] In 1633, "Widow Varnham's [a pensioner] petition was read desiring some relief towards her great necessity, by reason of her sickness and a great grief with a sore leg which cost her a great deal of money and was not yet well recovered". The churchwarden was ordered to give her twenty shillings.[41] Widow Tame, another pensioner, was reported in 1643 by the churchwarden to the Vestry as "being in a course of physic, desired to have their further help and was thankful to their former charity to her". The churchwarden was ordered not to see her in want and gave "at several times to Mr. Butler the apothecary for physic and to relieve her in her necessity £2–08–00".[42] Three years later, in 1646, Widow Tame "being in great necessity" was given "2 shillings a week for her maintenance and likewise to pay her surgeon for his care and recovery of her"; the total was £2.2s.6d.[43]

There is little hint from the records that a system of wise women, or of local, non-"professional" expertise was being tapped, with the possible exception of the reference to Mrs Tedman. The very poorest members of the community availed themselves of expert help, and the parish authorities do not seem to have objected to their seeking out the expertise available in the medical market-place. Of course, a term such as "surgeon" could carry a multitude of meanings (as can be seen from the medical advertisements of the time) in a period where licensing was slack, and variety, rather than uniformity, in medical education and knowledge the norm. However, the records do not tell us if the parish poor paid for lay medical expertise (this is not suprising as lay medicine was often practised in the contexts of the family, or of charity).

The help given by the parish to pay for medical aid was not given automatically or as of right. The poor had to petition for it, they usually had to spend their own money first before trying to get it back, and they frequently had to be seen to be penniless and in debt before any money would be given. For instance, when Widow Tame in 1646 asked for help, she had already been given fourteen shillings to redeem the clothes that she had had to pawn.[44]

[39] Ibid., 110, 111, 114.
[40] Ibid., 89; Vestry Minute Books, vol. 1: 110.
[41] Ibid., 1: 114; Account Books, 94.
[42] Ibid., 123; Vestry Minute Books, vol. 2: 1.
[43] Ibid., 20; Account Books, 129.
[44] Ibid., 129, reads one pound; Vestry Minute Books, vol. 2: 19.

The sick poor in St Bartholomew's Exchange

The parish did not always pay the high cost of medical treatments. In 1659 Widow Hall, one of the pensioners, had an accident and the churchwarden wrote in the Vestry book:

> I desire to know what they please to do about the great charge that had been disburst for widow Hall, who fell down her stairs and broke her arm and bruised her head and body ["bruised" in the seventeenth century had a much stronger sense than today], and what I should do with some moneys I found in her chamber which was sealed up by the overseers of the poor and left in my hands.

The lumping together of the high cost of treatment and the discovery of Widow Hall's money was no accident. Charles Younge, the churchwarden, continued:

> Twas referred wholly to the overseers of the poor and they were also desired to mediate with Mr. Thicknes in her behalf who required £6 for her cure. And they accordingly did speak with him but he would not bate any thing, so they paid him that sum out of her money and gave her the rest which was about £6 more out of which she was to pay the apothecary and the other charges to be borne by the parish.[45]

Here the parish seems to be making the arrangements for treatment, though it is not certain if the initiative came from it or Widow Hall herself: in other cases the poor themselves seem to have decided to embark on the course of treatment.

Though the poor account for 1659 was large (it brought in £302.19s.8d., of which £118.10s.3d. was carried to it from the previous year, with £168.04s.9d. being spent during the year) six pounds and more was a tidy sum for the parish and it is not suprising that Widow Hall had to pay the medical costs out of her own money—in any case, this was inevitable given the legal prerequisite for poor relief, which was destitution. One wonders if Churchwarden Younge just happened to find the money or if he deliberately searched for it. In the event, the parish did spend ten shillings for Dr Daughtrey and 11s.6d. for "necessaries"; it raised Widow Hall's pension for a number of weeks, paid her nurse 4s.6d. a week for four weeks, 3s. for six weeks, and 12d. for three weeks, making in all £1.17s.; and gave Mary Bulling 5s. for "keeping her since".[46]

What the parish paid for was a mixture of the two systems—of the parish poor caring for each other and of medicines and orthodox medical care. This, in fact, was the norm, especially when the case was protracted. From early on, the two systems were joined together. In 1598, the parish testified to the medicinal value of alcohol and "paid to the relief of a poore man which was fallen sick in the Royal Exchange about the 12 of January 1598, and for aqua vitae and 3 poor women to look to him, 20d."[47]

One way of illustrating the way in which the two systems ran side by side is to look at the case of Katharine Rumney, or Rumley. The related documents are summarized in the Appendix. Her father was a plasterer who did the occasional job for the parish. By 1647, he was a pensioner of the parish and both he and his wife, Goody Rumley,

[45] Ibid., 71.
[46] *Account Books*, 166.
[47] Ibid., 6.

received extra money when ill. The extracts from the Vestry Minute Books and the Account Books illustrate many themes already discussed: the extra payments for special needs and for care when death was imminent, relatives being paid to care for each other, the poor being paid for caring for one of their own, and the use of orthodox medicine. The case also illustrates what happened when one of the poor was taken to an institution. The sick poor in St Bartholomew's, even if very ill, normally were looked after in the parish. This was understandable, given the scarcity of hospitals and the model of the care of the sick within the family, which was favoured by the well-off. Katharine Rumney was one of the few exceptions, and was sent at different times to Bethlem, the only public institution for the mad in London, though there were private mad-houses that catered for those with money. A patient could stay at Bethlem for a maximum of one year, the charges to the parish were high, and Katharine Rumney's illness was probably episodic: in any case, she entered Bethlem several times and the parish seems to have taken extra care of her in the periods before she became a patient and after her discharge (see the Appendix).[48]

The care of the sick in the parish of St Bartholomew's seems so far to have been reasonably humane. But for those who did not belong to the parish, that is, who had not been born there or resident there for three years, the picture was far less rosy. The parish was often a fount of charity, whether, as in 1599, giving 6d. "to a poor man which went to the Bath", paying ten shillings to "Dr. Crumton for his opinion about Mr. Webbe's stone", giving 8d. "to one which had been Mr. Mapledon's maid which was gotten with child" or, in 1614, paying two shillings "to two poore turkes turned Christians", ten shillings "to Mr. Parker his son being borne within this parish for his relief in his extremity", and giving four shillings "to two poor men who came by patent [special permit] for relief".[49] The parish could also respond collectively to other people's disasters, as in 1675–76 when eighty-four parishioners (most of the parish) contributed £32.9s.6d. "towards the relief of the poor inhabitants of the town of Northampton burnt out by the late dreadful fire".[50] However, charity was either given to the parish's own, or to outsiders who were recognizably legitimate recipients. Those who were strangers to the parish and poor, if fit, would be whipped out of the parish. Those who were sick were kept in the parish cage, a covered pen, where only minimal care was given such as bales of straw for bedding. In St Bartholomew's, pregnant women were noted as being kept there, and many deaths occurred in the cages of other parishes. The sums laid out by St Bartholomew's on behalf of women in the cage were small: "paid to Mr. Knotsford per so much he laid upon a poor woman carried to the Cage, 5/3"; "Paid Ezekiell Cakebread for carriage of a woman in labour to the Cage, 12d., for straw 1/4, for relief 6d".[51] The Poor Laws, and custom, ensured that a sense of close-knit community existed between the parish and its poor. The frequent allusions to strange big-bellied women being moved out of the parish so that they did not become a charge upon it, and the refusal of relief to

[48] Not all of the monies paid to the Rumneys have been noted, my intention being to give a representative impression of the family's career as noted in the Account and Vestry books.
[49] *Account Books*, 6, 49.
[50] *Vestry Minute Books*, vol. 2: 128.
[51] *Account Books*, 74, 108, (1626, 1637).

The sick poor in St Bartholomew's Exchange

petitioners born or resident outside the parish, must all have helped to produce a sense of exclusiveness and hence inclusiveness.

The description of the parish of St Bartholomew can give only a limited picture of how parish poor in general were looked after. The work of Tim Wales on Norfolk, Margaret Pelling on Norwich, and Thomas Forbes on London can broaden it, and clearly more detailed work on parishes in London and elsewhere has to be carried out.

THE WIDER CONTEXT

At one level, this account of St Bartholomew's and its poor can complement studies of hospitals of the time. The clientele were the same—poor—as was the emphasis on regulating their lives. The parish acted as a smaller version of the hospital, but kept the sick poor in the community.[52]

This is the gloomy picture of the care of the sick. It worsens if one notes how often the pensioners in St Bartholomew's followed in the footsteps of their fathers, mothers, (and adoptive mothers) or husbands and remained caught in the poverty trap of seventeenth-century London (for instance, the two pensioners for 1676, in the last entry in the Vestry Minute Book, are Sara Hasard and Susan Chandler, whose mothers had also been pensioners). However, there are one to two brighter spots—money was expended on the care of the sick poor in the parish, even if death was the likely prognosis (maybe not a bright spot, just the bottom line for care and charity). The poor were paid to look after their own, when they could have been forced to do so for nothing, as happened in almshouses and hospitals. Finally, I seem to detect a sense of neighbourliness or family care, but one in which the care is paid for.

The gloomy picture has become the standard view of hospital care and parish poor relief in the hands of Michel Foucault and other historians. We see the hospital emerging in the eighteenth and nineteenth centuries from its small-scale origins in the early modern period and before, to serve as part of a two-fold image. The hospitals with their captive poor are depicted as growing at the expense of the "good" image of illness in the family setting, where the patient was in familiar surroundings and free from the domination of institutions and of doctors.[53] It may be that these contrasting pictures are both correct. But it would pay to be cautious. The contrast has been made between the eighteenth and nineteenth centuries and the period before, and between the hospital and the family. I am not convinced that enough is known about the seventeenth-century care of the sick in the family to be able to decide whether it really was a lost golden age—but that is another paper.

---

[52] The hospitals took in a greater variety of people, but the emphasis on residential qualification, poverty, and the policing of virtue was of the same nature as in the parishes. See *The Order of the Hospitals of King Henry the viii^th and King Edward the vi^th viz St Batholomew's Christ [Hospital]. Bridewell. St Thomas's*, London, 1557, pp. b7v, c6v-c7r, d1r-d2r, e1r-e1v. See also the *Orders and ordinances for the better government of the Hospital of Bartholomew the Lesse . . .*, London, 1652.

[53] On this see Michel Foucault, *The birth of the clinic: an archaeology of medical perception*, trans. A. M. Sheridan, London, Tavistock, 1973; Erwin Ackerknecht, *Medicine at the Paris Hospital 1794–1840*, Baltimore, MD, Johns Hopkins University Press, 1967. For a different view of the rise of the middle-class hospital in the late nineteenth century, see Morris Vogel, *The invention of the modern hospital*, Chicago University Press, 1980.

VIII

In the brief space left in this essay I shall look at sick people who were independent financially, as opposed to the dependent poor, and indicate that the same two systems of health care—lay and expert—were used, but in different ways, when independent, well-off people were ill. In other words, the structure of health care was analogous, if not the same in terms of quality, across the population.

The poor named in the records of St Bartholomew's remain silent. We do not know what they thought of the welfare provided by the parish, nor do we know what sort of care they gave each other—whether they made up medicines, performed medical procedures or whether they gave only simple nursing care.

The diaries, letters, autobiographies and other documents of the articulate, literate, population provide us with answers to these types of question and, of course, give a kind of history different from that which we can write about the poor.[54] In well-to-do households a great deal of lay medical expertise was put into practice. Often the medical expert seems to have been largely absent, being consulted only in cases of very severe illness. For example, only on such occasions was a doctor brought in from Wigan to care for the Blundell family of Crosby, a journey of about twenty-five miles. William Blundell (1620–98) had recourse to a family recipe book in which visitors were invited to write useful remedies for illness.[55] In his notebook he wrote:

> The best cure for a flux of blood is suppositories made of the fat of bacon put up betwixt every stool till you find the effect which will be complete in two days. If the bacon be roasted it is rather better than otherwise. This was told me by my old friend Mr. Price, the Protestant Bishop of Kildare, who had good experience of it.[56]

There was clearly a traffic in favourite remedies in early modern England. John Donne wrote "some shall wrap pils, and save a friends life so".[57] Lord Edmund Howard, son of the Duke of Norfolk, wrote in the 1530s to the Lady Lisle:

> Madame, so it is I have this night after midnight taken your medicine, for the which I heartily thank you, for it hath done me much good, and hath caused the stone to break, so that now I void much gravel. But for all that, your said medicine hath done me little honesty, for it made me piss my bed this night, for the which my wife hath sore beaten me, and saying it is children's parts to bepiss their bed. Ye hath made me such a pisser that I dare not this day go abroad, wherefore I beseech you to make mine excuse to my Lord and Master Treasurer.[58]

In 1538, Lord Lisle wrote to his wife that her "powder for the stone had saved two lives",[59] so the remedy—if it was the same—had good effect.

---

[54] For this type of medical history, see the essays by Beier, Lane, and Wear in Porter (ed.), op. cit., note 33 above; and Andrew Wear, 'Interfaces: perceptions of health and illness in early modern England', in Roy Porter and Andrew Wear (eds), *Problems and methods in the history of medicine*, London, Croom Helm, 1987.

[55] Margaret Blundell, *Cavalier letters of William Blundell to his friends 1620–98*, London, Longmans Green, 1933, 56–7.

[56] T. Ellison Gibson, *A cavalier's note-book*, London, Longmans, 1890, 193.

[57] John Donne, 'Upon Mr. Thomas Coryat's crudities', in *John Donne: complete poetry and selected prose*, ed. John Hayward, London, Nonesuch Press, 1962, 141.

[58] Muriel St Clare Byrne (ed.), *The Lisle letters*, 6 vols, University of Chicago Press, 1981, vol. 2: 499–500.

[59] Ibid., 500.

The sick poor in St Bartholomew's Exchange

The medical system of early modern England was an open one in which people moved from lay to medical expertise very easily. Physicians might write medical books for a popular audience, but they were not averse to learning about remedies from lay people—in a sense treating them as experts. Dr John Symcotts (1592?–1662) used remedies garnered from Lady Alston, Lady St Albans, Lady Harvey, Lady Luke, etc., and from "My sister Symcotts", "My brother Robert", and "My Brother Thomas".[60] Class was no bar. Symcotts reported the case of a patient suffering from a "purpuric condition during pregnancy": "A beggar woman told the patient that she would recover if she took shepherd's purse in her broth. Hence I ordered her a broth of plantain, periwinkle, shepherd's purse etc."[61] Symcotts used the remedy again in another case. He was not hostile to lay expertise and gave it credit, as when he wrote of the case of Goodwife Viccar of Sutton, "stricken with a palsy all one side . . . a woman gave her counsel to be close covered with 2 large sheep skins new taken off for 24 hours together. She endured 17 hours . . . and so was recovered"[62]

The gravest illnesses were envisaged as candidates for lay treatment. The large number of popular medical books published in the seventeenth century, although often written by physicians, gave detailed advice on how the public could treat serious illness. Although the reader might be warned that consulting a physician was best, the lack of means to pay for one, the distance from one, and the fact that medical skill was one of the attributes of an accomplished lady were given as reasons for publishing the advice. Yet many consulted physicians or surgeons—Pepys often did—and lay cure was frequently described with one eye to its sanction by the experts. Mrs Elizabeth Walker, whose "holy life" was set down by her husband, looked after sick neighbours as well as her husband:

> She had a competent measure both in physic and chyrurgery, which she attained with no small industry and labour and increased by experience. Her first and main stock she acquired from a brother in law and very able doctor of the London College . . . and was very freely communicative . . . and directed her what methods to proceed in for most common diseases, into which her poor neighbours might be incident, and she was very inquisitive of other doctors and had many books, Riverius, Culpepper, Bonettus etc. which she read . . . and good store of vomits, purges, sudorificks, cordials, pectorals.[63]

The two systems of community and expert care were intertwined right across English society from the poor to the rich. There is no further space to go into detail to demonstrate this, but if I am right, where does the parish, and its possible analogue the hospital, stand? Is parish and hospital care of the sick poor an anomaly in the seventeenth century, something that contrasts with family, neighbourly, and community care, and which, as it grew, would exchange "good" humane family care for the anonymity, and alienation of the institutional incarceration of populus and industrialized England?

[60] F. N. L. Poynter and W. J. Bishop, *A seventeenth-century doctor and his patients: John Symcotts, 1592–1622* (Bedfordshire Historical Record Society vol. 31, 1950), introduction, p. xxi.
[61] Ibid.,
[62] Ibid.,
[63] A. Walker, *The holy life of Mrs. Elizabeth Walker*, London, 1690, 177–8.

VIII

A way of seeing institutional care of the sick (whether in parishes or hospitals) in this period and freeing it a little from its repressive label is to make the point that nursing-homes, small hospitals or "ill-houses" (like seventeenth- and eighteenth-century mad-houses)[64] were dotted around England. They were not repositories for the poor but places where particular groups of patients went. Thomas Brockbank was cared for in a nurse's home when taken ill with smallpox as a student at Oxford in 1691, and then he recuperated in different lodgings:

> I sent for my apothecary Hopkins and he told me the smallpox were appearing on my face. I desir'd him to get a nurse for me which he did; and he accompanied me to her house . . . I grew very ill and not very sensible in the evening Sir Teasdale etc came to see me and immediately sent for Dr. Frie.[65]

As he recovered, he wrote:

> I was removed from my old quarters (widow Tipler's in Coach and Horses lane) to Henry Clinches in St. Clements for airing [a change of air was an important part of recovery from illness] where I stayed 1 month at 12/– the week. Here I purged and was cleans'd and lay on great expenses.[66]

A surgeon, Josias Nicholes of Deal in Kent, had a private hospital separate from his house in the late seventeenth century, "a hospitall for sick and wounded seamen" with twenty-three beds.[67] The London surgeon, Richard Wiseman, often had patients who came from outside London for treatment, especially his venereal patients for whom the treatment by salivation (using mercury) needed time and caution. It was quite usual for the patient to take lodgings nearby. One "woman of about 50 years of age, of an ill habit of body . . . was brought to me . . . She importuned me to put her in a course of salivation by unction, and took a lodging near me".[68] Wiseman wrote that, in general,

> Your patient ought to lodge near your house in a close warm chamber. If the season be cold the windows must be covered with blankets and the bed near the fire, and incompassed with a screen if the chamber be large. You ought also to have a strong healthy nurse, such as hath been accustomed to the employment, that she may in the absence of the chirurgeon know how to wash the patient's mouth and direct and encourage him in such rules as may be necessary in the time of salivating.[69]

Sometimes the patient stayed in the home of a medical man. One patient of Wiseman's lodged in an apothecary's house, and the apothecary invited Wiseman and

---

[64] A. Fessler, 'The management of lunacy in seventeenth-century England: an investigation of Quarter Sessions records', *Proc. Roy. Soc. Med., Section of the History of Medicine* 1956, **49**: 901–7; William Parry-Jones, *The trade in lunacy: a study of private madhouses in England in the eighteenth and nineteenth centuries*, London, Routledge & Kegan Paul, 1972.

[65] Thomas Brockbank, *The diary and letter book of the Rev. Thomas Brockbank 1671–1709*, ed. R. Trappes-Lomax, Manchester, Chetham Society, 1930, 36–7.

[66] Ibid., p. 39.

[67] Kent Archives Office, Canterbury Consistory Court. Probate inventories, PRC/27/33/160. I am grateful to Dr Richard Palmer of the Wellcome Institute for the History of Medicine for the information.

[68] Richard Wiseman, *Several chirurgicall treatises*, London, 1676, book 7: 48.

[69] Ibid., 11

The sick poor in St Bartholomew's Exchange

a physician to undertake his cure. In another case, "A man about 34 years old of a full body came to London and lodged himself and wife in the house of his physician, he being indisposed with an inflammation of his belly to his left groin".[70]

Clearly, although many illnesses and deaths happened at home, some took place in other people's homes where the patient had gone for cure. In the London parish of St Lawrence Jewry, the burial register noted the death in 1599 of "Julian Hopkins, a sojourner, lying at physic at Mr. Bratchs girdler".[71]

The needs of special groups like soldiers, sailors, travellers, young migrants, and seekers of specialized medical care in the metropolis could all be catered for in places that were like homes but which, in a functional sense, could also be seen as embryonic hospitals. The poor also had recourse, as I have pointed out, to this type of care and perhaps provided it on an organized basis. The parish clerk's memorandum book of the London parish of St Botolph without Aldgate has been uniquely preserved, and it gives us more details about parishioners than would normally be available from the registers, vestry or account books. Through this book, in the Social and Economic Study of Medieval London project, run by the Institute of Historical Research and the Museum of London, the activities have been traced of a woman known variously as "Ellen Wright", "Mother Wright", and "a widow", who from at least 1588 to 1599 was taking sick people and pregnant women into her house.[72] In 1588, a stillborn child, whose father came from Pembridge in Hertfordshire, was "born in the house of Ellen Wright, a widow dwelling in taynter yard";[73] in 1589, was christened Rose Saunders, whose father was "John Saunders, basket maker, dwelling within the house with Mother Wright" (he died of the flux in 1599 at Widow Wright's, so he was probably a lodger or relative).[74] Katherine Melton, whose father Thomas was a "sailor", was "born in the house of Mother Wright" in 1589.[75] In the next year, the daughter of Richard Graves "a musician dwelling in the parish of St. Ollifes in Hart Street" was stillborn—"This child being by him begotten of the body of a single woman named Marie Linch who was sometimes his servant and now lying at the house of Hellen Wright . . .".[76] Ellen Wright took in sick people, for in 1598 we read of "Thomas Evered of Bromfield in Essex gent being a bachelor who being troubled with a desease or cancer in his mouth called 'Nolie me tangere' and lying at the house of Ellen Wryght a widow . . . where he died. Aged 60."[77] The daughter of Henry Wootton, "a serving man" and another stranger to the parish, was still born in 1598: her mother "Isabell Wootton was delivered of said child in the house of Ellen Wright . . .".[78]

---

[70] Ibid., 26, 27. In the second case Wiseman added, "pretending he had over-heated his body by disorder in drinking".

[71] *The Register of St Lawrence Jewry, London, 1538–1676,* transcr. and ed. by A. W. Hughes-Clarke, London, Harleian Society, 1940, vol. 70, pt 1: 130.

[72] I am very grateful to Dr Derek Keene, the director of the project, for allowing me to use his material, and also to Dr Martha Carlin for her help.

[73] *Parish Clerks Memorandum Book for St. Botolph's* (microfilm in Guildhall Library), 17 December. 1588.

[74] Ibid, 12 October 1589; 8 February 1599.

[75] Ibid, 7 January 1589.

[76] Ibid, 10 November 1590.

[77] Ibid, 19 December 1598.

[78] Ibid, 26 February 1598.

VIII

Ellen Wright clearly took in outsiders whose occupations, or those of their mates, placed them in the lower ranks of society. We know of her activities only when there was a death, birth or stillbirth in her house, and she may well have had many clients unknown to us. In any case, she clearly built up a reputation and people were sent to her house when being treated or recuperating. In 1599:

> John Akenhead a tapster late dwelling at the sign of the greyhound in Southwalk who for some desease was to be cured by one Mr. Foster a chirurgian and did lie [was lodged at] at the house of Ellen Wryght a widow . . . where he died . . . years 25 . . . de morbo gallico [of syphilis].[79]

If the above reminds one of Wiseman's patients, the next one has similarities with that of Thomas Brockbank—Humphrey Page died of consumption and was buried on 8 July 1599. He was:

> Citizen and haberdasher of London whose dwelling was in St. Sweethins Lane in London who being a bachelor and being sick in hope to recover his health by changing the air [a typical treatment for consumption] was lodged at the house of Ellen Wryght a widow dwelling in a garden house. [Ellen Wryght's house was in a green and wooded part of the parish, ideal for good air] . . . Aged 25.[80]

There were clear inequalites in the care of the sick across society—one has only to remember how plague nurses came to be feared when the better-off were locked up in their houses and given a taste of the parish care that the poor habitually faced.[81] Nevertheless, health care, when seen in structural, if not in social, terms, appears similar for both rich and poor. Both had recourse to lay and to expert help in terms of treatment, care, and lodging. A certain degree of neighbourly, family-type care was given by the poor to one another, if on a commercial basis. Conversely, commercial, small-scale institutional care was not limited to the poor but was used by a large section of the population—not surprising in an England where relatively small nuclear families and population mobility were common. There is a slithering, ambiguous, and flexible scale running from the care of the sick in families to the care of the sick poor by parishes and institutions in which the same structural elements express themselves at different points along it. The easy dichotomies produced up to now by historians will have to be altered.

APPENDIX: THE RUMNEY FAMILY

Philip Rumney was a plasterer. "Goody" (possibly Margaret) Rumney was his wife, and Katharine (or Katherine) their daughter. In the following, "Ac."signifies the *Account Books* (note 3 above) and "v.", vol. 2 of the *Vestry Minute Books* (note 2 above), with the page numbers.

1647   Phillip: Pension five shillings per week; and, "at several times being in want and sick—18s." (Ac. 133; v.22)

1650   "Paid for Margaret Rumney before she went to Bethlem and since she came from thence with money for clothes and other thing in her sickness"—£11.3s. (This could be Goody

---

[79] Quoted by Forbes, op. cit., note 13 above, p. 92.
[80] *Memorandum Book*, 8 July, 1599.
[81] Of course, most of the well-to-do would have been able to afford to leave London at times of plague, and the sums given by St Bartholomew's to support well-off parishioners were quite high.

The sick poor in St Bartholomew's Exchange

Rumney.) "Margaret Rumney in Bethlem Hospital 5/– [per week] . . . £13.0.0". (Ac. 141; v. 30, 35)

Goody: "Allowed her by reason of sickness and other poor people of this parish—£4.4.0."

Phillip is made parish beadle, on probation. (Ac. 141; v. 30, 35)

1651 Phillip's rent is paid for a year: £2.

Goody: "for beds and other things—£1.0s.0d."; "paid Goody Rumney's pension for a year £1.6.0."

Katharine: "Paid Goody Rumney 3/– a week for her daughter £7.16.0". (v. 37, Ac. 144)

1652 Phillip: "Pension at 2s. per month and 4s. per month for 9 months—£2.4.0."

Katharine; "Paid Rumney for his daughter besides his pension at several times 18s." (Ac. 146)

1653 Phillip and Katharine: "Phillip Rumney being aged and his daughter distracted"—a pension of £2.12s.

Katharine: "Rumney's daughter being distracted, ordered to be carried to bedlam for her cure at the parish charge".

Among "Monies given to the poor in their sickness"; 2s.6d. to Rumney's wife.

Katharine: "To a nurse for keeping Rumney's daughter 15 days—5s.6d."; "To Rumney and his daughter being mad January 6th—6s.0d". "To Rumney 2/6 February 19th".

Goody: for nursing a foundling for 9 days—three shillings.

Katharine: "Paid and spent on the mad doctor for Rumney's daughter—1s.0d." (v.47, 48; Ac. 149, 150)

1654 Goody: "paid to the nurse for three weeks' keeping of Goody Rumney—9s.0d. Paid to the searchers and charges for her burial- -15s.8d."

Katharine: "For a bond warrant and other charges to get Rumney's daughter into Bethlem—6s.6d. For keeping her there 18 weeks and 3 days at 5s.0d. per week—£4.12s.0. Paid and spent in getting her out thence—1s.8d." (Ac. 152)

1655 To Phillip, a pension of £1.6s.

Katharine: "for her relief this year—£1.4s.6d."; "Paid at a meeting about Katharine Rumney—8d." (Ac. 154, 156). Vestry minutes have her in Bedlam (v. 52), and the churchwarden is ordered to relieve her as occasion serves (v. 55).

1656 Philip: "old Rumney was voted out of the warder's place" and he receives a pension and relief totalling £2.19s.6d. that year.

Katharine: "paid for Katharine Rumney's going to Ware [a place where foundlings were nursed]—3s.0d. For a pair of shoes for her—2s.6d. For four months there—£2.8s.0d. For coming home—4s.10d. and more given her for her relief and *attending her father*—£2.10s.6d. [total]—£5.8s.10d." She is given a pension of four shillings and noted as "distrat" in the vestry minutes.—£10.8s.0d. (highest by far)

Phillip: Widow hall (pensioner) and Nurse Pelter are given, "for their attendance on Goodman Rumney and Widow Bullin in their sickness—£6.5s.6d."; "Paid Widow Shorey for her relief—14s.6d. and for physick for her and Wells and Rumney in their sickness—20s.0d". (Ac. 157, 158: v, 57, 59)

1657 Phillip: "monthly pension for a year £1.6s.0d."; "Paid Mr Evans plasterer for mending Rumney's house and their vault emptying. £00.16.08d."

Phillip and Katharine: "their weekly pension for a year—£9.2s.0d."; "It was ordered that I [churchwarden] should pay what I think fit towards the maintenance of Goodman Rumney and his daughter."

Katharine: "Given old Rumney's daughter in her sickness—2s.0d." (Ac. 160, 161; v. 61)

1658 Phillip dies: "Paid nurse that tended Goody Rumney in his sickness—8s.0d."

Mr. Beale (later one of the poor) petitions successfully to be the tenant of Rumney's house at £3 per annum. The house, which belonged to the parish, to be repaired at its expense: £1.3s. (v. 66)

VIII

Katharine petitions at the vestry for maintenance and is given two shilings a month (v. 66), as well as 2s.6d. to buy shoes. "Paid a joiner that removed Katharine Rumney's goods and set them up—3s.0d." (Ac. 163; v. 66)

1659　Katharine: "3 months' pension at 2s.—6s.0d. 8 weeks' allowance besides at 12d.—8s.0d For 17 weeks' pension at 18d. before sent Bedlam—£1.5s.6d. For necessaries and people to watch her and other expenses before she could be admitted—£1.6s.0d. . . . For a bond and warrant—6s.0d. For carrying her to Bedlam and given the keepers—5s.6d. Paid William Godbie, Steward of Bedlam, for 21 weeks and 6 days for her keeping there at 5s. per week—£5.9s.6d. For a Bedlam gown, petticoats, waiscoats, neckcloths, shifts, porter etc.—£1.1s.6d. For a pair of hose and shoes—4s.6d. For necessaries weekly after she came out of Bedlam—16s.6d." (Ac. 167)

1660　To Katharine; a pension of 18d. per week—£3.18s.0d. (Widow Hasard's pension was two shillings per week) "To Susan Chandler and Margaret Ralsey for helping Katharine Rumney—6s.6d. [Ralsey was a pensioner, Chandler one of the poor.] To Mr Thicknes for Katharine Rumney —13s.6d. To [Katharine] at several times by order—£1.6s.0d." (Ac. 170)

1661　To Katharine, a pension totalling £3.18s. (Ac. 173)

1662　To Katharine; 16 weeks' pension at 18d. per week—£1.4s. "Paid and spent in getting Katharine Rumney in Bethlem and for a warrant and bond, and other charges—14s.9d. To Goodman Wells for looking to her 3 nights and days, meat and drink—8s.9d. and to Margaret Ralsey for looking to her 3 weeks—5s.0d." and "for 23 weeks and 2 days at 5s. per week in Bedlam—£5.16s.6d."; "Spent at several times for looking after Katharine Rumney, for washing her linen and other charges at Bedlam House at her coming forth—14s.10d."; "Paid for 3 yards 3/4 of cloth for Katharine Rumney to make her clothes when she was in Bethlem—£1.1s.7½d."; "For making Katharine Rumney's clothes £0.10.0."
"Paid Katharine Rumney for 13 weeks pension from Christmas to Our Lady Day she being very weak and ill new come forth of Bethlem 2s.6d. per week—£1.12s.6d. For sweeping the chimneys of Goody Hazard and Katharine Rumney—1s.0d. Paid Katharine Rumney's scores at Bendalls and Parsons at several times before she went to Bethlem—7s.9½d." [Parsons was one of the poor; she became a searcher and her husband was a pensioner] (Ac. 176, 177)

1663　To Katharine; a pension totaling £6.8s. for the year. (Ac. 180)

1664　To Katharine; a pension of £6.10s. "Paid to her [Susan Chandler] and several others for looking to Katharine Rumney £0.6.0" (Ac. 183, 184)

1665　To Katharine; a pension, totalling £5.10s. (Ac. 187)

1666, 1667　To Katharine; a pension totalling £13. (Susan Chandler and Margaret Ralsey receive £2.12s. and £4.18s. respectively). (Ac. 191)

1668, 1669　"Paid Katharine Rumney's rent £2.0.0"; "Paid for Katharine Rumney's shoes £0.5.0" (Ac. 192).

1670　To Katharine; a pension totaling £6.10s. (Ac. 194)

1671　"Paid Katharine Rumney for letting her blood 10s.6d."; a pension totalling £6.10s."Paid more to Katharine Rumney 4/6". (Ac. 195)

1672-3　"Paid for [Katharine's] rent 5s.0d."; a weekly pension at 2s.6d. per week for 4 weeks—ten shillings. Eight weeks' pension at 4s.6d. per week "when she lay sick—£1.16s.0d. Paid for a pair of sheets and a shift for her—10s.0d. Given her nurse 6d. Paid for a coffin for her 7s.0d. Paid for an apothecary for physick for her 2s.0d."

IX

The popularization of medicine in early modern England

Popular medicine in early modern England is not *terra incognita*. In the last few years there have been important studies of the social history of English medicine of this period. From them it is clear that there was a medical marketplace composed of many different types of practitioner, and it was not limited to the physicians, surgeons and apothecaries – the traditional objects of study of medical historians. At the same time, patients' actions and attitudes in relation to illness have been studied.[1] The overall impression produced by the new research is that in early modern England there was a largely unregulated open-market place in which the layperson and the patient had much more choice and power in relation to medical practitioners, and, indeed, that power was shown by the prevalence of lay and of self-treatment.

It would be easy to call this open medicine with its many different kinds of practitioner (and multiplicity of explanations for illness, for instance, religious and magical as well as naturalistic), popular. But popular in relation to what? Our use of the term implies a contrast: élite–popular, high–low culture, written–oral. The new picture of English medicine is one in which people at the time recognized distinctions, for instance, between the learned physician trained in the universities in the classical works of Hippocrates and Galen and the empiric or mountebank with his travelling show and cure-alls. Yet in practice those distinctions were often ignored. People used many different kinds of practitioner without being troubled about the distinctions between them. In this context and at this time, therefore, 'popular' has an ambiguous sense which it had lost by the nineteenth and twentieth centuries; when, in fact, the

Medicine in early modern England

growth of the academic study of the popular indicates that it was a proper category defined with the aid of its antitheses – by knowledge of what is not popular.

Another difficulty with the idea of popular medicine in the early modern period is that the term 'popular' has been made to do too much. It has encompassed the literate middle class, people like Pepys, as well as illiterate wise men and women. The oral culture of medicine can include Pepys being given word-of-mouth medical advice by friends for an illness as well as what we can reconstruct of the knowledge handed down by a succession of white witches to each other. This problem becomes immediately apparent when discussing popularized medicine, the topic of this chapter. Who was it who could read the books which brought medicine to a 'popular' audience? Clearly not the illiterate, the most 'popular' part of the population. Despite a putative educational revolution between 1558 and the 1640s, the poorest, lowest part of the population still remained illiterate. The higher social groups such as the gentry, yeomen, and merchants and shopkeepers increased their male literacy rates, while husbandmen, poor artisans, labourers and servants still had high illiteracy rates. It is true, as Keith Wrightson and Margaret Spufford have pointed out, that the need to be literate was felt by the poorest and that much of oral culture was in the process of being put into print.[2] Geographically, there was a wide variation in literacy rates; some parishes, especially where there was a school or a teacher, had rates of male illiteracy ranging as low as 28 to 40 per cent in the early 1640s, while other parishes had rates as high as 90 per cent. The distribution of literacy across the country varied enormously. As the testimonies of Richard Lowe and Thomas Tryon indicate, it was possible for the very poor to learn to read and write. Moreover, reading on its own was much more widely practised than reading and writing. Women were often taught only to read. And it is impossible to calculate rates of reading, as reading, unlike writing, leaves behind no record. However, despite the large gains in literacy in early modern England, half the population was probably illiterate in 1750[3] and there were still many whose culture was totally oral, though their numbers were declining. To be able to read popular medical books meant, therefore, that one belonged to a special section of society, the literate. The readership of popular medical books has to be seen in a restricted sense, and the term 'popular' used cautiously.

Medicine in early modern England

Despite these caveats is it possible to speak of popularized medicine in early modern England? At first sight, the answer must be yes. Many books were published in England in English (ably discussed by Paul Slack[4]), which digested, popularized, and made accessible the classical works of Hippocrates and Galen. This suggests a model of medical knowledge coming down in a diluted form from the top to the reading public. It also implies the existence of distinctions, for instance, between medical writer and reader, or between learned source and popular author. Another way of putting it is that the popularization of medical knowledge involves the movement or trickle down of that knowledge from high to low culture. As I have indicated there are problems with this view. In practice, distinctions were blurred in an open medical culture in which family members or patients themselves might treat the most serious medical, if not surgical, conditions and in which the patient, the family, neighbours, clergymen and their wives, wise men and women, midwives, uroscopists, herbalists, empirics, astrologers, tooth-drawers, lithotomists, as well as apothecaries, surgeons and physicians, were all able to provide care. The lack of effective regulation of medical practice also helped to blur distinctions and hierarchy among medical practitioners. The College of Physicians controlled medical practice only within London and seven miles around and its powers were whittled away during the seventeenth century.[5] In the rest of the country there was no licensing except for a sporadic form of ecclesiastical licensing. The State and the law, those creators and enforcers of distinctions, were absent from large areas of the medical marketplace.

In this chapter I shall bear in mind the paradox of distinctiveness and openness in early modern English medicine, and I shall be examining how it was expressed by the authors of popularized English medical books. Their perceptions of what they were doing are in terms of contemporary interests and problems and they place their work historically. In the final part of the chapter I shall range more widely to emphasize the point that popular and popularized medicine (the former provides the context for the latter) in this period were *sui generis* and very different from the nineteenth or twentieth centuries.

Medicine in early modern England

The popularization of learned medicine

In 1539 Sir Thomas Elyot in the introduction to his *Castell of Health*, one of the most popular and frequently reprinted guides to health, defended his right to publish a work in medicine even though he was not a physician.

> But yet one thing much greveth me, that notwithstand-
> inge I have ever honoured and specially favoured the
> revered College of approved Phisitions yet some of them
> hearing me spoken of, have sayd in dirision, that although
> I were pretely seene in storyes, yet being not learned in
> Phisicke, I have put in my books divers errours in presum-
> ing to write of hearbs and medicines.[6]

In his defence Sir Thomas spelled out how, before he had become twenty years old, a learned physician read to him 'the workes of Galen of temperaments, naturall faculties, the intro-duction of Johannicius with some of the Aphorismes of Hippocrates'.[7]

Clearly Elyot felt he could be as learned as an approved physician of the College. In other words, for an educated person the learning of the physicians was not esoteric and out of reach. The literature of medicine was accessible to those who were not trained in medicine. This is an important point, for the openness of medicine and the ability of laypeople to practise medicine depended partly on the denial of claims that only the medically educated could understand medical books. Indeed, as the main thrust of learned medicine's claim to expertise lay in the scholarly, book-based nature of the discipline, to deny others who were literate entry into this learning might not be credible. Although Galenic medicine was self-consciously based on a mixture of experience and book learning (the union of the empirical and dogmatic schools of Galen's time), it was difficult for the learned physicians to base their claims to a monopoly of expertise upon experience alone, for that pointed in the direc-tion of the empirics and quacks, their hated enemies. There-fore, the best they could do against Sir Thomas Elyot was to point to his errors in transmitting the knowledge he had gained from books – his scholarly errors.

The list of authors that Elyot went on to read for himself comprised the great and the good in medicine:

Medicine in early modern England

And afterward by myne owne study I read over in order the more part of the works of Hippocrates, Galen, Oribasius, Paulus, Celius, Alexander Trallianus, Celsus, Plinius the one and the other, wyth Discorides. Nor did I omit to reade the long Canons of Avicenna, the commentaries of Averrois, the practises of Isake, Haliabbas, Rasis, Mesue, and also the more part of them which were their aggregators and followers.[8]

It is worth leaving Sir Thomas for a moment to consider the wider context of the learned medicine that he refers to. Learned medicine, the medicine of Hippocrates and especially of Galen, was undergoing popularization before and during the Renaissance. Printing alone had diffused medical knowledge more widely. Within learned medicine knowledge was also being diluted. In the Renaissance the methodical reduction of knowledge into compendia was in fashion among university medical men. For instance, the *Institutionum Medicinae* (1555) of the German humanist physician Leonard Fuchs gave an orderly, compartmentalized account of medical theory – the elements, qualities, humours, the parts of the body, its actions, then the non-naturals, the causes of illness, account of fevers, brief descriptions from head to toe of the ills of the body, and a discussion of signs and diagnosis. Other works such as the *Medicina Universa* of Giovanni Battista Da Monte (1587) and the *Methodi Vitandorum Errorum* (1603) of Sanctorio Sanctorio structured medical knowledge in more complex ways using models drawn from Galen's medical philosophy.[9] The gist of Greek and Arabic medicine could be read in one volume and the reader was spared having to use the large multi-volume folios of the Junta edition of Galen's work. Andrew Boorde, the sometime suffragan bishop of Chichester who travelled widely in Europe in search of medical education, wrote in his *Breviary of Health* (1547) that 'every man now a dayes is desirous to rede brefe and compediouse matters'[10] as in his own work. It was not only in the Renaissance that the process of abstracting past medical learning had taken place. In the Middle Ages the aggregators whom Elyot mentions produced compilations and abstracts of classical and Arabic medical texts. And before them in Elyot's list of authorities Pliny appealed to a lay popular readership, while others like Oribasius, Alexander of Tralles and Avicenna produced compendia of learned medicine. Galen himself had synthesized previous medical writings. Since Greek times, therefore, popularization in the sense of making medical knowledge available in easier and more accessible forms had been taking place. The difference between lay and medical readerships was not clear-cut. Although much of this was 'popularization' for a medical readership it was not exclusively so. Galen expected his patients to be as learned in medicine as he was and this view of a shared medical culture continued through to the eighteenth century.[11] The sources of medical knowledge could also be lay and popular. Galen showed no professional hesitation in incorporating folk remedies into his writings. This fits a model of culture that was to last to the Enlightenment in which élite culture found no difficulty in borrowing from oral, popular culture – indeed, there are examples in seventeenth-century England of doctors as well as patients using folk remedies.[12] Learned medicine was always composed of different levels of complexity, and the boundaries between it and popular medicine were more permeable than they might appear at first sight. This is even more so in popularized medicine, the learned medicine available to the public at large.

To come back to Elyot's introduction. After defending himself against the College of Physicians he moved to the attack. Despite never having been 'to Montpellier, Padua nor Salern' yet, he wrote, he had found for himself 'something in Phisick, whereby I have taken no little profit concerning myne owne health'.[13] In other words, universities are not essential for a knowledge of medicine. Elyot then explained that he wrote so that 'men observing a good order in diet, and preventing the great causes of sickness they should of those maladies the sooner be cured'.[14] Empirics sold cure-all remedies, but the mark of the physicians was that they offered advice on diet and regimen as well as remedies tailored to the individual. Elyot is saying that a special part of the physicians' expertise can be written about by a layperson. Moreover, the literate public should share this knowledge. In the next sentence Elyot goes on to justify writing his book in English rather than in Latin, the language of the learned. This was the *sine qua non* of a popular medical book and was often deemed worthy of comment (or excuse if the author came from the ranks of the learned physicians):

Medicine in early modern England

But if Phisitions be angry, that I have written phisicke in English, let them remember that the Greeks wrote in Greeke, that Romaines in Latin, Avicenna, and the other in Arabicke, which were their owne proper and maternall tongues.[15]

And then Elyot adds bitterly:

And if they had bene as much attached with envey and covertise as some nowe seem to be, they would have devised some particular language with a strange cypher or forme of letters, wherein they would have written their science, which language or letters no man should have knowen, that had not professed and practised Phisicke: but those, although they were Paynims and Jewes, yet in this part of charity, they far surmounted us Christians, that they would not have so necessary a knowledge as phisicke is, to be hid from them, which would be studious about it.[16]

The learned physicians had invested time and money mastering Latin medical books at university, and Latin clearly helped to protect their trade. As John Securis, a Salisbury physician who had been a pupil of the staunch Galenist Sylvius in Paris, put it in 1566:

If Englyshe Bookes could make men cunnying Physitions, then pouchemakers, threshers, ploughmen and coblers mought be Physitions as well as the best yf they can reade.[17]

From English books Securis immediately went on to make a general complaint that in actual fact anyone was allowed to practise medicine. This brings out nicely the point that the assumption of a monopoly of practice through learning and Latin had no connection with the real world, despite the physicians' wishes and claims that only those with learning and Latin should be allowed to practise. Securis wrote:

Then wer it a great foly for us to bestow so much labour and study all our lyfe in the scholes and universities, to breake oure braynes in readyng so many authours . . . yea and to the greatest follye of all were to precede in any

Medicine in early modern England

degree [i.e. take a degree] in the Universities with our great coste and charges, when a syr John Lacke latin a pedler, a weaver, and oftentymes a presumptuous woman, shall take uppon them (yea and are permytted) to mynister Medicine to all menne, in every place, and at all tymes. *O tempora, O mores* . . . and so, many tymes not only hinder and defraud us of our lawful stipende and gaynes: but (which is worst of all and to much to be lamented) shall put many in hasarde of their lyfe . . .[18]

In Elyot's introduction to his *Castell of Health* we find some of the recurrent themes of popularized English medicine in the sixteenth and seventeenth centuries: a wish to appear respectable and learned, a confidence in one's own experience and knowledge, and the desire to make medical knowledge available to a wider number of people.

How wide varied with the author. Elyot wrote for the reasonably well-to-do with servants; they could use his advice to look after their own health or as an act of Christian charity to help the poor. Nicholas Culpeper in the middle of the seventeenth century, with a much more radical approach (discussed below), reached out to a larger audience, though it had its limits for, apart from interest and price, literacy formed a natural barrier to true popularization. Another common theme hinted at by Elyot and which was used to justify popularization is the image of a medical establishment mean and monopolistic, against which the author fights the good fight. The learned physician had been associated with expense, greed and covetousness from the Middle Ages and these qualities could be countered by the Christian one of the altruistic charitable care of the sick.

But not all writers who wrote in the vernacular were against learned medicine. James Hart, John Cotta and James Primrose were staunch Galenists who wrote treatises in English in the first half of the seventeenth century that warned people away from empirics, women practitioners, 'parson-physicians' and the other rivals to the learned physicians. James Hart, a Northampton puritan physician, wrote an extremely strong condemnation of these rivals in the introduction to his *KAINIKH, or the Diet of the Diseased* (1633), yet he went on to disseminate the secrets of his fellow physicians to the general public. He was clearly aware that Latin was the trade language of the learned physicians. He wrote that he did not set down lists of remedies (he

Medicine in early modern England

was concerned with diet for the sick) because the public could not be instructed to relate the remedies to the constitutions and ills of individual patients (the mark of the learned physician):

Those remedies therefore are to be sought for in the learned workes and volumes (which Empiricks and all sorts of ignorant Physitians are never able to attaine unto, and by consequent unfit to practise this profession) of the judicious and learned Physitians of all ages; and can by none but by a judicious understanding, trained up in that profession, be duly as they ought accomodated to several individuall parties; *observatis observandis*, with due observation of all the several circumstances of time, place, person etc. Hence then may easily be evinced the error and ignorance of such as divulge abroad in the vulgar tongue, their rare secrets (as they call them) against any disease whatsoever. I doe not deny, but they may sometimes be seconded by some prosperous and successful issue in some: but that is by hap and hazard (as we say) *as the blinde man throwes his staff*... But when I see the world use these aright, they have already, then shall I be both ready and willing to communicate further what I know. My earnest care and indeavour hath ever bin since my first setting upon this profession, is, and ever, I hope, shall be to benefit the publike: but by such a course I should rather abouse than benefit any.[19]

The force of Hart's language was designed perhaps to show that he had not broken ranks with his learned colleagues. But he did give advice on diet in English to English readers. He justified this by referring to his desire 'to doe the common-wealth most service'[20] – a typical wish of the puritan godly. He also pointed out that classical advice on diet for the sick had not been based on English experience but 'according to that countrey and climat of Greece, . . . the which how farre it differeth, even at this day, from the diet of this our Iland both in sicknesse and in health, thou who have travelled into those countries, and the learned Physitian are best able to judge'.[21] The sense of Englishness was a potent reason for going beyond foreign authority, however learned. Hart's final motive for publishing was to give the public the information that would enable them to protect themselves. He stated that he wrote 'so people may the better be enabled to detect and discover the ignorance and unsufficiency of many ignorant persons intruding upon the practice of this profession, and to prevent posture'. In general, 'My purpose is only to teach the simple ignorant sort of people, whose credulous simplicity is too often exposed as a prey to every cheating and ignorant asse'.[22] This sense of protecting and educating the public can be found in continental works such as Laurent Joubert's *Erreurs populaires au fait de la medicine et regime de santé* (1578) which Hart quoted extensively, and in the attack on uroscopists and other empirics by the Dutch physician Peter van Foreest in his *De Incerto, Fallaci Urinarum Judicio* (1589) which Hart translated as *The Arraignment of Urines* in 1623. Hart's Northampton colleague John Cotta also wrote in defence of learned medicine and attacked other practitioners.[23]

Out of this wish to protect the public medical knowledge became popularized. James Primrose originally published his book on *Popular Errors* in Latin (1638), but when in 1651 his friend Robert Wittie translated it into English, Wittie wrote that he did so because he was especially concerned that gentle-women who practised charitable medicine for the poor should learn of their errors from the book.[24] These writers were seeking to re-educate their readers away from popular practitioners and practices and turn them to learned medicine, and to do this they used the demotic instrument of the vernacular to reach their readers, and so made more permeable the barriers set around learned medicine.

However, appeals to national and demotic sentiment more often served to justify a move away from learned medicine. Timothie Bright, a Cambridge physician later turned clergy-man, extolled the virtues of native English remedies. Bright was a Cambridge physician who had put in eleven years of study for his MD and had published various works in Latin. But the College of Physicians was no friend and threatened him with prison for practising without its licence in London. He was a rebel within the ranks of learned medicine. At a time of intense national feeling Bright argued in his *Treatise Wherein is Declared the Sufficience of English Medicines* (1580) that God's providence ensured that every country produced within its borders the remedies for the diseases that were native to it. The remedies of the classical and Arabic authorities could work in Greece and Asia but only English remedies could be effective for English diseases in English bodies with English constitutions.

Medicine in early modern England

(Significantly, William Harrison in his nationalistic *Description of England* (1586–7) expressed the same sentiment.[25]) As Bright put it:

> The whole art of physic hath been taken partly from the Greeks and partly from the Arabians. And as precepts of the art, so likewise the means and instruments wherewith for the most part the precepts of the same art are executed: which hath bred this error in times past, now by a tradition received, that all the duty of a physician touching restoring of health, is to be performed by the same remedies, not in kind only, but even especially with those which the Grecian and Arabian masters used, who wrote not for us, but for their Greeks and Arabics, tempering their medicines to their estates.[26]

Not only should medicine be written in the local language, but its remedies were also to be local. In this way, the Anglicization of medicine was breaking the hegemony of learned medicine.

Phillip Barrough, who was licensed by Cambridge University to practise both surgery and medicine, also tried to break away to some extent from classical authority. His *Method of Physick* (1583) deals with diseases and their remedies in the traditional head-to-toe order and has additional sections on fevers, tumours, venereal disease and the making of remedies. It was a comprehensive handbook of medicine.

Barrough discussed why he wrote the book. He clearly had a religious view of the duties of a physician: 'shall not the physition looke to have a shrewd checke at Gods hand, if he either hath proudly denied his helpe to the poore, or negligently visited them?'[27] This view of uncharitable physicians who might prefer 'lying fame and vile lucre'[28] made it easier to argue that patients could treat themselves. Barrough, like other English Protestant writers,[29] stressed that the body was of God's workmanship and had to be kept in good order: 'What can be more excellent than to be able to maintaine and keepe in order that best workmanship of God, and (which is more) to correct, reforme and amend it . . . And seeing there is nothing given unto us of God more acceptable than the health of the body, how honourably must we thinke of the means by which it is continued, and restored if lost?'[30] Barrough castigated those who did not look after their own bodies so that their bodies 'have been nothing else but storehouses and mansions of disease' and they had become like 'an evil and negligent tenant' though 'God had bestowed their bodies upon them as gorgeous palaces or mansion houses, wherein the mind may dwell with pleasure and delight'.[31]

This strong religious sentiment helped Barrough to argue for self-help and treatment. He wrote that 'it behoveth every man to be cunning in his own constitution, and to know so much as may serve to forestall the coming of many ordinary diseases which commonly light upon the ignorant: yea and sometime to be able to chafe away a malady when it hath already caught hold of the body'.[32] In a sense, the physician was not needed for 'every man may judge best of his owne bodie, and preserve the declinings and alterations of the same'. More practically, Barrough pointed out that physicians were not always available when needed – an often repeated complaint used to justify such books as Stephen Bradwell's *Help for Suddain Accidents Endangering Life* (1633) and Thomas Brugis's *The Marrow of Phisicke* (1640).

The type of medicine Barrough wrote about was self-consciously aimed at the lay reader. He extolled the virtues of experience and wrote that it is not enough to read the books of Galen, for 'when they shall go into the commonwealth to practice . . . they shall meet diseases that Galen never dreamt of'. The realization of the imperfection of the art of medicine should lead the physician to accept 'that as experience was the ancient beginner of Physicke, so that now it is the true and sincere accomplisher of the perfection of the same'.[33] The emphasis on experience, especially experience not available in books or to Galen, was a liberation from authority. A stress on experience and the aim of a popular readership often went together.

A practical advantage was that experience might exclude theory and could be synonymous with remedies and treatments. In other words, the text was simpler and the reader could get more quickly to the bits that mattered – what to do about the illness. Barrough's book, in fact, was reasonably learned as well as being compendious; it had Latin marginalia and was in the tradition of the Latin *practica* or vade-mecums on therapeutics[34] which lay at the simpler end of the spectrum of difficulty in learned medicine. It gave a very brief description of the disease, its signs, and cause and then concentrated on its treatment. As Burrough put it:

I have (good reader) for thy benefit collected out of sundry Authors, as it were a breviary or abridgement of Physick, and together with those deductions, I have enterlaced experiments of mine owne, which by long use and practise I have observed to be true. Throughout the whole book I have bin more curious in prescribing the sundrie curations and waies to helpe the disease, then in explaining the nature of them: my reason was, because if my books should come to the hands of the unlearned, a little would suffice (the former being more necessarie).[35]

Nationalism, religion, an emphasis on experience all led to the popularization of learned medicine, and to the conclusion that patients could treat themselves – which, of course, reflected what happened anyway. What we have are attempts to break down the barriers erected by learned medicine. Nationalism, religion, and experience all helped in this because of their concern with, and appeal to, the population at large.

Radical alternatives

As we have seen, the sense of anger with physicians was a motive for popularization. This was particularly so in the case of books on medicine for the poor where the Christian sense of charity was a powerful vehicle for this anger. Robert Pemel in his ΠΤΩΧΟΦΑΡΜΑΚΟΝ *or Help for the Poor* (1650) gave as his main reason for publishing 'these hard times, wherein the poor have scarse bread to eat, much less money to go to the Physition or Chirurgion'.[36] One of the celebratory poems to Pemel's work castigated physicians for their 'love of large reward' which made them deaf to the cries of the poor who 'hath no gold to grease their fists'.[37] Lancelot Coelson, 'student in Physick and Astrology', in his *The Poormans Physician and Chyrurgian Containing Above Three Hundred Rare and Choice Receipts . . . . Published for the Publique Good* (1656) referred to 'the insolency and Pride' of Greek and Roman physicians[38] and asked that 'the Physicians of our times may have contrary spirits humble, meek and lowly, visiting even the poorest of Patients when help is required, for the life of the most miserable vassal is as dear in the sight of God, as the life of the most renowned Monarch'.[39] Thomas Cocke, in his *Kitchen Physick: Or, Advice to the Poor* (1676), rather than giving low-cost medical receipts as did Pemel and Coelson, instead proferred advice on the appropriate diet for particular disorders. He deplored the fact that physicians would not visit the poor, so that neighbours and friends had to go on their behalf to get advice.[40] The poor, he reported, said 'Physick and Physicians are only made for rich men, and wait on Princes, and receive gifts of kings, but never thanks, not prayers from him who hath no other fee'.[41] There is a clear ideological and political force in these statements.

The Civil War and Protectorate was the time when the political desire to break down the barriers to medical knowledge and provision was at its most intense. Charles Webster has fully explored the calls and projects for medical reform in his magisterial *The Great Instauration*. It is clear that a Christian charitable approach that emphasized the needs of the poor came to be united with a theoretical approach at variance with Galenic medicine.[42] The latter was often based on Paracelsian, chemical, and/or astrological ideas. Galenic medicine was not only attacked because of the greed of its practitioners, but medical reformers like Noah Biggs (1651) and the Leveller William Walwyn (1669)[43] also bitterly criticized its procedures which they saw as cruel and ineffective. In other words, the arguments for medicine to be open to all were given added force by the existence of alternative medical theories. Popularization, therefore, could take place in the context of theory change. Nicholas Culpeper exemplifies the more politically pointed characteristics of the Civil War period as well as some of the earlier facets of the medical popularizer, and it is worth having a brief look at his reasons for popularizing medicine.[44]

Culpeper had fought in the Civil War on Parliament's side and had been wounded. He was clearly a political radical. In 1649 he wrote:

God gave Tyrants in his Wrath, and will take them away in his Displeasure. The Prize which We now, and They (all the Nations in Europe) within a few years shall play for is THE LIBERTY OF THE SUBJECT.[45]

Medicine in early modern England

This comes from the introduction to Culpeper's unauthorized translation into English of the College of Physicians' pharmacopoeia. He quickly descends to particulars. Priests, physicians, and lawyers most infringe the liberty of the Commonwealth.[46] He castigates the pride, ignorance, fearfulness, uncharitableness, and greed of the physicians:

> Would it not pity a man to see whol estates wasted in Physick, ('all a man hath spent upon Physicians') both body and soul consumed upon outlandish rubbish? . . . Is it handsom and wel beseeming a Common-wealth to see a doctor ride in State, in Plush with a footcloath, and not a grain of Wit, [knowledge] but what was in print before he was born? Send for them into a Visited House [with plague], they will answer, they dare not come. How many honest poor souls have been so cast away, will be known when the Lord shall come to make Inquisition for Blood [will try felonies, crimes deserving execution]. Send for them to a poor mans house who is not able to give them their Fee, then they will not come, and the poor Creature for whom Christ died must forfeit his life for want of money.[47]

Culpeper was perhaps a Leveller; he was certainly concerned, as his contemporary biographer assures us, to provide cheap remedies for the poor, culled from native herbs and not from expensive foreign products.[48] As Culpeper wrote, plagiarizing Timothie Bright word for word, God provided animals with remedies, so he would not forsake another part of his creation – human beings – by not providing them with remedies for their illnesses wherever they lived.[49] Culpeper's motives for publishing and making available medical knowledge to a wide public were both political and religious (the two are almost inseparable in this period) and a sense of charity was prominent. He wrote that the good of his country and the needs of the poor motivated his translation of the London pharmacopoeia of the College of Physicians:

> Pure pitty to the Commonality of England (I assure you) was the motive, the prevailing argument that set my brain and pen a work upon this subject, many of whom to my

31

knowledg have perished either for want of money to see a Physitian, or want of knowledg of a remedy happily growing in the garden.'[50]

Culpeper called himself 'Student in Astrology and Physick' and joined Christian charity to an astrological–chemical medical system; he saw it as his calling (bestowed by God) to provide this medical knowledge for the poor. It would, however, be ahistorical to compare Culpeper with a figure from later popular medicine, railing against medical authority and putting forward an idiosyncratic medical system underpinned by a populist and religiously based medical ethic alien to orthodox medicine. Criticism of orthodox medicine for its monopolistic, closed tendencies had already been expressed by popularizers such as Elyot and Burrough. Moreover, Culpeper was writing at a time when religious values, such as a stress on charity, were the orthodoxy and were dominating discussion of the nation's affairs. This was also a time when the Galenic consensus within learned medicine was crumbling, and it was unclear what was to be the future foundation of learned medicine. But, in any case, Culpeper himself publicized Galenic medicine in his *Treatise of the Fevers, the Method of which was Galens* (published in *Culpeper's Last Legacy* 1655) and he was involved in the commercial enterprise of translating Latin medical texts written by Galenists or by mildly radical continental medical writers.[51] Despite appearances, Culpeper was reasonably typical of his time.

In terms of this chapter, Culpeper illustrates the paradox of openness and of distinctions that informs much of popular medicine. When replying to a possible charge that by translating the pharmacopoeia, and setting out the virtues and uses of the remedies 'thereby fellows will be induced to the practise of Physick',[52] Culpeper wrote:

All the Nation are already Physitians, If you ayl any thing, every one you meet, whether man or woman will prescribe you a medicine for it. Now whether this book thus translated will make them more ignorant or more knowing any one that hath but a grain of understanding more than a horse may easily judge.[53]

But Culpeper quickly departed from the assertion of the complete openness and universality of medical practice among the

English. He pointed out to the apothecaries that it was in their interest that he had made their work available to a larger public.

> . . . . it tends to the advancement of their trade, if they have not wit enough to know that private men cannot make up most of these compositions themselves, but knowinge the vertues of the vertues of them, will resort the more to them for physick, they deserve the name of a Company of Dunces.[54]

Not everyone could be an apothecary to their ills. Distinctions did after all exist, medicine was not open in all senses to all.

Another way of seeing the paradox is to consider Culpeper's uncertainty in his *Directory for Midwives* (1651) as to who was educating whom. He noted that he had been called by God to correct error, but he added that if a midwife thought he had got anything wrong then she should tell him and he would amend it.[55] The distinctions of knowledge both exist and do not exist in English popularized medicine of this period.

Conclusion

There is much else to English popularized medicine than the authors I have mentioned. For example, books were written publicizing the virtues of spas, often with the aim of attracting more customers. Examples of cures were advertised and medical theories set out that explained the reasons why the particular waters worked. The openness of English medical culture is here apparent, for the writings were aimed at the customers, the patients, to persuade them to come to the spas, rather than at the physicians who would then recommend the spas to their patients. William Turner in the sixteenth century hoped his work on the 'Bath of Baeth' would inform 'the manie in the North partes, which being diseased with sore diseases would gladly come to the bath of Baeth, if they knewe that there were any there, whereby they might be holped'. In a nationalistic vein, Turner added that these Northerners 'know not whether there be any [baths] in the Realme or no . . . therefore I thought good to showe the vertues of our own Bathes, for if they be able to help mennes diseases, what shall men need to goe into farre countrys to seke that remedie there which they may have here at home?[56] In the seventeenth century Michael Stanhope, Robert Wittie, Robert Pierce, and others extolled the virtues of Knaresborough, Scarborough and Bath.[57] The promotional literature on the spas (often of a high technical level) illustrates the desire to make a medical facility available to the largest number of people possible who could afford it, and shows commerce joined with medical popularization.

There were other means of popularizing medicine. Advertisements in the form of posters or bills not only advertised the services of a practitioner but also conveyed something of his or her work. But what interested people probably more than anything else were medical recipes. They were what made you better. Women were especially concerned with them. They were often the main providers of medical care and, lacking the learned theory of the physicians, they depended heavily on prescriptions. Gervase Markham, who wrote a series of how-to books (fishing, fowling, farming, the care of horses), discussed in his *English Hous-wife* (1615) the 'inward and outward Vertues which ought to be in a complete Woman'. These were: 'her skill in Physick, Surgery, Cookery, Extraction of Oyles, Banquetting stuffe, Ordering of Great Feasts, preserving of all sorts of Wines, conceited Secrets, Distillations, Perfumes, ordering of Wool, Hemp, Flax, making Cloth and Dying, the knowledge of Dayries, Office of Malting of Oates, their excellent uses in a Family, of Brewing, Baking and all other things belonging to a Household'.[58] Before the intense specialization in the provision of services and products ushered in by the consumer revolution of the early eighteenth century and then by the Industrial Revolution, the household produced many of its own goods and services – even if as with physick, surgery, or brewing they were also commercially available. In a sense, the material conditions of life in principle enabled anyone to be a distiller, brewer, textile maker, baker, etc., just as anyone could practise medicine or surgery – if the money and the apparatus were available. Markham's housewife was a well-to-do one.

Markham did make the usual nod in the direction of the physicians:

> the depth and secrets of this most excellent Art of Physick, are far beyond the capacity of the most skilful woman, as lodging only in the breast of learned professors, yet that our House-wife may from them receive some ordinary

Medicine in early modern England

rules and medicines, which may avail for the benefit of her Family is (in our common experience) no derogation at all to that worthy Art. Neither do I intend here to load her mind with all the Symptomes, accidents and effects which go before or after every sickness as though I would have her assume the name of a Practitioner, but only relate unto her some approved medicines, and old doctrines, which have been gathered together, by two excellent and experienced Physitians, and in a Manuscript given to a great Countess of this land . . .[59]

Despite his patronizing tone Markham went on to give directions and recipes for the housewife to deal with the most serious illnesses such as plague, frenzy, and the different types of fever.

The large number of manuscript collections, often put together with recipes for food and cosmetics, indicates that people were not merely passive readers of medical knowledge but took an active interest in bringing it together. The collections tended to be indiscriminate and eclectic, illustrating a lack of concern with keeping to particular sources and types of medical knowledge (hence showing again that the categories 'popular' and 'popularized' were at this time ambiguous and indeterminate). The published collections of remedies often laid more stress on who had put the collection together (often a royal or noble figure) than on their medical provenance.

William Blundell and his family got their visitors to give them the details of any effective remedies which they then wrote into a book.[60] Lady Ranelagh, Robert Boyle's sister, was probably the compiler of a manuscript collection from the late seventeenth century. As well as describing how to make sugar cakes, 'Lady Essex a Cream Cheese', the collection also gave prescriptions for serious illnesses. Some are from lay people, 'Mrs Rodgers. A drink for the Rickets which never yet failed', others were from learned medicine as Dr Denham's remedy for the gout, 'commended by Galen, Avicen and Fallopius'; while yet others were from Paracelsians, the rivals of learned medicine, as 'Quercetans [Quercetanus'] Decoction for the jaundice'.[61] All types of medicine are present here without distinction.

There were some forms of medicine which did not come from lay, learned, or radical medicine. Recipe no. 617 reads:

Medicine in early modern England

A Receipt by way of Charm from Ague. Our Saviour Jesus
Christ seeing the Cross. He had a Agony upon him; the
Jews asked him art thou afraid and He said I am not afraid
nor have I an Ague, All those that fear the Name of Christ
and wear the Name of Christ about them shall have no
Ague, Amen, Sweet Jesus, Sweet Jesus, Sweet Jesus. Amen
Sweet Jesus, Amen. This to be sewed in a black silk and put
to the pitt of the Stomach an hour before the fitt comes
and not seen by the party but worn till all in pieces.[62]

Keith Thomas in his *Religion and the Decline of Magic* has charted
the prevalence of religious and magical healing. Not only were
wise men and women thick on the ground, offering to discover
witchcraft causing illness, and selling amulets and charms, but
the established Church also proffered means to cure illness. In
times of plague, prayer and atonement were institutionalized in
national days of prayer to God to withdraw his anger and
punishment. Godly ministers like William Perkins at the beginning of the seventeenth century not only taught (in effect,
popularizing) that God in his providence brought illness and
could take it away, but also taught what was the best type of
medicine that the ill should use (in his case, Galenic). Certainly,
magic and then religion were to decline in significance as the
Enlightenment began, but in the earlier part of our period the
existence of witchcraft, magic, and religion, all recognized by
the State and the law, meant that there were other bodies of
medical knowledge and other medical practices and practitioners that reinforced the paradox of distinction and openness. Religion, and even witchcraft and magic, the tools of
Satan, the necessary antithesis of God, in principle crossed all
social boundaries. Their effectiveness and existence were, in
terms of theological doctrine and law, universal, not popular or
élite, not high or low culture. Of course, condemnations of
witchcraft and magic did use social categories – their practitioners in England were often taken to be poor or ignorant. In
the same socially stigmatizing way, the learned physicians castigated the ignorance of empirics, 'vagabundes and ronagetes'[63]
who proffered medical care. However, the openness of English
medicine helps to drown the significance of these voices and
the existence of religious and other supernatural means of
causing and treating illness increases the eclectic and open

Medicine in early modern England

sense of medicine. Popular and popularized medicine are categories that, in this time, one should indeed be cautious about.

Notes

1. Roy Porter (ed.), *Patients and Practitioners. Lay Perceptions of Medicine in Pre-industrial Society* (Cambridge: Cambridge University Press, 1985); Lucinda McCray Beier, *Sufferers and Healers. The Experience of Illness in Seventeenth Century England* (London: Routledge, 1987); Roy Porter and Dorothy Porter, *In Sickness and in Health. The British Experience 1650–1850* (London: Fourth Estate, 1988); Dorothy and Roy Porter, *Patient's Progress. Doctors and Doctoring in Eighteenth Century England* (Oxford: Polity Press, 1989); Doreen G. Nagy, *Popular Medicine in Seventeenth Century England* (Bowling Green, Ohio: Bowling Green State University Popular Press, 1988). Also on medical practitioners, see Margaret Pelling and Charles Webster, 'Medical Practitioners' in Charles Webster (ed.), *Health, Medicine and Mortality in the Sixteenth Century* (Cambridge: Cambridge University Press, 1979), 164–235; on French popularized medicine, see Andrew Wear, 'Popularized Ideas of Health and Illness in Seventeenth-Century France', *Seventeenth Century French Studies*, I (1986), 229–42. On German Lutheran popular medicine, especially women's care of children, see Steven Ozment, *When Fathers Ruled: Family Life in Reformation Europe* (Cambridge Mass: Harvard University Press, 1983).

2. On literacy, see Lawrence Stone, 'The Educational Revolution in England 1560–1640', *Past and Present*, 28 (1964), 41–80; David Cressy, *Literacy and the Social Order* (Cambridge: Cambridge University Press, 1980); Margaret Spufford, *Small Books and Pleasant Histories* (London: Methuen, 1981, chap. 2); Keith Wrightson, *English Society 1580–1680* (London: Hutchinson, 1982), 183–99; Peter Laslett *The World We Have Lost – Further Explored* (London: Methuen, 1983), 228–37.

3. Laslett, *The World We Have Lost – Further Explored*, pp. 232–3, states that after 1753 a little over 60% of males and 40% of females were literate. His figures are drawn from Roger Schofield's study of the consequences of the Hardwick Marriage Act of 1753 where, for the first time, both bridegroom and bride had to sign the marriage register or leave their mark.

4. Paul Slack, 'Mirrors of Health and Treasures of Poor Men: The Uses of the Vernacular Medical Literature of Tudor England' in Charles Webster (ed.), *Health, Medicine and Mortality in the Sixteenth Century* (Cambridge: Cambridge University Press, 1979), 237–73.

5. On the College of Physicians, see George N. Clark, *A History of the Royal College of Physicians* (Oxford: Clarendon Press, 1964–6), 2 vols; Harold J. Cook, *The Decline of the Old Medical Regime in Stuart London* (Ithaca and London: Cornell University Press, 1986).

6. Sir Thomas Elyot, *The Castel of Health* (London, 1580), sig. A 3r. Here and elsewhere I have often used editions of early modern works that are later than the first.

Medicine in early modern England

7. ibid., sig. A 3v.
8. ibid., sig. A 3v.
9. On Renaissance medical method, see N.W. Gilbert, *Renaissance Concepts of Method* (New York: Columbia University Press, 1960; W.P.D. Wightman '*Quid Sit Methodus?* Method in Sixteenth Century Teaching and Discovery', *J. Hist. Med. 19* (1964), 360–76; Andrew Wear, 'Galen in the Renaissance' in V. Nutton (ed.) *Galen: Problems and Prospects* (London: Wellcome Institute for the History of Medicine, 1981), 229–62; *idem*, 'Explorations in Renaissance Writings on the Practice of Medicine' in A. Wear, R.K. French, I.M. Lonie (eds), *The Medical Renaissance of the Sixteenth Century* (Cambridge: Cambridge University Press, 1985), 118–45; Jerome Bylebyl, 'Teaching *Methodus Medendi* in the Renaissance' in Fridolf Kudlein and Richard J. Durling (eds), *Galen's Method of Healing* (Leiden: E.J. Brill, 1991), 157–89.
10. Andrew Boorde, *The Breviary of Health* (London, 1547), sig. A 6r.
11. For an influential analysis of this culture in the later period, see N. Jewson, 'Medical Knowledge and the Patronage System in Eighteenth-Century England', *Sociology* 8 (1974), 369–85; also R. Porter, 'Laymen, Doctors and Medical Knowledge in the *Gentleman's Magazine*' in Roy Porter (ed.), *Patients and Practitioners* (1985), 282–314; Andrew Wear, 'The Meanings of Illness in Early Modern England' in Yosio Kawakita and Shizu Sakai (eds.), *Patient–Doctor Relations in History* (Tokyo: Ishiyaku Euro American, forthcoming); on Galen and patients' medical knowledge, see Galen, *De Optimo Medico Cognoscendo*, ed. Albert Iskander (Berlin: *Medicorum Graecorum Supplementum Orientale* 4, Berlin Academy of Sciences, 1988).
12. On Galen's eclectic use of sources for his knowledge of drugs, see Vivian Nutton, 'The Drug Trade in Antiquity', *Journal of the Royal Society of Medicine 78* (1985), 138–45. Reprinted in Vivian Nutton, *From Democedes to Harvey: Studies in the History of Medicine* (London: Variorum Reprints, 1981), chap. 9. The early modern reader of Galen could see how he noted lay medical practice; for instance, he set down how a 'plebeius' prepared and used fumitory either as a cathartic or as a strengthening medicine, Galen (1625), *De Simplicium Medicamentorum Facultatibus* in *Galeni Opera*, vol. 5, Venice: Junta, p. 49 v. An example from the sixteenth century comes from Thomas Cogan (1584) *The Haven of Health*: of chamomile he wrote 'And this medicine I learned of a countrey man for an Ague, which I have proved true in many though it fayled in some. Take a handful of Cammomill, washe it cleane and bruise it a little, and seeth it in a pint of Ale, till halfe be wasted, scumme it well and straine it, and drinke it an houre before the fit, and if you thinke it better put in Sugar, cover you warme and procure heate, so doing three daies together fasting' (my edition London, 1612, pp. 68–9).
13. Elyot, *Castell of Health* sig. A 3v.
14. ibid., sig. A 4r.
15. ibid., sig. A 4r.
16. ibid., sig. A 4r.

Medicine in early modern England

17. John Securis, *A Detection and Querimonie of the Daily Enormities and Abuses Committed in Physick* (London, 1566), sig. B 2r-v.

18. ibid., sig. B 2v.

19. James Hart, *KΛINIKH Or the Diet of the Diseased* (London, 1633), 26–7.

20. ibid., p. 24.

21. ibid., p. 25.

22. ibid., p. 26.

23. John Cotta, *A Short Discoverie of the Unobserved Dangers of Severall Sorts of Ignorant and Unconsiderable Practisers of Physicke in England* (London, 1612).

24. James Primrose, *Popular Errours or the Errours of the People in Matter of Physick* (London, 1651), trans. Robert Wittie: Wittie's Epistle Dedicatory to Lady Frances Stickland sig. A 3v.

25. William Harrison, *The Description of England*, ed. Georges Edelen (Ithaca: Folger Shakespeare Library, Cornell University Press, 1968), chap. 20, pp. 265–8.

26. Timothie Bright, (1580) *A Treatise Wherein is Declared the Sufficiencie of English Medicines. For Cure of all Diseases, Cured with Medicine* (London, 1580), 47.

27. Phillip Barrough, *Method of Physick* (London, 1634), sig. A 5r.

28. ibid., sig. A 6r.

29. See Andrew Wear, 'Puritan Perceptions of Illness in Seventeenth Century England' in Roy Porter (ed.), *Patients and Practitioners, Lay Perceptions of Medicine in Pre-industrial Society* (Cambridge: Cambridge University Press, 1985), 55–99 esp. 61–3.

30. Barrough, *Method of Physick*, sig. A 6r.

31. ibid., sig. A 7r.

32. ibid., sig. A 7v.

33. ibid., sig. A 6r.

34. On the *practica* see Andrew Wear, 'Explorations in Renaissance Writings on the Practice of Medicine' in A. Wear, R.K. French and I.M. Lonie (eds), *The Medical Renaissance of the Sixteenth Century* (Cambridge: Cambridge University Press, 1985), 118–45.

35. Barrough, *Method of Physick*, sig. A 7r.

36. Robert Pemel, ΠΤΩΧΟΦΑPMAKON, *Or Help for the Poor* (London, 1650), sig. A 2v.

37. ibid., sig. A 3r.

38. Lancelot Coelson, *The Poormans Physician and Chyrurgian* (London, 1656), sig. A 4v.

39. ibid., sig. A 5r.

40. Thomas Cocke, *Kitchen Physick: Or, Advice to the Poor* (London, 1676), 10.

41. ibid., p. 8.

42. Charles Webster, *The Great Instauration* (London: Duckworth, 1975), esp. pp. 245–323; Webster's conclusions of a puritan-Paracelsian-reform of medicine nexus must still stand for the period after 1640 or slightly before, despite Peter Elmer's revisionist thesis in his 'Medicine, Religion and the Puritan Revolution' in Roger French

Medicine in early modern England

and Andrew Wear (eds), *The Medical Revolution of the Seventeenth Century* (Cambridge, Cambridge University Press, 1989), 10–45. However, puritans, in the period before the Laudian reforms when they felt they constituted the real Church of England, often took a conservative Galenic line (see James Hart, John Cotta, William Perkins, William Gouge).

43. Noah Biggs, *Mataeotechnia Medicinae Praxews. The Vanity of the Craft of Physick* (London, 1651); William Walwyn, *Physick for Families: Or the New Way of Physick* (London, 1669).

44. On Culpeper, see F.N.L. Poynter, 'Nicholas Culpeper and his Books', *Journal of the History of Medicine*, 17 (1962), 152–67; *idem*, 'Nicholas Culpeper and the Paracelsians' in Allen G. Debus (ed.), *Science, Medicine and Society in the Renaissance: Essays to Honor Walter Pagel* 2 vols (New York: American Elsevier, 1972), vol. 1, 201–20; Charles Webster, *The Great Instauration*, 267–73 *et passim*.

45. Nicholas Culpeper, (1649) *A Physical Directory or a Translation of the London Dispensary Made by the College of Physicians* (London, 1649), sig. A 1r.

46. ibid., sig. A 1r.

47. ibid., sig. A 1v. The quotation 'all a man[sic] hath spent upon Physicians' is from Mark 5, 25–7: 'And a certain woman, which had an issue of blood twelve years. And had suffered many things of many physicians, and had spent all she had and was nothing bettered, but rather grew worse. When she had heard of Jesus, came in the press behind and touched his garment.'

48. Anonymous, 'The Life of the Admired Physician and Astrologer of our Times, Mr Nicholas Culpeper' in Nicholas Culpeper, *Culpepers School of Physick* (London, 1659), sig. C 4r.

49. Culpeper, *School of Physick*, 1–49.

50. Culpeper, *A Physical Directory*, 314–24.

51. Abdiah Cole in the 1660s was advertising his series of books making up 'The Physicians Library' which included texts by Sennert, Riverius, Plater, Bartholinus, Riolan, Veslingius, Fernel, etc., some of which were claimed to be translated by Culpeper. Culpeper's biographer in *The School of Physick* wrote that a member of the College of Physicians agreed 'That he [Culpeper] was not onely for Gallen and Hypocrates, but he knew how to correct and moderate the tyrannies of Paracelsus', sig. C 4v. How far this was put in to make Culpeper acceptable to a wide variety of readers and how far it represents Culpeper's own position is unclear.

52. Culpeper, *A Physical Directory*, sig. A 2r.

53. ibid., sig. A 2v.

54. ibid., sig. A 2v.

55. Nicholas Culpeper, *A Directory of Midwives Or a Guide for Women* (London, 1681), sig. A 4r-v.

56. William Turner, *The Rare Treasor of the Englishe Bathes* in Thomas Vicary, *The Englishemans Treasure* (London, 1586), 105.

57. Michael Stanhope, *Cures Without Care . . . Mineral Waters near Knaresborow . . .* (London, 1632); Robert Wittie (1660) *Scarborough Spaw*; Robert Pierce, *Memoirs of the Bath* (Bristol, 1697).

Medicine in early modern England

58. Gervase Markham, *The English Hous-Wife* (London, 1653), titlepage. On women and medicine, see the works by Beier, Nagy, the Porters, and Ozment in note I, and Patricia Crawford, 'The Sucking Child: Adult Attitudes to Child Care in the First Years of Life in Seventeenth Century England', *Continuity and Change*, I (1986), 23–51 and *idem* 'The Construction and Experience of Maternity in Seventeenth Century England' in Valerie Fildes (ed.), *Women as Mothers in Pre-industrial England: Essays in Memory of Dorothy Mclaren* (London: Routledge, 1990), 3–38.

59. Markham, *The English Hous-Wife*, 4.

60. T. Ellison Gibson, (1880) *A Cavalier's Note-Book* (London, 1880), 244–6.

61. 'Collection of 712 Medical Receipts with some Cooking Recipes', *Wellcome MS 1340, Boyle Family*, nos 234, 240, 85, 631, 101.

62. ibid., no. 617.

63. Boorde, *Breviary of Health*, sig. 7v.

X

Medical practice in late seventeenth- and early eighteenth-century England: continuity and union

INTRODUCTION

To argue that medicine did not change, or changed slowly, in the second half of the seventeenth century and the beginning of the eighteenth century may appear perverse. After all, as the chapters in this book demonstrate, change was taking place all around medicine and moreover, the institutions and groupings within medicine were changing. But what of medical practice? Here also the different medical sects, the Galenists, Paracelsians, empiricists, chemists, iatrochemists, iatromathematicians had their own particular theories and remedies. Yet there was underlying unity that implied a lack of change both in medical theory and practice. This unity was the consequence of a need by medical practitioners to be understood by patients, to relate to their expectations and hence to attract their trade. Commerce, in other words, could transcend apparent theoretical or institutional differences.

MEDICAL THEORY

It appears obvious that medicine changed radically in this period. The chemical, corpuscular, experimental and mathematical developments in science came to be united in different ways to provide new theoretical bases for medicine. The non-mathematical, non-mechanical, qualitative–humoral system of the ancients seems to have been replaced. For instance, George Cheyne orders his *New Theory of Continual Fevers* using the language of 'Postulata', 'Lemma' and 'Scholium', and having

I would like to thank the members of the Cambridge conference, Peter Burke and Vivian Nutton, for their very helpful comments, and the Carnegie Trust for Scotland for a grant in aid of this research.

postulated 'that the whole body is nothing but a congeries of canals' he wrote in *Lemma* 1:

Let there be a greater distractile cylindrical canal, whose orifice is ABCD, through which a giv'n quantity of liquor passes in a giv'n time; and a lesser one EFGH . . .[1]

When giving practical advice Cheyne also applied ideas from the corpuscular philosophy, recommending for instance 'a large draught of warm water-gruel, or a warm small Mountain-wine whey, as an antidote against the nitrous effluvia, suck'd into the body'.[2]

The contrast therefore seems great between Cheyne and someone like Thomas Venner writing at the beginning of the seventeenth century. Venner used 'common sense' qualitative terms. His description of air contrasts with the apparent hard objectivity of Cheyne:

Therefore touching the knowledge of the goodness of the air, it must be considered that it be not vaporous, moist or putrid, nor too hot, or too cold, nor over-moist, or dry: for a vaporous, cloudy, gross or putrid air doth cause rheums, annoy the lungs, corrupt the humors, infect, the heart, deicet the spirits.[3]

The move from the qualitative, subjective, system of ancient and renaissance natural philosophy to the quantitative and objective world of the seventeenth century has been often and variously retold by historians of science. Yet in the case of medicine there is some doubt that we have the same story. The successes of the mechanical philosophy were rarely practical, and medicine in the end is practical. The mortality rate did not fall dramatically in this period nor can the small and ephemeral rise in the expectation of life after 1690 be attributed to medical advance (or even to increased prosperity).[4] Nor did medicine, through the new science, have any new technical apparatus (apart possibly from the microscope) that gave hope for cure.

The change that occurred, therefore, was theoretical and ideological and other historians in this book have been looking at its details. I want to argue, however, first that the new philosophy (which might have led to changes in practice), despite its empiricism was as speculative as the Aristotelian–Galenic when it came to describing the hidden happen-

---

[1] George Cheyne, *A New Theory of Acute and Slow Continu'd Fevers . . . To which is Prefix'd an Essay concerning the Improvements in the Theory of Medicine*, 3rd edn (London, 1722), pp. 7–8. On Cheyne's Newtonianism and his changes of stance within it see Anita Guerrini, 'James Keill, George Cheyne, and Newtonian Physiology, 1690–1740', *Journal of the History of Biology*, XVIII, 247–66, and her chapter in this book.

[2] George Cheyne, *An Essay of Health and Long Life* (London, 1724), pp. 10–11.

[3] Thomas Venner, *Via Recta ad Vitam Longam: Or, a plaine philosophicall demonstration of the nature, faculties and effects of all such things as by way of nourishments make for the preservation of health . . .* (London, 1628), p. 2.

[4] See E.A. Wrigley and R.S. Schofield, *The Population History of England 1541–1871* (London, 1981), pp. 234–6, 412–17.

ings of nature, for instance the sharp penetrating shape of acid particles, or the workings of a disease or medicine inside the depths of the
body. The need to show oneself as an educated, rational, physician and
to attract fee-paying patients made it inevitable that physicians continued to use what, in terms of the experimental and empirical approach of the late seventeenth century, were essentially speculations.
Medical theory, of whatever type, in its structure often fulfilled the
classical requirements of rational medicine (that is relating effects to
cause or, as in the practice of medicine which forms the second part of
this chapter, paying attention to a patient's constitution, regimen,
indications, changing condition and applying remedies to symptoms in
a rational way). But, as I argue, these, the central ideological defences
of the learned physician against the empiric, cannot always be differentiated from empirical practice.

Thomas Willis in his preface to his work on fermentation compared
the three natural philosophies of his time: the Aristotelian, the 'Epicu-
rean' or mechanical, and the chemical. The first had no 'peculiar
respect to the more secret recesses of nature, it salves the appearance of
things, that 'tis almost the same thing, to say a thing consists of wood
and stones as a body of four elements'. The second:

doth happily and very ingeniously disintangle some difficult knots of the sciences, and
dark riddles, certainly it deserves no light praise: but because it rather supposes than
demonstrates its principles and teaches of what figure those elements of bodies may be,
not what they have been, and also induces notions extremely subtle, and remote from
the sense, and which do not sufficiently quadrate with the phenomena of nature, when
we descend to particulars, it pleases me to give my sentence for the third opinion
before-mentioned, which is of the Chymists . . . affirming all bodies to consist of spirit,
sulphur, salt, water and earth.[5]

For Willis the chemists' philosophy was the *via media*, neither too
obvious nor too far from sense (though he did admit that 'the atomical
and our spagyric principles' could merge, the latter into the former as
long as the atoms or conceptions are real). His principles had to be
apparent to the senses:

I mean by the name of principles not simple and wholly uncompounded entities, but
such kind of substances only, into which physical things are resolved as it were into
parts lastly sensible. By the intestine motion and combinations of these, bodies are
begot and increase.[6]

Despite this protestation of empirical virtue, Willis could not remain
unsullied by the temptations of rationalism (in the general Galenic
sense). He naturally wanted to go from effects to causes. Take the
example of Peruvian bark, the new wonder drug for fevers. He ad-

[5] Thomas Willis, *Dr. Willis's Practice of Physick, Being the Whole Works* . . . (English
translation of Latin original) (London, 1684), p. 2.   [6] *Ibid.*, p. 2.

mitted that 'it is not to be dissembled, that 'tis very difficult to explicate the causes of these kinds of effects and the manner of working (of the bark)'. As a clinician he noted that the bark seemed to stay in the blood because, although the first bout of fever might still occur after taking the bark, it often stopped the second or third bout. From this he made up the story (or extremely weak inference) that the particles of the bark produce in the blood 'a certain new fermentation, by which, whilst the particles of the blood are continually agitated, they are wholly hindred, that they cannot heap up any excrementitious matter, or enter into feverish turgescencies'. He also noted that fever could return, because the bark was 'too sparingly given' and the 'venom repullulates, and the old poison, thought to have been exploded, is at length brought into act'.[7]

Despite his wish to keep to observables, Willis inevitably fell back upon his imagination when discussing the hidden happenings of the body. There was little difference in structure between Willis's story of what took place in the body and earlier humoral stories. William Clowes in the sixteenth century wrote confidently of quicksilver and its effect on syphilis:

But yet this I do know assuredly, that . . . it will resolve and molify: and it openeth the body, and provoketh sweat and emptieth the cause of this disease, sometimes sensible and sometimes insensible, and the blood thereby is purged from infection, and all the parts of the body is cleansed from superfluous humors, so that good humors are bred, and they do return again unto their natural cause and disposition, as we daily see by experience.[8]

The ability to tell the story from the seen (the effects) to the unseen (the causes) was from Greek times and up to and beyond the seventeenth century, the mark of the rational (and expensive) physician whose knowledge of causes set him apart from the crowd of empirics and quacks. As Daniel Coxe, the defender of the London College of Physicians against the apothecaries, wrote, the knowledge of causes was taken to mean better medical practice:

Then as for the cure of diseases, it seems highly probable that they who are best acquainted with the causes and symptoms of diseases will apply medicines more properly than others that cannot so well distinguish although possessed of the same remedies.[9]

[7] *Ibid.*, pp. 72–3.
[8] William Clowes, *A Briefe and Necessarie Treatise Touching the Cure of the Disease Called Morbus Gallicus* . . . (London, 1585), p. 25v.
[9] Daniel Cox, *A Discourse, Wherein the Interest of the Patient in Reference to Physick and Physicians is Soberly Debated, Many Abuses of the Apothecaries in the Preparing of their Medicines are detected* . . . (London, 1669), p. 77. Harold J. Cook writes in *The Decline of the Old Medical Regime in Stuart London* (Ithaca and London, 1986), pp. 167–70 that Cox was one of a group of experimental physicians who were trying to make the College more empirical, his language, nevertheless, often expressed the traditional, rational, virtues.

There was tension between the rational and the empirical even for that most empirical of English physicians, Thomas Sydenham. He was certainly suspicious of theory:

He that in physick shall lay down fundamental maxims and from thence drawing consequence and raising dispute shall reduce it into the regular form of a science has indeed done something to enlarge the art of talking . . . And he that thinks he came to be skild in diseases by studying the doctrine of the humors, that the notions of obstructions and putrefaction assists him in the cure of fevers, or that by the acquaintance he had with sulphur and mercury he was into this useful discovery, that what medicines and regimen as certainly kill in the latter end of some fevers as they cure in others, may as rationally believe that his cook owes his skill in roasting and boiling to his study of the elements and that his speculations about fire and water have taught him that the same seething liquors that boils the egg hard makes the hen tender.[10]

Sydenham developed this philosophical position when he tried to study illnesses by observation alone. However, in his practice he made the jump 'into the hidden causes of things'.[11] I will return to this case, but one look at Sydenham's advice to a patient of his, John Locke, shows him as an oldfashioned rationalist.

You may not in the least doubt but that a steady persisting in the use of the following directions (grounded not an opinion but uninterrupted experience) will at last effect your desired cause. First, therefore, in order to the diverting and subduing also the ichorose matter 'twill be requisite to take your pills twice a week as for example every Thursday and Sunday about 4 o'clock in the morning and your clyster in the intermitting days about six, constantly till you are well. In the next place, foreasmuch as there is wanting in bodies broken with business and dispirited upon the before mentioned accounts, that stock of natural heat which should bring the matter quickly to digestion 'twill be highly necessary that you cherish yourself as much as can be going to bed very early at night, even at 8 o'clock.[12]

Sydenham may have known by experience that his method would work (the pills, the clyster, the sleep) but the diverting and subduing of the 'ichorose matter' and the natural heat and its digestive power were hidden, theoretical matters. Nevertheless, patients, even one like John Locke, needed to be given reasons for remedies and what better way of explaining things, honorary virtuoso to virtuoso, than by using the language of traditional humoral medicine.

The problem for physicians who wanted to base their work on experience alone was that they might have ended up like Willis and Sydenham reasoning about events in the body during illness or therapy which often could not be known by observation or experiment. This

---

[10] In Kenneth Dewhurst, *Dr Thomas Sydenham (1624–1689), His Life and Original Writings* (Berkeley and Los Angeles, 1966), p. 81.
[11] *Ibid.*, p. 81: 'But proud man, not content with that knowledge he was capable of and was useful to him, would needs penetrate into the hidden causes of things, lay down principles and establish maxims to him self about the operations of nature.'   [12] *Ibid.*, p. 167–8.

was less of a problem for writers like Cheyne who easily moved from general principles (mechanical or chemical) in physiology, pathology and finally to treatment. William Cole's discussion of apoplexy in *A Physico-Medical Essay* (1689)[13] is a good example of this. Cole began with general corpuscular theory mixed with anatomical findings to explain brain function and disfunction; he used the bills of mortality to discover the prevalent seasons for the condition and finally, having arrived at the view that cold changed the brain's tone so that particles in the air could enter it to cause apoplexy, he produced a rational treatment for it. However, as Cheyne acknowledged, the logical progress from fundamentals to specifics could be interrupted, though his certainty in the former remained undiminished:

Perhaps my manner of explaining some great and fundamental truths, and a few of the consequences I draw by my method, may be defective: And perhaps, from some of the links being dropt, and from faults in the wording, the chain of the reasoning may not be always clear and strong; but I am sure the foundation is solid and just.[14]

Whether a physician was an empiricist or rationalist (the latter did, of course, allow empirical data to enter into the argument) there does seem to have been a major difficulty for each in the new medicine of the later seventeenth and early eighteenth centuries. The principles of the new medicine, derived as they were from the physical sciences, were abstract and non-biological as Boerhaave put it:

Nothing is more evident that the general rules which are deduced from mechanical experiments; but nothing is more uncertain than what mechanicians assert from those general rules concerning the human body.[15]

The empiricist needed to give a rational account of the working of an illness or a treatment to satisfy the reader or patient, but in so doing could fall from his philosophical position. Again, as Boerhaave wrote, although reasoning (and here he meant reasoning in the traditional medical sense of describing hidden causes for effects) together with the collecting of facts formed the basis of physic, it was nevertheless suspect:

The art of physic was anciently established (1.) by a faithful collection of facts observed, whose effects were (2.) afterwards explained, and their causes assigned by

[13] William Cole, *A Physico-Medical Essay Concerning the Late Frequency of Apoplexies* (Oxford, 1689).
[14] George Cheyne, *An Essay on Regimen* (London, 1740), Preface, p. VII. Dr John Henry (private communication) suggests that Cheyne may have meant by 'fundamental truths' the findings of the senses, which all proponents of the new science took to be fundamental rather than fundamental, theoretical, ideas. The context of the passage and the first chapter where the body is described as 'an hydraulic machine', as if it was an indisputable truth, inclines me to remain with the latter interpretation.
[15] H. Boerhaave, *Academical Lectures on the Theory of Physic*, 6 vols. (London, 1742–6), I, p. 47.

the assistance of reason; the first carries conviction along with it, and is indisputable; nothing being more certain than demonstration from experience, but the latter is more dubious and uncertain; since every sect may explain the causes of particular effects upon different hypotheses.[16]

The tensions produced by the application of the teachings of one sect, those of the mechanical philosophers, to medicine, can be seen in the history of eighteenth-century medicine: the rise and fall of different systems, and descriptions of diseases based upon symptoms rather than causes. Instead of using hindsight and giving as a reason for this the absence from the eighteenth century of organic chemistry, bio-chemistry, neurobiology, molecular biology and the other disciplines that span the gap between the physical sciences and the body, I want to briefly look at other types of reasons for difficulties faced by physicians in the period of the new science.

If one takes the long view and contrasts the later part of the seventeenth century with the centuries immediately before, it becomes apparent that in certain respects there was no such thing as a new medicine. The picture of the physical world may have been trans-formed. The same did not happen for medicine despite appearances. The preservation of health was discussed in terms of the six non-naturals both in the renaissance and the eighteenth century.[17] It made sense for both humoralist and mechanist, given the conditions of life, to see health in terms of one's food, drink, exercise and passions. The fact that today this still applies is no reason to be blind to such categories. In disease, the language used to describe the secret happenings in the body was the same for both the late seventeenth century and the period before. Despite the impression of objectivity, the use of analogy and metaphor to create the images of fight, defence, penetration, expressing the movement from symptom to cause – were the same for the two periods. Here is Cheyne on sulphur as a remedy for gout:

By its agreeable taste and lightness on the stomach . . . its tenacity, ropiness and elasticity; the smallness of its parts; their efficacy in destroying the mischief of all saline particles, with their natural warmth, join'd to the activity of its acid salt, (making it a kind of natural soap) it enters the small vessels, where no other dilutent, hitherto known, can come; cleanses their insides from the foulness that sticks to them; imbibes and retains all the gouty salts, and carries them out of the body by perspiration; softens, smooths and relaxes the parch'd and stiffn'd fibres; and by leaving some of its oily parts on their surfaces sheaths and defends them from the points of the salts afterwards introduc'd.[18]

---

[16] *Ibid.*, p. 42.
[17] On the non-naturals see L. J. Rather, 'The Six Things Non-Natural: A Note on the Origins and Fate of a Doctrine and a Phrase', *Clio Medica*, III, (1968), 337–47; P. Niebyl 'The Non-Naturals', *Bulletin of the History of Medicine*, XLIII (1971), 486–92.
[18] George Cheyne, *An Essay of the True Nature and Due Methods of Treating the Gout* (London, 1723), p. 39.

There are several points to be made about this sort of language. First of all it was qualitative, the only difference is that instead of the humors and herbs of the sixteenth century we have chemicals. A theory, even one as powerful as the mechanical or corpuscular, could not immediately overcome a deeply rooted way of describing substances. (Its practitioners might have stated that they were not yet at the stage where they could dispense with such language.) Sir John Floyer explicitly recognized in *The Preternatural State of Animal Humours Described by their Sensible Qualities* (1696) that the new philosophy, particularly experimental chemistry, still had a place for the perception of qualities and that as the title of another book of his had it, one could discover 'the Virtues of vegetables, minerals and animals by their tastes and smells'.[19] The public had to use their own taste, smell and sight when deciding what was good meat, fish or water. We still sometimes do this today, but public health bodies and scientific methods and analysis have replaced subjective judgement. In the seventeenth and eighteenth centuries the qualities of things were matters of everyday importance. So Cheyne would have been able to take his audience along with him when he wrote:

All other things being equal, vegetables and animals of a strong, poignant, aromatic and hot taste, are harder to digest than those of a milder, softer and more insipid taste.[20]

In the case of illness, patient, relative and doctor also had to use a qualitative evaluation of the state of the patient's body. Cheyne's description of the hidden effects of sulphur on gout was a narrative, a story of courageous deeds in the body, and it was couched in qualitative terms. On both these counts it was accessible to the patient, in fact Cheyne's treatise was ostensibly written for a patient. This accessibility has been discussed recently by Jewson and Porter (and in a forthcoming article by Nicolson).[21] But let me add a caveat before going overboard for the open market-place theory of the medical world of the eighteenth century where patient dictated financially to the doctor and where the latter had to tailor his explanations to the understanding of the former. One can imagine Cheyne giving bits of the above

---

[19] Sir John Floyer, Φαρμακο-Βαϐανος *Or the Touch-Stone of Medicines. Discovering the Virtues of Vegetables, Minerals, and Animals by their Tastes and Smells*, 2 vols. (London, 1687–91).

[20] Cheyne, *An Essay of Health and Long Life*, p. 26.

[21] N.D. Jewson, 'Medical Knowledge and the Patronage System in 18th Century England', *Sociology*, VIII (1974), 269–285; Roy Porter, 'Laymen, Doctors and Medical Knowledge in the Eighteenth Century: The Evidence of the *Gentleman's Magazine*', in Roy Porter (ed.), *Patients and Practitioners. Lay Perceptions of Medicine in Pre-industrial Society* (Cambridge, 1985), pp. 283–314. Malcolm Nicolson, 'The Metastatic Theory of Pathogenesis and the Professional Interests of the Eighteenth Century Physician', *Medical History*, (forthcoming).

explanation when treating a patient with sulphur but, although the explanation in its form and much of its content was accessible to the patient, being part of a common experience (a story structure and qualitative description), the tone of the story presupposes an unravelling, an explanation of complex workings – as such it is specialized knowledged possessed by the physician alone. (There are no contradictions here: just think of the status of the Homeric poet and the popularity of his stories.)

Nevertheless, it was probably the need to be understood by the patient that led to the graphic, qualitative element in medical theory. A part may also have been played by the poorly regulated market composed of wise women, herbalists, empirics, astrologers, apothecaries, chemists, barber–surgeons, physicians, as well as those less clearly defined as practitioners: the self-help patients, family members, neighbours, clergymen. As long as physicians competed in this type of market, they could not afford to mystify their clients by going overboard for chemical or Newtonian medicine. Instead, they had the best of both worlds: the cachet of a fashionable new theory, but expressed in a language which reflected how illness had traditionally been perceived (and still is by many lay people today).

MEDICAL PRACTICE

If medical theory, as it related to illness and therapy, did not change in its basic structure, what of medical practice? Again, at first sight, the answer is easy. If we follow some recent historians who have reflected in their work the 'professional' and occupational divides in medicine, and take at face value the rhetoric of the London College of Physicians against the empirics, or of traditional Galenists against empiricists influenced by the 'new science', then clearly there was great change and disunity in the world of late seventeenth-century medicine, and this had its counterpart in the relatively recent changes in theory (Paracelsian, chemical, mechanical).[22] At one level this picture cannot

---

[22] See, for instance, Theodore M. Brown, 'The College of Physicians and the Acceptance of Iatromechanism in England 1665–1695, *Bulletin of the History of Medicine*, XIVL (1970), 12–30; Theodore M. Brown, 'Physiology and the Mechanical Philosophy in Mid-Seventeenth Century England', *Bulletin of the History of Medicine*, LI (1977) 25–54; Michael Hunter, *Science and Society in Restoration England* (Cambridge, 1981) is wide-ranging and subtle but still gives great emphasis to institutions, especially the Royal Society; see also the valuable new work by Harold J. Cook, *The Decline of the Old Medical Regime in Stuart London*. The large amount of work on the Royal Society and, to a lesser extent, on the College of Physicians has perhaps put too much emphasis on the growth and internal struggles of institutions, and on lines of demarcation.

be denied. But underlying this diversity there was some unity in medical practice (and at this point my focus moves from the question of change to that of its approximate opposite, unity).

Diversity fits a medical market-place where medical authority and licensing was not strong enough to impose uniformity. But a market-place, if it deals in one commodity (here health, or cure of disease) must show not only diversity but unity, the outward differences which make the goods attractive conceal underlying similarities, otherwise how could customers recognize them in the first place and make comparisons? Patients certainly moved easily between different types of practitioner and ignored the rhetoric that sought to demonstrate that the members of a particular group were the sole practitioners of proper medicine. In about 1652 Willis described the case of Mrs White of Pusey who 'has suffered from the spitting of thick and yellow coloured matter in which there were sometimes blood-stained flecks'. He noted that she had dipped into the medical market-place (which by extension included self-help and the family):

She has so far tried many remedies during the summer from her brother, a learned doctor; she also began studying medicine, and recently has taken from empiric women many remedies which are said to be good for phthisis. Since the disease grows worse she begs me and her brother to prescribe some method of cure, if this be possible.[23]

The easy movement of the sufferer from one type of practitioner to another may indicate that the differences between practitioners were more real to the providers of health than to the buyers. Certainly, the patient often was seen as a poor judge of the quality of medical practice. Daniel Turner wrote in *The Modern Quack, or the Physical Imposter Detected* (1718) that his purpose was:

to set before Mens Eyes the great Danger they incur by meddling with any Medicines (let their titles be never so specious) sold in divers Parts of this City at Tradesmens Shops and which are indeed not other than so many *Baits* laid to defraud them farther, that no great or powerful Medicine can be prepar'd but that if taken in this way of publick *Advertisement* in *News-papers*, or distributed by Bills, either given into their Hands, or posted upon Posts, altho' the nicest Directions that can be are delivered therewith, yet will the same be liable to do more Harm than Good.[24]

It was not only the 'Common People' who lacked judgement and had to be warned:

---

[23] Kenneth Dewhurst, (ed.), *Willis's Oxford Casebook (1650–52)* (Oxford, 1981), p. 147. Dewhurst points out that Willis had mixed views about empirics: he 'warned that a quack's remedies are "like a sword in a blind man's hand"' (p. 41) but he also thought that empirics' remedies could be better than a physician's (p. 50); Willis himself early on worked as a 'piss prophet' or uroscopist at Abingdon market (p. 128).

[24] Daniel Turner, *The Modern Quack, Or the Physical Imposter Detected* (London, 1718), p. a2v.

The Common People did I say? I might, I think, have included all Orders and Degrees of Men, since we find oftentimes those of great Fortunes, and as great a Share of Understanding in other Matters, have been in this way impos'd on as much as others.[25]

Rhetoric such as this can bear a different intepretation: it shows that the buyers of health were not impressed by the differences in medical practice. If this was the case, what were the common structures in medical practice that allowed patients to move across different parts of the market? Clearly it was not a structure based upon theory, at least as expressed in the different viewpoints of Galenists, astrologers, Paracelsians, chemists and iatrochemists. Although, as noted above, underneath the surface of new theories there can be discerned the same type of qualitative narrative that had helped to make sense of the inner happenings of the body. There were probably two structures. One is banal but important. People wanted remedies and all types of practitioners offered them. In the end all practitioners were nostrum pedlers. The second common structure was the wrapping around the remedies. Practitioners rationalized about their remedies and made them appear appropriate and attractive to buyers. How this was done varied in elaboration, the most expensive and thick wrapping being of the 'rational' physician who tailored the remedy to the niceties of the patient's constitution, others might imitate the 'rational' physician, but use less time and care over the fit between remedy and patient or they might advertise their wares by appealing to experience and authority. The language in which this was expressed could vary according to the practitioner's theoretical standpoint. Another way of putting it is that all practitioners gave out remedies and that the empiric was a bit of a rationalist and vice versa.

THE PHYSICIAN'S PRACTICE

James Clegg, the dissenting Derbyshire minister and physician, wrote in his diary on 28 of August 1723 about the case of his daughter Margaret who on the 19th 'was seized with a violent pain in her stomach and bowels, which was attended by frequent and painful vomiting of green and yellow choler, this continued about 3 days'. The structure of Clegg's treatment is significant. He responded not only to the general condition, but also to the day-to-day state of his daughter, and he also tried to foresee complications. He attempted to deal with both the causes of the illness (clearing the choler and absorbing the acid) and with its symptoms (settling the stomach, quietening pain):

[25] Ibid., p. a2v.

I endeavoured to clear her stomach of it (choler) by giving her frequently to drink a decoction of camomile and tea, and chicken broth but her pain still continued and vehement sickness. After the vomiting staid, I then gave her a little Diacodium, but very little to compose her spirits, settle her stomach and procure sleep. She rested better but awakened very sick and thus continued two days more. I ordered a cooling clyster for she was very hot and restless her pulse quick, breath very short. The clyster brought nothing away, in the evening I ordered another which gave only one stool, hard greenish and very foetid. Her fever increased, I had before ordered and continued to give her powder of crabs claws, oyster shells and nutmeg with sugar to absorb the acid and sweeten the juices in her stomach. On the Saturday the pain in her belly being violent I gave her about one scruple and a half of Rhubarb in powder in syrup of July flowers to procure a passage and gentle discharge. On the day following she had a stool and found ease but it continued not long . . . her fever increased, her pulse quick, breath short . . . On the Monday morning another stool, loose but not very large, at noon she parted with much wind and found some ease. She was restless and hot and in frequent sweats. I feared a diorrhea and to prevent it gave her the white decoction with tormentil root . . . but on Monday night . . . she grew much worse her tongue faltered her pulse quicker but weaker the phlegm disturbed her she sweat much and slumbered, but awakened sick. Thus she continued til about '6 a clock and then departed.[26]

In some ways this is a very empirical piece of description. It has a Hippocratic air about it, it notes the pulse, breath, stools, etc. as well as the other symptoms. It is rational in so far as there seem to be reasons for the treatment ('a cooling clyster for she was very hot and restless . . .'), and at very stage of the illness Clegg responded with treatment for the changing symptoms. The attempt to give rational treatment, whether in the strong form to causes or more weakly to symptoms, was significant especially in the eyes of physicians. Cheyne praised the 'Medicina philosophica seu rationalis' where the virtues and uses of medicines were known and adjusted to the causes of a particular illness so that 'the best natural philosopher will . . . ever be the best physician'.[27] Whether Clegg was rational in the sense of attacking the causes rather than the symptoms of the illness is a moot question. I am possibly stretching a point by taking choler and acid to be the causes of the illness in Clegg's mind, though I suspect they were.

Clegg could also have been rational in another sense. He may have seen his daughter's symptoms as the indications of her constitution during the illness. Indications were crucial for the Galenic *methodus medendi* and helped to differentiate learned medicine from that of the empirics by stressing that as indications varied from person to person the care had to be tailored to the individual and not to the illness. (The indications would include the patient's normal constitution, the time

[26] James Clegg, *The Diary of James Clegg of Chapel en le Firth 1708–1755*, ed. Vanessa S. Doe, part I, (Derbyshire Record Soc. II, 1978), pp. 19–20.
[27] George Cheyne, *The Natural Method of Cureing of the Diseases of the Body and the Disorders of the Mind depending on the Body* (London, 1742), pp. 64–5.

of year as well as the changing state of the patient.) Richard Browne, a licentiate of the College of Physicians, saw the difference between the ways in which physicians and empirics treated their patients in this way:

their general directions for such their trash ['the pills and elixirs of our quacks'] are sufficiently exploded. For it requires the deliberate and particular consideration of the best physician, whether to purge his patient at all, and (if requisite) with what sort of physic, and when to terminate the dose. Of how many murders then must they be guilty that let fly their poisonous, ill prepared and worse proportioned doses at a venture among the multitude, upon their own and their poor deluded patients small discretion when and how to take them.[28]

Despite such propaganda for the physicians it may not be unfair to compare their practice with that of the empirics. In some ways Clegg was practising as an empiric, as did many other much more learned physicians. What Clegg was doing was to give a nostrum for each particular stage of the illness, just as an empiric gave a single nostrum to cover all the stages of the illness. Moreover, the treatments that Clegg gave at the different stages of his daughter's illness were pretty standard ones – for instance, cooling clysters and testaceous powders. If one looks at his general practice we find him giving similar standard treatments, with little individual tailoring. Clegg's practice was a busy one, he often had to travel miles across country to visit patients and he could not be with them during all the stages of their illness as he could with his daughter. On 24 September 1728 he wrote:

Visited Mrs Waterhouse at Martinside she is afflicted with an hysteric asthma. I prescribed gum ammoniac in Vin(egar) Solu(tion) and spermacelis after bleeding. Visited Mrs Swan at Waley Bridge. She was in an intermitting fever. I ordered an electuary of the bark and a julep. I was called thence to Mrs Barber at Malcoff and found her in a fever, took some blood and gave her a vomit which answered well.[29]

In the following days he saw Mrs Barber again, but gave no details of her illness or treatment. What we have here resembles, in a sense, the practice of a modern G.P., with little time available for patients and a preference for standard treatments.

Some apothecaries apparently argued that they could tell from previous experience of a physician's prescribing practice what he would order for any one case, that in other words, physicians had standard treatments:

I have heard several of the apothecaries confidently (not to say impudently) affirm they were so thoroughly acquainted with such mens practice, naming some eminent

[28] Richard Browne, *The Cure of Old Age and Preservation of Youth by Roger Bacon* . . . *Translated out of Latin; with Annotations* . . . (London, 1683), p. 91.

[29] Clegg, *Diary*, I, p. 42.

physicians that if they knew the case they would lay a wager they did exactly predict before they took pen in hand what they would prescribe.[30]

Daniel Coxe, defending rational medicine wrote, rather unconvincingly:

the knowledge they derive from doctors prescripts is very uncertain, and fallacious: it being absolutely impossible for the best physician to calculate a medicine that shall be proper for all that are, or shall be subject to any one disease, unless he were possessor of the Univeral Remedy. So great is the variety of complexions, so many are the complications of distempers and so infinite the variations of circumstances: all of which the judicious physician attends to, and which few apothecaries are capable of comprehending.[31]

Yet with no statistically-based clinical trials, rational medicine was a lottery, just like the empirics' nostrum. Moreover, the value of particular treatments for particular constitutions would often be a matter of subjective judgement and controversy despite general rules such as the cure by contrary. Clegg illustrated this, and also how the provincial physician could disagree (and be ignored) by his London superiors, when he wrote on 10 September 1725:

I was desired by my dear and good friend Mrs Elizab. Bagshaw to visit her second son Adam then dangerously ill of the small pox in London . . . Found the young man very full of smallpox of a bad kind under the care of a London physician called Knapp. The second fever came on the day after we came there. Dr Mead was called in. Blisters were applied to his arms, unseasonably as I thought, a strangury succeeded. Cordials were given but no sleeping potions were administered, nor could I prevail to have them. The fever continued to rise much on Friday. He had been without stool 12 to 13 days. I urged the necessity of clysters, but no stool could be procured tho' many were administered. On Saturday a delirium . . . and on the 19th Lords day morning . . . he expired.[32]

One can understand why people collected successful remedies and noted the sequence of remedies used in particular cases, (in other words the methods of cure). Traditional rational medicine, which emphasized the individuality of each case, could produce uncertainty; one could not easily use past cases as a guide to future ones as each case was supposed to be unique. But the ties with rational medicine were often broken, if unconsciously. The collections of John Hall and James Cook on successful cases, *Select Observations on English Bodies of Eminent Persons in Disparate Diseases* (1679), were published for instruction and imitation – despite the authors' seeming orthodoxy. Sydenham, of course, saw methods of cure as the solution to the problem of being a rational physician who did not want to go beyond

[30] Daniel Cox, *A Discourse*, pp. 75–6.   [31] *Ibid.*, pp. 74–5.
[32] Clegg, *Diary*, I, p. 22.

X

experience. Sometimes lay people noted down successful cures and remedies. In 1681, William Blundell, who had recovered from a 'violent cold' ordered his servant, Walter Thelwall, to write down all the medicines that he had been given by his doctor and by the 'elder Lady Bradshaigh': After listing the medicines Thelwall wrote:

My master's opinion of these several things in particular is here to be inserted for further use, viz. That the spirits first named, of which twenty-six drops were put into a small cap of barley water and beer or into barley water alone, had no apparent effect, although he doth not much doubt but the secret effect might be good. That the like might be said of the pills . . . although it seemed that they did somewhat assuage his cough, which was extremely violent. The Lohoch, a liquor like a syrup, did apparently bring up phlegm, and was well liked. The lozenges were pleasant and did sometimes stop the cough. Barley water . . .[33]

Here we have less the holistic sense of a method of cure, more that of remedies being sampled one by one, in other words an empirical approach very close to that of the empirics. There is really very little difference between a nostrum touted in an empiric's bill and one of Blundell's remedies:

The elder Lady Bradshaigh sent my master a bottle containing as we guess, about one ounce of balsam, which in her letter she calls (if we read it aright) balsam of sulphur. Her Ladyship then saith that it is an approved cure for a cough; that she had it from Sir Peter Brooks that it had cured him of a most violent cough, and that the Lady Ossory had sent it to him.[34]

Apart from the commercial note the advertisement below had essentially the same message as Lady Bradshaigh's letter:

Doctor John Turner his most excellent lozenges approved by Doctor George Bowls, and many others to excel the best and most approved lozenges which have been heretofore made by any other person whatsoever, for the preventing and curing of consumptions, coughs of all sorts, pthisics, putrified and corrupted lungs . . . You may take two or three of them at night.[35]

In both cases the remedy was to be used regardless of the type of patient (in terms of complexion, way of life, stage of illness, etc.), but they employed a common wrapping, experience and authority ('approved cure', 'approved lozenges', Sir Peter Brookes, Lady Ossory, Doctor George Bowls).

Some historians have presented the rise of empirics in the second half of the seventeenth century as a sudden disjunction in the practice of medicine. Certainly contemporaries were aware of their increase, and historians have rightly emphasized their effect on orthodox physicians and have given increased consumer spending and national prosperity

---

[33] T. Ellison Gibson, *A Cavalier's Note-Book* (London, 1880), pp. 245–6.   [34] *Ibid.*, p. 244.
[35] Advertisement in British Library collection of medical advertisements c.112 fo. 9.

as one of the main reasons for the explosion in the numbers.[36] However, empirics had been around from the sixteenth century and before as had physicians' diatribes against them.[37] Moreover, there is no evidence that patients' expectation of treatment underwent a radical change at this time despite what one reads from self-serving defences of the College of Physicians. What is likely, I would argue, is that the medicine of the empirics was acceptable to many patients because this is what occurred in their experience when they were treated by physicians: each stage of their illness was cured by a remedy, (whereas for the physician the treatment was a response to the changing state of the patient), the difference was that the empiric offered to cure the whole illness with one remedy. Empiric medicine was also familiar because it was analogous to the centuries-old practice of offering remedies to family and friends; indeed it is worth remembering that family remedies were sometimes equated with empirical medicine, and that physicians were seen as attacking both. The young law student, Dudley Ryder, noted that his cousin:

talked also about empiric medicines, which he said he begun to have a much better opinion of, for he recovered his daughter by some of them given him by a gentlewoman, after all that the doctor could prescribe had proved useless and ineffectual. But the doctors had made it their business to decry all this kind of receipts which are in the hands of private persons and thereby made persons of good sense and thought afraid to use any of them, though no doubt there may be very good receipts lodged in private hands.[38]

---

[36] See S.H. Holbrook, *The Golden Age of Quackery* (New York, 1959); Eric Jameson, *The Natural History of Quackery* (London, 1961); W.F. Bynum and Roy Porter (eds.), *Medical Fringe and Medical Orthodoxy 1750–1850* (London, 1986). On the increase in consumerism in the eighteenth century see G. Holmes, *Augustan England: Professions, State, and Society 1680–1730* (London, 1982); N. McKendrick, J. Brewer and H.J. Plumb, *The Birth of a Consumer Society* (London, 1982).

[37] For instance, the Frankfurt physician Johann Hartmann Beyer, wrote that 'mad, deaf, toothless witches, priests, barbers, porters, Jews, murderers, and criminals who deserve the cross, and also people who are bereft of reason, are all rich with remedies . . .', in Girolamo Capivaccio, *Pratica Medica* (Frankfurt, 1594) sig. 4v. See also the attack on empirics and uroscopists in J. Langius, *Epistolarum Medicinalium* (Frankfurt, 1589) p. 999; P. Forestus, *De Incerto, Fallaci Urinarium Judicio* (Leyden, 1589). William Clowes, *A Briefe . . . Treatise . . . Morbus Gallicus*, pp. 9–10 writes of how 'in these days, it is the more lamentable to see how so famous an art, and the true professors of the same, are thus spurned at, trodden down, embaced and defaced, through the wicked behaviour and counterfeit gloses of the afore named rude rable of obscure and imperfect experimenters and such prating peasants and ignorant asses'. Specifically, he condemned the 'cosinage and lewd crafts of one Valentine Rarsworme of Smalcade' and 'his adherents commonly called quacksalvers, mountebanks, landlopers, fugitives and other masterless makeshifts, the very spawn and frie of blind boldness and ignorance'.

[38] Dudley Ryder, *The Diary of Dudley Ryder 1715–1716*, ed. William Matthews (London, 1939), pp. 276–7.

X

I would argue that because there was, and had been for centuries a multiplicity of practitioners of various types, so there were no clearly defined boundaries between rational medicine and that of the empirics. But before discussing this further it is worth saying more about the nature of rational, orthodox medicine.

In a sense, time, rather than education or philosophy, was the criterion that served to distinguish physicians from empirics. The more time one could devote to a patient the more one could be a rational physician. But time was expensive and probably only physicians with rich clients could go into a very great deal of detail and study the patient's way of life and symptoms. However, the practice of John Symcotts and that of the surgeons Joseph Binne and Richard Wiseman shows that ordinary practitioners could give time and consideration to a patient.[39] Sir Edmund King was one such expensive physician, his case-book is full of rich and noble clients. In November 1679 he wrote down the details of a patient: 'A fine young lady aged about 22 florid complexion . . . beautiful and a widow. Had laboured under violent paines in her stomach and sides for a year and a half'. He noted her previous treatments, she had been 'through many courses of physic, with several Doctors, abundance of stools, several waters, without relief also bitter drinks'. He also let her tell him her idiosyncrasies, 'purging made her worse', and on another visit listed what brought on the pain:

1. fasting too long. 2. eating too much. 3. tea after dinner. 4. apple pie or apples. 5. chocolate ill made.[40]

All this information would need time to be elicited, but as the patient could give her views to the doctor she presumably felt happier for the personal attention, the doctor richer, whilst the norms of rational physic would have been fulfilled. Of course, not all physicians would go along with this and the doctor–patient interview has never been the easiest thing to manage even in the early eighteenth century, which recent historical work tells us was a time of patient power. For instance, on 13 June 1716 Dudley Ryder wrote, 'Intended to go to Dr Wadsworth about the pain in my arm, which is not yet gone, and also to talk with him about my whole constitution.' The next day he went to see Dr Wadsworth 'I intended to talk with the Doctor about my whole

---

[39] F.N.L. Poynter and W.J. Bishop, *A Seventeenth Century Doctor and His Patients: John Symcotts 1592?–1662* (Bedfordshire Historical Record Soc. XXXI, 1950); Joseph Binne, 'Chirurgical Observations 1633–1663', B.L. Sloane MS. 153; Richard Wiseman, *Severall Chirurgical Treatises* (London, 1676).

[40] Sir Henry King, 'Medical Cases and Receipts', B.L. Sloane MS. 1589, fos. 144, 146.

constitution, about the cold bath and Tunbridge and Bath waters. But when I came to talk with him I was at a loss what to say'.[41]

It may be a little unhistorical to talk of patient dominance in the doctor–patient relationship at this time, possibly we may be introducing modern concerns too much into the past. Yet there is no doubt that patients knew about rational medicine and spoke its language (Ryder's 'whole constitution'). A patient wrote to Sir Hans Sloane:

> I have been free from that complaint which I made to you at that time but cannot get rid of a very great heat, especially in my hands and feet which is very uneasy to me, and more than all the rest my tongue is grown worse than when I was in town, though not so bad as it has been sometimes, I have taken the bark as you ordered, and now drink the asses milk, I am weak and have very little appetite and no good sleeper. Pray Sir be so obliging as to think over this account of a crazy constitution.[42]

The reference to some of the non-naturals (appetite, sleep, constitution) tells us that patients had also been educated into the ways of rational medicine. The parenthetical and pathetic 'though not so bad as it has been sometimes' also tells us that anxiety and hope do not disappear even when the patient pays the doctor and apparently dominates the relationship (the binary opposition of dominance/subordination seems too simple here, and one can doubt the applicability of the Jewson thesis at the psychological level of the doctor–patient relationship as opposed to its financial and contractual aspects).

The large number of correspondents to Sir Hans Sloane, patients, their relatives and doctors who asked for medical advice seem to speak the language of rational medicine. Lay people used fewer technical terms, but many of the correspondents tried to give an account of the case which included the general condition of the patient and the various stages of the illness and the treatments used at each stage.

A representative example of how an orthodox practitioner saw a case is Charles Kimberley's report to Sloane of his patient, Mr Isted:

> I found his blood very firie, his pulse very regular, no thirst, a little clamminess in his tongue, urine good in quantity. His chief complaints were little wandering pains . . . and a great inclination towards sweat. I encouraged a gentle perspiration to the 20th but found no other alteration in any particular than his being tired with his confinement. On the 22nd I gave him a purge with manna, which worked very well, his pains still the same, leaving stiffness behind them. I have debarred him malt liquors and all seasoned meats. His chief drink is wine and Bristol waters and the wood decoction of your prescribing. Upon some little irregularity in the non-nat(ura)ls he has had a looseness, I think, not to his disadvanatage. His appetite is very good and what he eats gives him no uneasiness. His blood is foul and abounds with acid salts. Mercurial

[41] Ryder, *Diary*, p. 256, p. 257.
[42] Sir Hans Sloane, 'Medical Correspondence', B.L. Sloane MS. 4075, fos. 340–1. I am currently researching Sloane's medical correspondence.

purges by breaking the viscid cohaesions of the blood and attracting those salts might be of great service; but I doubt not you are very well acquainted with the prejudice Mr. Isted has conceived against them.[43]

The description of pulse, urine, the use of diet as a form of treatment all point to Kimberley being a rational physician. His description of the blood and its acid salts and the effect of mercury on them is one of the infrequent uses in the letters of the new science when rationalizing about the effects of remedies.

Patients, however, could move easily between rational and empiric medicine. John Evelyn wrote in 1703 to Sloane about his piles. He wrote that he was greatly troubled with them though:

Now is being look'd upon as a slight infirmity amongst my visitant neighbours, everyone is ready to recommend their remedies, as ointments of the ashes of oak. The bones of green fish calcind to a fine powder, and inwardly sulphurous lozenges etc. But none of these do stay them [the piles] from their periodic descend.

Evelyn then requested from Sloane what was really a nostrum, but he fully realized that he had to supply the details required by a rational physician.

If therefore you have any topiq [topical medicine] which might hinder them from falling down, it would be a mighty soulieyoument [?] to a weary octogenerius: I have always been naturally costive which by straining I believe irritates: but lenitive electuary relieves me, when my belly is hard and ponderous. I have in the meantime a good appetite and eat of everything that is tender; shellfish from the sea weekly, and of my own ponds. But my ill digestion makes me cautious. My urine which for 3 or 4 years past was as pale as clear water, is of late come to be of a landuble colour, nor have I been sensible of nephritic pains. In the morning I now and then drink a glass of meath made with birch-water: sometimes Grewell.[44]

In his next letter Evelyn discussed the success of Sloane's remedies; he did not see them as a method of cure but as a separate number of items which might or might not have an effect. He wrote: 'nor do either the liniment or sulphur lozenges keep up their swelling at the constant period', whilst after bleeding 'That night (or evening rather) the piles descended with great pain'.[45]

So far I have tried to show that, although both patient and doctor knew what rational medicine entailed, nevertheless, in structural terms it could appear to merge with the medicine practiced by the empirics. I now turn to them.

[43] Ibid., fo. 353.   [44] Ibid., fo. 94.   [45] Ibid., fo. 96.

THE EMPIRICS' MEDICINE

Harold Cook has indicated in his recent book how Royal Society empiricists were taken to be close to empirics. Also Michael Hunter has noted how:

Thomas Wharton, Censor of the College . . . fulminated against 'this new upturned brood of Vertuosis' with their 'Jesuitisme and policy, English books, Experiments, and receipts in phisick', who were likely to influence all the families of Note in England'; he linked them with 'the swarmes of quackes, mountebacks, chymists, Apothecares, surgions' who were ruinous to our old and settled and approved practice of physick.[46]

Historians such as Harold Cook, Theodore Brown and Michael Hunter who have concentrated on institutional quarrels and, in this case on the spleen of the old guard in the College of Physicians and on the reform of the College, have given us valuable insights.[47] But it would be a pity if institutional history was our only entry into the world of physicians and empirics, as the recent work of Porter, Barry, Bynum and Loudon on empirics demonstrates there is more to be said than that.[48] My argument is that physicians and empirics were closer than has been suggested (the very fact that they competed with each other is a sign of closeness). I have sketched how the physicians in their rational practice may have been nearer than they thought to empirics. Is it possible to argue that empirics were, at times, approaching the rational practice, or at least, the rhetoric of the physicians?

I do not want to overturn completely the received idea of the empiric. Certainly, if one reads their bills or adverts they made outrageous claims, though so did an orthodox physician every time he undertook a cure. And the stigma of quack or mountebank was so real at the time that empirics sought to avoid it. One bill, headed by a magnificent coat of arms stated: 'There is lately come to London, an Italian Doctor, who never was any Stage-Quack or Mountebanck, who has been very successful in the speedy cures of these following Distempers Viz.'[49] R. Clark, 'Chymist' acknowledged that there was a prejudice against medicines sold by advertising, but he pointed to the similar practice of the College of Physicians:

I am very sensible People are averst against Medicines, that are publish'd by way of Bills, yet several Ingenious Men, and some Colledg Physicians have done, and still do the same by Medicines that have been successful for many years.[50]

[46] Hunter, *Science and Society in Restoration England*, p. 138.   [47] See note 22.
[48] See their essays in Bynum and Porter (eds.), *Medical Fringe and Medical Orthodoxy 1750–1850*.   [49] In *Medical Advertisements*.
[50] R. Clark, *Vermiculars Destroyed, With an Historical Account of Worms* . . . (London, 1690), p. 31.

However, some empirics, men such as William Salmon, 'the Ring-Leader or king of the Quacks', published books and entered the world of learning. Salmon,[51] who began as an assistant to a mountebank, came to practice medicine and astrology at the gate of St Bartholomews Hospital and sold 'an antidote against the plague and all pestilential Venom', 'Family pills' and an *Elixir Vitae*. He was attacked in 1700 in a broadsheet: 'The Churchyards and Burying places are everywhere ample witnesses of your travels.' Salmon published books on herbal remedies, on chemistry for medicine and medical case studies.[52] There was clearly a commercial motive in publishing. His *Medicina Practica: Or the Practical Physitian* (1707) gave his address at the Blue Boar and advertised his 'Balsam de Chili': 'It is an excellent balsam differing from that of Peru ... but no way inferior in virtues and excellency as the several experiments lately made of it by several learned physicians in the curing of diseases have given sufficient proof'. He claimed it cured pains, ulcers, bruises, coughs, epilepsy, apoplexy, convulsions, palsies, it killed worms, cured ruptures, dissolved soft stones, eased colic, griping, provoked menstruation, opened obstructions of the liver, etc.[53] Yet when one comes to the main body of the book it is clear that what we have is rational medicine with a strong commercial pitch. In cases of hysteria he advised:

> To quiet the irregular and turbulent motion of the Spirit and hysteric fumes the following things are fit to be done. First the stomach, and whole region of the abdomen are to be bathed with *Powers of Amber*, or *Pennyroyal* ... Secondly, the nostrils are to be often touched with *Postestates Cornu Cervi* ... Moreover, our *Tinctura Hysterica* should be at convenient times given in a little wine ... The third intention of cure, is to sweeten the acid salts and juices of the body, for which purpose there is certainly nothing more powerful and admirable than our *Spiritus Universalis* (which see in our *Phyl Medic Lib.* 2 cap 2) given twice a day ... or instead of this, *Volatile Sal Armoniack* ... Some possibly may prescribe preparations of Pearls, Coral, Amber, Crabs Eyes etc. [often prescribed], but these things (though after a very long using may do some good, yet) being fixt Alcalies, do not immediately enter into the mass of blood, and are therefore to be laid aside ... The fourth indication is to evacuate the morbific cause, or peccant humor, which you may most completely accomplish with my *Pilulae Mirabiles*.[54]

The Latin *Phyl Medic* Lib 2 cap 2 was a nice touch. Clearly Salmon was imitating the rational physicians; he was also using the more up to date reasoning – the acids and alkalies. So here we have a small paradox: an empiric, who employed the new philosophy but who also used the

[51] Daniel Turner, *The Modern Quack or, the Physical Imposter Detected* (London, 1718), p. 79.
[52] C.J.S. Thompson, *The Quacks of Old London* (London, 1928), pp. 126–31.
[53] William Salmon, *Medicina Practica: Or the Practical Physitian* (London, 1707), p. B1V–B2V.
[54] *Ibid.*, p. 62–3.

language of traditional Galenic medicine, 'peccant humour', 'intention' and 'indication' (he was slightly confused about the last) and who gave a story of what was going on in the body to account for the symptoms and to justify the treatment. If profit was really motivating Salmon, then we are being told what, in Salmon's judgement, it was that people wanted to read: a bit of the new (chemistry) and a bit of the old (reasoned medicine). Both theories were mixed at will without contradiction, both provided good advertising copy. Salmon used them to wrap up his remedies for prospective buyers and to describe how the medicines could intervene in the inner happenings of the body (only a College Physician or pedantic historian would point out Salmon's inconsistency in using two apparently different theories – the fact that they could be mixed was a sign of their underlying unity discussed earlier).

Daniel Turner's sour view of the 'learned' empiric betrays the fact that a little learning was good for trade:

You will say probably 'that some of these People who put out Bills and print Advertisements, must surely be able Men, for that they publish Books concerning the Distemper and apply solely or chiefly to the study thereof'. I grant they do indeed put up for Authors, and set forth Books, but were yourselves judges of the Subject they debate you would need no greater Evidence of their Ignorance, as well as evil Design; for tho' they have some tolerable good Books to Steal from or Plunder, yet so wretchedly unskill'd are they in both terms of Art and Method, that they have only jumbled up a heap of incoherent Matter, interlarded with false Latin, flat Nonsense, or Sense inspired, which is only fit to amuse poor ignorant People, who are ready to take for granted, that he who can write a book, must . . . be some great Scholar.[55]

Quacks certainly used the authority of scholarship to sell their wares, but by labelling their works as 'flat Nonsense', Turner side-stepped a major point: the *meaning* of the quacks' books and bills must have appealed to customers and in much the same way as Turner's own learned medicine. R. Clark, 'living at the Golden Ball in Devonshire Street' in his *Vermiculars Destroyed, with an Historical Account of Worms: Collected of the Best Authors, as well Ancient as Modern. And Experiments By that Admirable Invention of the Microscope*, advertised his powder, plaister and ointment. He did so in the context of appearing learned and citing authors in the best text-book fashion, up to date with accounts of microscopical experiments and careful of his readers' healths. On the last he gave full accounts of 'the diagnostic signs of worms', of the 'signs of health', and the following section of his very detailed instructions for taking the 'Pulvis benedictus' might have

[55] Turner, *The Modern Quack*, p. 85.

been approved by a College doctor (though not in all respects, the patient deciding his constitution may have been disagreeable):

So great is the difference in Constitutions, that it is impossible to propose any one Dose for all, though of an age; when a child of five or six years of age will, and do often take three Papers, and shall have with it no more stool than a man that takes the same quantity, therefore I would advise you to begin with a low dose, till you know the strength of your constitution, and keep that dose as gives only two or three stools.[56]

Anthony Daffy, 'student in physick' acknowledged the cultural and theoretical signposts of seventeenth-century medicine: God, experience, Nature, equilibrium of the temperament, the differences in constitutions and noxious humours. Yet, in his advertisement for his 'Elixir Salutatis' he had the best of both worlds, a medicine that could relate to all the above concepts and yet was still a nostrum powerful enough to transcend all the distinctions of rational medicine and therefore was useful for everyone. (This was commercially important, as the drink would not be limited, for instance, to young female phlegmatics, but could be sold to everyone.) Daffy described 'his health-bringing Drink' as:

A famous CORDIAL DRINK, Found out by Providence of the Almighty, and (for above Twenty years) Experienced by myself and diverse persons (whose names are at most of their Desires here inserted) a most Excellent Preservative of Mankind.

A SECRET

Far beyond any Medicament yet known, and is found so agreeable to Nature that it effects all its Operations, as Nature would have it, and as a virtual Expedient proposed by her, for reducing all her Extreams unto an Equal Temper; the same being fitted into all *Ages, Sexes, Complexions*, and *Constitutions*, and highly fortifying Nature against any Noxious humour, involving or offending the *Noble Parts*.[57]

The surgeon, John Marten who could be called an empiric also advertised his 'anti-venereal pills' in his *Treatise of all the Degrees and Symptoms of the Venereal Disease in both Sexes* (sixth edn 1708?) He titilated his readers with case-histories, but the structure of his treatment (relating it to symptoms and the changing state of the body) was no different from what the College physician would have done in a different disease (venereal disease was often left to surgeons).

The public probably were attracted by some aspects of rational medicine as they were by those of empiric medicine. The need to cater for the public, a desire for status and a belief that their medicines

---

[56] Clark, *Vermiculars Destroyed*, p. 27.
[57] Broadsheet in Wellcome Institute Library, Cabinet of seventeenth-century empirics' broadsheets.

deserved to be used in the best possible way – and this should not be underestimated – were probably all reasons that led empirics towards rational medicine.

The empirical virtuosi, whom Harold Cook has rightly seen as close to the empirics, could also at times approach rational practice. Sydenham, in the letter to Locke mentioned earlier, set out a very traditional and rational view of the case. As well as discussing the cause of the illness, 'the ichorose matter', etc. Sydenham considered:

Your age, ill habit of body and approach of winter concurring, it comes to pass that the distemper you complain of yields not so soon to remedies as it would do under contrary circumstances.[58]

He also discussed what foods and drink Locke should have or avoid. The emphasis on constitution, season, food and drink together with the discussion of the causes of the illness shows that in a case where the physician felt he should talk with, or in this example write to, a patient (and a friend) at length, the old structures of rational, traditional, medicine took over.

Another virtuoso, Robert Boyle, certainly published his favourite remedies and felt that one could learn from the shops of the chemists and from traders.[59] Yet the people who took his remedies wanted instructions if not reasons. Anne Conway in 1664 wrote to her husband that she wanted him to get directions from Boyle as to when one of his remedies should be taken, how long for, how much, and in what 'vehicle' and if it was good for scorbutical distempers as well for her headaches.[60] The need to know the dosage was a direct echo of rational medicine which sought to tailor remedies to the individual's constitution and illness. In today's medical practice the instructions on the bottle of pills, although they may make us feel they are addressed to us as individuals, usually make distinctions only between large groups such as adults or children. However, all types of medical practitioners (Galenists, empiricists, empirics) took some account of the desire of patients to have individualized remedies or at least doses (the special language used to extol 'universal' remedies reinforces the point). One of Salmon's bills advertising his 'family pills' recommended them to

[58] Dewhurst, *Sydenham*, p. 167.
[59] See R. Boyle, *Medicinal Experiments: Or, a Collection of Choice and Safe Remedies; Of the Reconcileableness of Specific Medicines to the Corpuscular Philosophy; The Advantages of the Use of Simple Medicines* in Robert Boyle, *The Works*, 6 vols. ed. Thomas Birch (London, 1772), V; and part 2 of *Some Considerations Touching the Usefulness of Experimental Natural Philosophy*, in Boyle, *Works*, II.
[60] Marjorie Hope Nicolson (ed.), *Conway Letters* (London, 1930), pp. 229–30.

'Travellers, Soldiers, Seamen, and such like who cannot attend a Cure, but are forced to go about their business'. The recognition that people wanted, if possible, the individualized therapy of a 'cure' was paralleled by Salmon's instructions as to dosage. He made them as individualistic as possible by detailing how and when they could be taken, by splitting up the age categories and by giving the patient scope to find his or her own dosage level:

The way of using the Pills. These Pills may either be swallowed down alone, or taken in the Pap of an Apple or Honey, or a stewed Prune, or a little Syrup, or a Water with a little Beer, Ale, Wine, Broth, as every one likes best, and so taken early in the Morning, or late at Night going to Bed, with out Observation of any other Order, only taking heed of Cold. From two years old, to three or four, you may give one Pill: From four Years old to ten, you may give two or three: From ten to sixteen you may give three or four: and from sixteen Years of Age to threescore and upwards you may safely give five or six Pills; you may begin with a little Dose first, and so encrease it as you find the Body is in strength.[61]

Boyle himself used a variety of remedies for the different stages and symptoms of his own illness. The structure of his treatment was probably very similar to that found in King or Clegg. In the Meditation 'Upon his reviewing and tacking together the several bills, filed up in the apothecary's shop' he wrote:

Either my curiosity, Sophronia, or my value of health, has made it my custom, when I have passed through a course of physic, to review the particulars it consisted of; that taking notice by what remedies I found most good, and by what, little or none; if I should fall into the like distemper for the future, I might derive some advantage from my past experience. In compliance with this custom, as I was this day reviewing and putting together the doctor's several prescriptions sent me back by the apothecary; Good God! said I, in my self, what a multitude of unpleasant medicines I have been ordered to take! the very numbering, and reading them, were able to discompose me, and make me almost sick, though the taking of them helped to make me well. And certainly, if when I was about to enter into a course of physic, all these loathsome medicines, and uneasy prescriptions, had been presented to me together as things I must take, and comply with, I should have utterly despaired of a recovery . . . But then, although I now see these troublesome prescriptions all at once, I did not use them so, but took only one or two harsh remedies in one day, and thereby was enabled to bear them, especially being assisted by moderate intervals of respite, and supported by other seasonable cordials.[62]

It is interesting that Boyle employed, in a very orthodox manner, both doctor and apothecary, who clearly treated him in a step by step way. The empiricist/empiric was also there, taking no risks with empirics' nostrums but learning in the safest possible way (and in the most rational, as well as empirical) – from his own constitution.

61 Broadsheet in Wellcome Institute Library, Broadsheet Cabinet.
62 R. Boyle, *Occasional Reflections*, section 2, meditation xv, in *Works*, II, pp. 381–2.

CONCLUSION

The new philosophy did not, and could not, alter traditional rational ways of thinking about illness and the effects of medicines – although the terms in which the explanations were couched, of course, did change radically. Without the ideological force that a successful new philosophy of medicine could exert (as Newton's work did for the physical sciences) in producing uniformity, medicine was free to enjoy all the variations that there could be between rationalism and the practice of empirics. This was no period between paradigms, where a hundred medical flowers could blossom until the new paradigm asserted itself. Variety had been the norm in English medical practice for centuries; it was perhaps heightened by an increasingly commercialized market-place, but the significant point is that people were at ease with the two extremes of the medical market-place. One reason for this is that perhaps they had more in common with each other than we might think.

In some ways this was still the time of the *longue durée* in medicine, despite evidence to the contrary from the other contributions in this book. Although theory changed it was still expressed in such a way that it spoke to patients and so attracted their trade. The warring factions in the medical market-place probably exaggerated their differences; all the groups had in common remedies and some degree of rationale or advertising to justify them. Moreover, we know that patients in actual fact frequently moved with ease from one type of practitioner to another.[63] What change there was came at bottom, not from new scientific theories but from commercial developments in the market. This was a time when Lockyer's Pills were sold wholesale on an organized basis in different towns, and George Jones's 'Tincture of the Sun', his Balsam and Electuary were sold by his 'trusty Friends' such as Mr John Ashtone, postmaster of Warrington, Richard Ballard Esq., mayor of Monmouth, Mr Joseph Russel, postmaster of Arundel, Mr John Holm, barber chirurgeon of Penrith in Cumberland and by many others in over fifty places spread across the country.[64] Given such

---

[63] See the essays in Porter, *Patients and Practitioners*. A typical story of patient mobility is in John Marten, *A Treatise of all the Degrees and Symptoms of the Venereal Disease in Both Sexes*, 6th edn (London, 1708?), pp. 142–3; a gentleman of fifty-four years contracted a gonorrhoea, was treated at a hospital for many weeks but the advice and treatments had no effect. He went to 'an eminent physician' but 'with as little success' and was 'at last recommended to me'. The possibility that the 'history' was made up by Marten, makes it even more typical.

[64] In Wellcome Institute Library, Broadsheet Cabinet. The Jones advertisement was probably written in 1675.

X

commercial developments, and the growth of an urban group of
practitioners centred around the chemists' shops and warehouses, it is
not surprising that emphasis was being placed on the remedy rather
than the process of cure. But the public, or rather the literate public,[65]
still desired the appearance of individualized prescribing. In all this, the
new scientific theories formed part of the rhetoric used to differentiate
medical groups and served the same function as humoral medicine, to
make sense of illness, but in a deep sense they altered little. Change in
medical practice in this period was slow, just as change in many of the
material practices of life was slow.

[65] Little is known, or can be, of the way in which practitioners related to the expectations of
illiterate patients.

XI

Epistemology and learned medicine in early modern England

Preface

This paper poses the question as to whether and how far it is possible to talk of epistemology in relation to a learned tradition in medicine, when that tradition is well established and is concerned to emphasize the unchanging nature of its knowledge in the struggles against its competitors in the medical market place. Some of the discussion bears upon the question of why learned medicine came to die out in England, but this issue is not the main focus of the paper.

I have not spelled out modern-day historiographic categories (for instance, epistemic or sociological, or to use more old-fashioned terms from the history of science and medicine, internal or external). They express dichotomies which for the sixteenth and seventeenth centuries are not historically grounded. (For instance, a sixteenth-century divine or politician would not have agreed that a point of religious doctrine was a matter either of epistemology or sociology – even if the latter could have been recognized at the time – though it might be seen as a blend of both. Our modern scholarly traditions and disciplinary rivalries mean that one or the other tend to be given priority.)

Introduction

The epistemology of Western learned or scholarly medicine was not completely successful; it did not produce knowledge of such certainty as to kill off all other rivals in the medical market place. It is also doubtful if in early modern Europe learned medicine was using epistemology in any heuristic sense to create new knowledge. Nevertheless, it is perhaps possible to see a kind of epistemology at work when patients' symptoms were being related to already established explanatory categories, and epistemology was certainly part of the rhetoric used by learned physicians to do down the opposition – they claimed that they possessed the correct epistemology whilst empirics and others did not.

152

In this paper I want to try to bridge the gap that usually exists between philosophers and historians. Discussion of epistemology is often carried out in terms of the discrete categories of philosophers, such as 'observation', 'reason', etc. and their various amplifications in which everyone, it is assumed, is a rational being, or at least possessing an equal amount of reason. Historians, well aware of the diversity of people and of the uses to which appeals to reason can be put, tend to ignore such epistemological discussions; at least they ignore their details and look only to their effects. I have a sympathy with this latter approach, but in the case of learned medicine consideration of epistemology is at the heart of its claims to be the best form of medicine and the nature of its epistemology cannot be ignored. First, the connection between epistemology and the wider world is worth considering in the broadest of terms.

Learned or scholarly medicine in Europe was born in classical times without any protection or privilege, except insofar as it shared in the power and status of literate culture. Despite the claims of this type of medicine to possess the most certain form of knowledge, neither Greek states nor Roman governments recognized any such claims, for instance, by instituting a system of licensing of medical practitioners or any other measure of protection for learned medicine. In the Middle Ages and Renaissance learned medicine did become more culturally defined and perhaps its epistemological claims came to be more recognized. It was taught in the universities and given some special status by limited local licensing by city colleges of medicine or by Spain's Protomedicato.[1] Epistemology did not play a totally successful role in the career of learned medicine. If epistemology is concerned with how certain knowledge is acquired then it is clear that not everyone from the classical period to the end of the sixteenth century was convinced that medicine had acquired such knowledge. Other systems of healing and other epistemologies managed to compete

---

[1]   See, for instance, Nancy Siraisi, *Medieval and Early Renaissance Medicine* (Chicago: Chicago University Press, 1990); Katharine Park, *Doctors and Medicine in Early Renaissance Florence* (Princeton: Princeton University Press, 1985); Richard Palmer, *The Studio of Venice and its Graduates in the Sixteenth Century* (Padua: Edizioni Lint, 1983); Andrew W. Russell (ed.), *The Town and State Physician in Europe from the Middle Ages to the Enlightenment* (Wolfenbüttel: Wolfenbütteler Forschungen, 1981), vol. 17; Luis Garcia-Ballester, Michael R. McVaugh and Augustin Rubio-Vela, *Medical Licensing and Learning in Fourteenth-Century Valencia*, Transactions of the American Philosophical Society, vol. 79 (Philadelphia: American Philosophical Society, 1989), part 6; J.T. Lanning, *The Royal Protomedicato: The Regulation of the Medical Profession in the Spanish Empire* (Durham: Duke University Press, 1985); Sir George Clark, *A History of the Royal College of Physicians of London*, 2 vols. (Oxford: Clarendon Press, 1964), vol. 1.

successfully with learned medicine, with the medicine of Galen and his followers.[2]

At this point I want to argue, slightly pedantically, that one reading of epistemology, the art of acquiring certain knowledge, is that there is a necessary connection between certainty and the assent of people to that certainty. The acid test of certain knowledge was, as Aristotle argued, that once it was demonstrated or laid out to view then everyone would immediately agree with it.[3] What I am doing here, of course, is trying to show that on philosophical grounds there is a connection between *epistēmē*, certain knowledge, and people or the world at large – rather than imposing the connection.

Of course, not everyone is a philosopher, and Galen for instance could, and did, blame his patients and his medical rivals for not being as educated as he was and thus failing to be convinced by his arguments and conclusions.[4] In other words, despite the belief by some philosophers that *a priori* everyone should be able to recognize and agree to certain knowledge, it might be, as Plato would argue, that most people's minds were too clouded and only the few could achieve such recognition.

Here it seems to me we have two positions. First, it is in the nature of certain knowledge that it is certain only if it is acceded to by all, and if this immediate perception, whether by the mind or eye, does not occur, then it is not certain knowledge (this latter, converse, view, although it logically follows, for obvious reasons was not popular with many philosophers). Second, that failure to agree to what someone puts forward as certain knowledge may not necessarily invalidate such knowledge, but may be the result of the ignorance, obtuseness and blindness of the general population – this view was popular with philosophers (and medical, legal and religious writers), even if by holding this opinion the universal power, to produce assent, inherent in certain knowledge was adversely affected. I suspect that many learned

---

2   On the diversity of the medical market place see Siraisi and Park (note 1); Roy Porter (ed.), *Patients and Practitioners. Lay Perceptions of Medicine in Pre-industrial Society* (Cambridge: Cambridge University Press, 1985); Lucinda McCray Beier, *Sufferers and Healers. The Experience of Illness in Seventeenth-century England* (London: Routledge, 1987); Vivian Nutton, 'Healers in the Medical Market Place: Towards a Social History of Graeco-Roman Medicine', and Katharine Park, 'Medicine and Society in Medieval Europe', in Andrew Wear (ed.), *Medicine in Society. Historical Essays* (Cambridge: Cambridge University Press, 1992), pp. 15–58 and 59–90.

3   See Aristotle, *Posterior Analytics* 71b17–72b4.

4   For example in Galen, *On Examinations by which the Best Physicians are Recognised*, edition of the Arabic version with English translation and commentary by Albert Z. Iskendar (Berlin: Medicorum Graecorum Supplementum Orientale, Academie-Verlag Berlin, 1988).

traditions in many different societies exhibit this tension between the belief that their knowledge is so certain that everyone should agree with it and the realization that in practice not everyone does. Institutionally, the result is that learned traditions make universalistic claims but also have a sense of being an exclusive group with everyone within them sharing and agreeing to a set of accepted propositions, whilst the rest of the world outside has yet to be convinced (as in the case of the learned physicians of sixteenth- and early seventeenth-century England). At different times such groups might feel beleaguered or they might derive a sense of power from their exclusiveness as does, for instance, the medical profession in the twentieth century.

I hope I have made the point that there is a reasonably natural connection between epistemology and people. Other chapters explore in detail the epistemological bases of Western learned medicine. But for the purposes of my chapter I want to point out that classical medicine did not make as strong claims as did classical philosophy to certainty. The perennial debate as to whether medicine was a science, that is concerned with knowledge, or an art or techne is one sign of this. Another is the Hippocratic recognition, echoed throughout the centuries, that there is a multiplicity of experience in medicine, some of it fallacious.

Learned medicine did, however, have an epistemological standpoint. Galen's epistemology was a blend of the empirical and the rational, for Galen believed that one without the other led to the excesses of the empiricists and the methodists. I leave it to others to discuss Galen's heuristic use of experience and reason. For learned medicine in the sixteenth century, that is Galenic medicine, there is no doubt that what was crucial was accepting Galen's doctrines rather than developing new fundamental theories by experience or reason.[5] The humanist revival of the *prisca medicina* of the Greeks brought with it a great emphasis on orthodoxy (one can also find the same with the arrival of the 'new Galen' in the Middle Ages).[6] Innovation within learned medicine did occur, but only in one or two areas such as anatomy, where new observational knowledge contradicted Galen's observations but not his physiological

---

[5] Walter Pagel, 'Medical Humanism – a Historical Necessity in the Era of the Renaissance', in F. Maddison, M. Pelling and C. Webster (eds.), *Essays on the Life and Work of Thomas Linacre* c. *1460–1524* (Oxford: Oxford University Press, 1977), pp. 375–86; Vivian Nutton, 'John Caius and the Linacre Tradition', *Medical History*, 23 (1979), 373–91; Andrew Wear, 'Galen in the Renaissance', in V. Nutton (ed.), *Galen: Problems and Prospects* (London: Wellcome Institute for the History of Medicine, 1981), pp. 229–56.

[6] See Luis García-Ballester, 'Arnau de Vilanova (c. 1240–1311) y la reforma de los estudios médicos en Montpellier (1309): el Hippócrates latino y la introducción del nuevo Galeno', *Dynamis*, 2 (1982), 97–158.

theories of the body, or in relation to diseases such as syphilis and plague. The great effort of the learned physicians lay in trying to get rid of uncertainty in the application of Galen's medicine to the myriad differences that existed among patients. Their different environments and life-styles all had to be taken into account together with their ill conditions or ill constitutions when aetiology and therapy were being considered. Da Monte at Padua, especially, was concerned with the enterprise of making Galenic medicine more methodical.[7] The popularity of tables setting out aspects of Galenic medicine (with the most general categories on the left of the page and then moving by inclusive brackets to more detailed headings on the right of the page) is a sign of this interest in reducing learned medicine to method and hence to greater certainty. But such tables are also to be found at this time in other learned traditions such as law and were not confined only to medicine.[8]

In a sense, the learned traditions of the Renaissance were at a stage where new fundamental knowledge was not the issue. Rather the emphasis lay in being true to the past and in ordering past knowledge in the best possible way. (Here, comparisons with other learned traditions would be interesting.) However, within learned medicine there was some room for creativity and for personally acquiring knowledge, and this is discussed below.

Early modern England

A discussion of epistemology and learned medicine in sixteenth-century England could also apply to much of Europe. However, compared to Italy England was a backwater; it was not a major centre for the renaissance of medicine. It did possess a few good humanist scholars like John Caius though much of medical knowledge was transmitted in English and not in Latin books, and in the seventeenth century William Harvey gave England a reputation in anatomy.

[7]   See A. Wear, 'Contingency and Logic in Renaissance Anatomy and Physiology', unpublished Ph.D. thesis, London University (1973), pp. 175–243; Donald G. Bates, 'Sydenham and the Medical Meaning of "Method" ', *Bulletin of the History of Medicine*, 51 (1977), 324–38; A. Wear (note 5), pp. 238–45; Jerome Bylebyl, 'Teaching *Methodus Medendi* in the Renaissance', in F. Kudlein and Richard J. Durling (eds.), *Galen's Method of Healing* (Leiden: E.J. Brill, 1991), pp. 157–89.

[8]   K.J. Höltgen, 'Synoptische Tabellen in der Medizinischen Literatur und die Logik Agricolas und Ramus', *Sudhoffs Archiv*, 49 (1965), 371–90; more generally N.W. Gilbert, *Renaissance Concepts of Method* (New York: Columbia University Press, 1960); W.J Ong, *Ramus' Method and the Decay of Dialogue* (Cambridge, Mass.: Harvard University Press, 1958).

It also had the College of Physicians of London, founded on the model of the Italian city college of medicine, which had limited and not very effective powers of overseeing medical practice in London and seven miles around. The College often seemed beleaguered. In the sixteenth century politicians like the Secretary of State Francis Walsingham and at times Elizabeth herself interfered with the College's policing of unlicensed practice in London. In the seventeenth century its powers to prosecute illicit practice began to be circumscribed by the courts and by the beginning of the eighteenth century the apothecaries had acquired the right to practise.[9] Essentially, there was an open medical market place in early modern England, and learned medicine was one amongst many groups which offered medical services.

This was a context in which claims to exclusiveness of knowledge, to having the right answers, was balanced by the fact that the medical culture of the time encouraged an eclectic mix of views. What I want to do is to analyse some of the ways in which epistemology was used by the learned physicians in their war against their medical opponents. But first it is worth considering in a general way the use or otherwise of epistemology in medicine at this time.

Authority, reason and experience

In 1628 the Bath physician Tobias Venner produced one of the many health advice books. His *Via Recta ad Vitam Longam* was:

a plaine Philosophicall demonstration of the Nature, faculties and effects of all such things as by way of nourishment make for the preservation of health, with divers necessary dieticall; as also of the true use and effects of sleepe, exercise, excretions and pertubations, with just applications to every age, constitution of body and time of yeare.[10]

Venner was offering advice on hygiene or the preservation of health, something which the learned physicians took pride in claiming was lacking in their opponents, the empirics, who treated patients only when they became ill.[11]

Venner was a good Galenist, but he had his own opinions. The learned physicians did not have to follow authority slavishly. Galen had

---

[9] See Sir George Clark (note 1), and especially Harold J. Cook, *The Decline of the Old Medical Regime in Stuart London* (Ithaca and London: Cornell University Press, 1986).

[10] Tobias Venner, *Via Recta ad Vitam Longam* (London, 1628), title page.

[11] On the views of learned physicians on empirics and their stress on regimen see Harold J. Cook, 'The New Philosophy and Medicine in Seventeenth-Century England', in David Lindberg and Robert Westman (eds.), *Reappraisals of the Scientific Revolution* (Cambridge: Cambridge University Press, 1990), pp. 396–436.

commended pig's flesh, but Venner disagreed and set up his own criteria of what made for good nourishment:

Swines flesh, because of the strong and abundant nourishment that it yeeldeth, as also of the likenesse that it hath unto mans flesh both in savour and taste, is of Galen and other of the ancient Physicians, commended above all other kindes of flesh in nourishing the body. But in my opinion, the choice of flesh is rather to be taken, from an odoriferous pleasantnesse of the same, laudable substance, good temperature, easie concoction, and goodnesse of iuyce that it breedeth, then from the strongnesses of nourishment that it giveth, or the aforesaid. In respect of all which, Veale, Mutton, Steere or Heyfer Beefe are to be preferred before Porke. (p. 50)

All the criteria here are subjective ones. This, of course, fits the subjective basis of Western learned medicine – its four humours were made up of the different combinations of the qualities hot, cold, dry and wet which are all perceived by the senses. Galen judged pig's meat to be like man's flesh 'both in savour and taste' (the epistemology of cannibalism). Likewise, Venner's criteria were also subjective and based on the senses: 'odoriferous pleasantnesse' is clear enough whilst 'laudable substance', 'good temperature', 'easie concoction' and 'goodnesse of iuyce' are assessments dependent on personal judgement or experience, even if they had some theoretical grounding, for instance, on what 'good temperature' or temperament might be. The subjective experiential element that lay at the heart of Galenic medicine allowed different subjective criteria of, in this case, the goodness of pig's flesh, to be easily substituted. It also meant that, using such criteria, everyone could judge of the goodness of pig meat. An expert like Venner declared what sort of meat was good, but he used language which was held in common with his readers. After all, the goodness of meat, fish, water and so on was something that everyone had to decide daily for themselves. There were no water boards to guarantee the purity of water, and the inspection of markets was not very effective.

But what Venner did was to use this language and also more specialized terminology in areas which his readership would not normally have entered. He was able, as an expert, to make statements about what happened inside the body when particular foods were eaten. He wrote:

But seeing that Porke is of hard digestion, and in substance more grosse than convenient, it is not good for them that be aged, that are grosse, that have weake stomackes, that live at ease, or are any wayes unsound of body. For in such it causeth obstructions of the mesaraicke veines, liver and reines, the Gowte and Dropsie, especially if they shall be cold and moyst by constitution; for unto them is Porke very greatly hurtfull, because in them it is wholly converted into crude and phlegmaticke humors. Wherefore let such as are phelegmaticke, aged or subject unto obstructions, that leade a studious life or have queasie stomackes, altogether abstaine from the use of Porke. (pp. 50–1)

From the possibly common experience that pork is difficult to digest Venner then proceeded to hidden events taking place within the body. He imagines what pork does inside the body: his story is shaped by Galen's theory of digestion (food is concocted in the stomach into chyle which then travels through the mesenteric veins to the liver to be altered into blood) and his conclusions about the effect of pork on phlegmatic constitutions and upon the aged are conditioned by Galenic humoral theories. Yet the reader is given the sense that Venner has really seen what is happening in the body. The anatomical references help to do this for they signify observable structures. In a sense, here we have authority and pre-established theories being used in a reasonably creative and lively way to give the impression that the author has actual (experienced?) knowledge of what he is stating is going on in the body.

Paradoxically, Venner is using Galenic epistemology, the mix of the empirical and the rational, to describe the effect of pork in the body; but he is doing so not in the way we normally think of epistemology being used, that is to discover and establish new knowledge. Instead, Venner is creating knowledge but from old knowledge. And I suspect that this applied to most of learned medicine at this time – inevitably so.

What is striking about Venner's account of the healthiness of pig meat is how his judgement of what is the case appears authoritative. The experiential-subjective basis of the qualitative system in natural philosophy and medicine meant that ultimately each individual had through their senses the capacity to judge the nature of the world and of all living things in it (obviously keeping within the broad theoretical framework of qualities, elements and humours).

Perhaps there is also, as well as the mix of the personal and the Galenic, another aspect to Venner's account. Aphoristic, declaratory, knowledge had a long history going back to the Hippocratics. This type of knowledge is often expressed without any hints as to its origin. Here is Venner on birds:

The Black-bird or Owle that is fat, is greatly commended for pleasantnesse of taste, lightnesse of digestion and goodnesse of nourishment. The Thrush that is of a darke reddish colour, is of the same nature: they are best in the winter, and are convenient for every age and constitution of the body, especially for the phlegmaticke. (p. 60)

Common experience, oral tradition, personal experience and learned authority could be involved in such aphoristic knowledge. Some of this knowledge we tend to call received wisdom, for instance the often repeated view that marshy ground was unhealthy which now has the support of modern historical demographers.[12] However, what is significant is that these pieces of discrete knowledge do not usually disclose how they were arrived at. Their epistemic origins lie hidden.

William Vaughan, an unsuccessful colonizer of Newfoundland and a writer on health matters, wrote in his *Directions for Health* (1617) of the healthiness of water and asked, 'What is the nature of Fountaine-Water?' He answered:

Fountaine-water is the best water for preservation of health: But you must observe, of what side it springs, for if it comes from the East, it excels the rest as well in moysture and thinnesse of substance, as in pleasant smel, and it doth moderately comfort the spirits: Contrariwise those fountaines which spring out of rockes, towards the North, and which have the Sunne backward, are of a hard digestion, and nothing so pure as the other.[13]

Vaughan gave some rationalizations or explanations: fountain waters from the east are thinner and of pleasanter smell, whilst from the north are hard to digest and not so pure. But on the basic points of why fountain water was healthiest and of why the east was better than the north there was no real explanation of how these conclusions were arrived at. This type of declaratory knowledge was very common in learned medicine in the early modern period. It can be found at the centre of curative medicine, in its remedies. The lists of remedies in books on practical medicine are usually presented baldly, as a list of ingredients without any rationale for their use. What was important was the recipe itself, but how it came about, or how it was known that it was successful, was often not discussed. At a popular level there were a large number of books published which gave the remedies collected by the nobility, by royalty or by famous doctors. Again, there was no explanation of why they worked in particular diseases. All one has is the name of the condition and a number of remedies for it. Leonard Sowerby in *The Ladies Dispensatory* (1652), which was concerned to list simples rather than medicines 'compounded by a hodge podge of sophisticated Drugs',[14] advised 'for those which spit and vomite Bloud' one or other of the following simple remedies:

[12] See Mary Dobson, '"Marsh Fever": A Geography of Malaria in England', *Journal of Historical Geography*, 6 (1980), 359–89; also see Mary Dobson, 'The Last Hiccup of the Old Demographic Regime: Population Stagnation and Decline in Late Seventeenth and Early Eighteenth-Century England', *Continuity and Change*, 4 (1989), 395–428.
[13] William Vaughan, *Directions for Health*, 5th edition (London, 1617), p. 24.
[14] Leonard Sowerby, *The Ladies Dispensatory* (London, 1652), 'To the Reader', p. A4r.

160

Reere Eggs supped
Ashes of Harts – horne washed, and drunk with Gum Dragant
Water Betony drunk
Juyce of wild Time the weight of two drachms drunk in vinegar
Dung of a wild she goate mingled with wine, or water, drunk
Purslaine well boyled eaten. (p. 62)

Or, of special concern to Ladies, 'to cause standing of the yard' one had
the choice of:

Costus drunk in honied wine
Saffron drunk
Lin-Seed taken with hony and peper
Boyled Turnips eaten
Rocket much eaten
Seed of Rocket eaten. (p. 19)

Sowerby wrote that he had followed Gerard with Johnson, Goraeus and
Fuchs, and had no objection against 'my Authour Dioscorides' (p. A4r).
Their authoritative experience or learning gave validity to the remedies.
Of course, more learned writers might give the qualitative degree of
heat, cold, moisture or dryness of an illness and provide for it a remedy
of an appropriate degree of a contrary quality (the cure by contrary
quality). But even here a writer could always disagree with tradition and
use his personal, subjective judgement to define anew the quality of a
remedy – something which in any case he would have to do with newly
discovered medicines, for instance, from the New World. In practice,
only simples or remedies with very few ingredients could be allotted a
specific qualitative degree (on a scale of one to four). In the case of
polypharmacy or compound drugs the system broke down and the total
mix of ingredients was usually presented simply as a cure for a condition
without any analysis or rationalization of why it worked. What was
important was the recipe itself. In this sense, it was a piece of aphoristic
knowledge, and there were very many pieces of such knowledge as the
lists of compound remedies appear endless.

It seems to me that in learned medicine in the early modern period we
have a situation in which the desire to remain orthodox and to stay
within the bounds of Galenic doctrine is very strong. The Renaissance
saw a concerted move to get a 'purer' Galen into medicine, purged of
Arabic and medieval Latin barbarisms. And if the period of 'Galen
worship'[15] waned after the 1530s, by and large what innovations there

[15] Marie Boas, *The Scientific Renaissance 1450–1630* (London: Collins, 1962), p. 135; for
the philological results see R.J. Durling, 'A Chronological Census of the Renaissance
Editions and Translations of Galen', *Journal of the Warburg and Courtauld Institutes*, 24
(1961), 230–305.

were within learned medicine were produced using Galen's theories and concepts. The shared admiration for classical medicine and the pressures of competition in the medical market place produced cohesion and conformity within learned medicine (though there were some exceptions).[16]

Now, what I have noted above about the existence of people creating personal knowledge in terms of the qualitative–humoral nature of things and their use of an aphoristic style of knowledge means that there was space within learned medicine for independent ways of gaining and expressing knowledge. On the whole, it was second-order knowledge dependent on a pre-existing Galenic framework, but it allowed the physician (and lay people, for they also made qualitative judgements) to feel that by using their senses they could assess for themselves the nature of illnesses, foods and the world around them. The aphoristic type of knowledge, whether derived from folk wisdom, personal experience or tradition and authority, did not threaten Galenic medicine. It was too brief and usually contained no theoretical statements, though theory might be implied. By the manner in which it was presented it could equally be new or ancient knowledge, and this may have given early modern writers, again, the feeling that they could contribute in a substantial way to learned medicine.

In other words, learned medicine in this period was not a rigid orthodoxy; there was flexibility, for instance, in creating narratives of what was going on inside the body, and in giving people the feeling that they could personally contribute to medical knowledge through their senses, and by adding pieces of information in an aphoristic, unargued way. Of course, the reason why this could happen without conflicting greatly with learned medicine lay in Galen's development of a qualitative medicine based on the senses and his openness to folk wisdom especially in the case of remedies. Another reason, and this may be worth comparative consideration, is that the personal–sensory basis of medical knowledge reflects the material conditions of life from the Greeks to the early modern period. Technology was simple, and in everyday life the senses were the main means of assessing the environment, food and people's ill or healthy conditions. But I have perhaps stressed the creative side to learned medicine too much. Orthodoxy and claims to know more than the opposition are characteristic of early modern medicine in England. The emphasis lay on pre-existing knowledge

---

[16] Exceptions relate to plague where a contagionist rather than a miasmatic theory began to be accepted by learned physicians and to the use of concepts of occult qualities and of the power of the 'total substance' of a remedy which, although discussed by Galen, were frowned upon by the majority of Renaissance learned physicians.

taught over a long period of time at university, and only if a practitioner
was initiated into this knowledge could he become a learned physician.

Epistemology and learned medicine

Most diseases and conditions had names. They were known. In the
heyday of a learned medical tradition it would have been surprising if it
had been otherwise. (Though as I write this I sense a tautology!) Lay
people were also confident that they could diagnose and name diseases.
In London, old women, often pensioners of the parishes, acted as
'searchers of the dead' and diagnosed the causes of death amongst
London's citizens for the bills of mortality. The published books of
remedies and the private manuscript collections were aimed at or
produced by lay people, especially women, and referred to the whole
range of illnesses. The medical culture of the time, both lay and learned,
did not lack confidence in diagnosing or naming an illness. (And where
doubts might exist there were sophisticated fail-safe procedures – a
patient might be labelled hypochondriac – in the modern sense – as the
seventeenth-century Nonconformist minister Richard Baxter found to
his cost.)[17] Or the case might be seen as being caused by witchcraft, a
practice which Thomas Ady in 1655 castigated as 'a cloak for Physicians
ignorance . . . when he cannot find the nature of the Disease, he saith the
Party is bewitched').[18]

Of course, the learned physicians sought to differentiate their skill
from that of empirics and lay people. Learned medicine was presented
as the best possible type of medical knowledge, but as also complex and
full of difficulty. Galenic physicians like John Cotta and his Northampton colleague James Hart[19] stressed that the learning to be gained
from study in the universities alone provided the required degree of
knowledge and discernment to properly 'work the system', that is to
make use of the holistic potential of learned medicine.

The learned physicians stressed how they took into account many
more factors than did empirics. For instance, the differences between
diseases had to be considered along with the constitution, age and life-

---

[17] See Andrew Wear, 'Puritan Perceptions of Illness', in R. Porter (ed.), *Patients and
Practitioners: Lay Perceptions of Medicine in Pre-Industrial Society* (Cambridge: Cambridge University Press, 1985), p. 95.

[18] Thomas Ady, *A Candle in the Dark: Or, A Treatise Concerning the Nature of Witches and
Witchcraft* (London, 1655), p. 115.

[19] John Cotta, *A Short Discoverie of the Unobserved Dangers of Severall Sorts of Ignorant and
Unconsiderate Practisers of Physike in England* (London, 1612); James Hart, *Kliniki, or
Diet of the Diseased* (1633); see also John Securis, *A Detection and Querimonie of the
Daily Enormities and Abuses Committed in Physick* (London, 1566).

XI

style of the individual patient. I am going to refer extensively to the work of an obscure but learned physician, Eleazar Dunk, as it gives a typical but detailed account of knowledge and medicine. In a letter published in 1606 he set out how the learned physician should think about a case when he defended the physicians against the empirics:

First the learned Physician is to search out the proper signes of this disease, and by them to distinguish it from others that hath some affinity with it: then he looketh into the cause of it ... he examineth the naturall constitution of the patient, his present state of body, his former course of life, his age, his strength, the time of the disease, the season of the yeare etc he considereth the qualities and quantity of the humours; from whence the matter of the disease floweth ... by what passages it moveth, whether swiftly, or slowly ... Out of an advised consideration of all these, first a diet is to be appointed: this cannot be the same in every one that laboureth of this sicknesse, but it requireth great variety and alteration agreeable to the foresaid circumstances. Then follow with the consultations of the meanes of the cure: what kind of evacuation is fittest whether opening a veine ...[20]

The learned physician's trademark was that he took into account the patient, and that it was the individual patient and not the disease that had to be treated, so that one remedy could not cure all who suffered from the same disease.

Such a view was also held by the highest in the land, James I, who in *A Counterblaste to Tobacco* (1604) wrote:

Yea, not onely will a skilfull and wary Physician be carefull to use no cure but that which is fit for that sort of disease, but will also consider all other circumstances, & make the remedies sutable therunto; as the temperature of the clime where the Patient is, the constitution of the Planets, the time of the Moone, the season of the yeere, the age and complexion of the Patient, and the present state of his body, in strength or weakness: For one cure must not euer be used for the selfsame disease, but according to the varying of any of the foresaid circumstances, that sort of remedy must bevsed which is fittest for the same.[21]

Dunk believed that empirics could be confused or mistaken about all the stages of diagnosis and treatment. His attack on empirics for their poor diagnosis allows us to learn what he saw as good diagnosis, especially the knowledge that was required in making it:

Diseases are knowen and distinguished by their signes ... because they [empirics] are ignorant, they must needs fall often into this fault [of wrongful diagnosis]. This is seldome discovered but when rationall Physicians have opportunity to look into their practise; then they see the disease taken to be in

[20] Eleazar Dunk, *The Copy of a Letter Written by E.D. Doctour of Physicke to a Gentleman, by whom It was Published* (London, 1606), p. 24.
[21] James I of England and VI of Scotland, *A Counterblast to Tobacco*, in *The Workes of the Most High and Mighty Prince, James* (London, 1616), p. 219.

the liver, when it is in the lungs or kidneis; to be in the heart, when it is in the head or mouth of the stomacke; to be in the brest, when it is winde in the stomache extending that region: and many such. What though they can judge of the gout, the palsie and the dropsie? So can simple women doe: but to judge rightly of the causes and the differences of these diseases, of the manifold differences of Agues, of simple and compound sicknesses and of sundry diseases of the head; that requireth Arte, which is not in any Empiricke. (pp. 25–6)

In therapy the empiric could also go wrong. As in the case of diagnosis some of the mistakes occur because of the greater complexity of learned medicine, with its many distinctions and differences. In a sense, learned medicine offered more possibilities in diagnosis, more courses of action in therapeutics and especially greater precision (at least in the eyes of learned physicians like Dunk):

Hence is a broad gate opened to a large field of medicines of sundry sorts, ointments, plaisters, syrups, potions etc. Some of these are very hot and much opening; some very cold and binding. In the use of these, and also of all the former things [Dunk had been describing bleeding, purging and fomentations], the Empirike is plunged into many doubts, and the patient into as many dangers: if he take away too little blood, he taketh not away the disease; if too much, he taketh away life: if he purgeth when he should open a veine, or doth this when that is required, he committeth a pernicious errour: if he iudgeth not rightly of the humour abounding, of the complexion etc. (of which only Arte is the competent iudge) he can attempt nothing in the cure safely, nor so much as appoint a fit diet. (p. 25)

Dunk continued in this vein, and the reader may well wonder if in reality the learned physician exercised such fine judgement as Dunk claimed. (See my 'Conclusion' for some comments on this.)

How did the learned physician avoid all these pitfalls? Where did he gain the necessary knowledge? Dunk answered, 'in the great variety of these doubts, difficulties and distinctions there is a necessary use of sound judgement, confirmed by long study and profound knowledge both in Philosophy and Physicke' (p. 25). Learning, reading and study was what constituted the 'Arte'. In relating to diseases and their differences Dunk wrote that 'the eye can not discerne colours but by the light, nor Physicians diseases but by learning'. The remedy of bleeding also led to 'doubts and difficulties as require much reading and deepe knowledge' (p. 27). Study made the physician. Dunk's little treatise *The Copy of a Letter Written by E.D. Doctour of Physicke to a Gentleman, by whom It was Published* pointed in its title page to the crucial role of study 'wherein is plainly prooved that the practise of all those which have not beene brought up in the Grammar and University, is alwayes confused, commonly dangerous and often Deadly'.

Two questions need to be answered. Can we talk of epistemology in this context, and why did English learned physicians so emphasize their learning? If epistemology is the creation of new knowledge then I do not think that epistemology is involved in the learned physician's view of medical knowledge. However, that may be to rely too much on a modern view of epistemology which stresses new knowledge discovered especially through experience (though the use of reason or the mind obviously is not precluded, especially in relation to the classical period). Dunk's physician was taught; he learned from books. Empirics, on the other hand, 'learn by our perils, and they trie experiments by our death'. And he added:

Experience alone, with a little helpe of nature maketh men skilfull in mechanickall trades, in merchandise, and in other kinds of buying and selling; but the deepe knowledge conteined in the liberall sciences, and in other learning arising out of them, requireth much reading, long study, great meditation; and after the theorie or speculation of them is obteined, then practise and experience confirmeth and establisheth them: but without the former, the latter is weake, larne and maimed. (p. 32f.)

No nonsense here about the falsifying power of experience. In fact, experience is there to bolster learning – the expectation is that it will confirm it. Although Dunk recognized that Galen required both 'learning and Experience', and so could conclude 'therefore the best Empiricke is but a lame and left-legged Physician' (p. 33), he clearly gave priority to learning which alone taught the method of medicine, that is which taught the system of medical knowledge: 'It is a full consent of all learned in Physicke or Philosophy, That nothing can be happily done in the Art of Physicke without method and order: and it is as true that experience can not teach this method' (p. 33).

John Cotta's *A Short Discoverie of the Unobserved Dangers of Severall Sorts of Ignorent and Unconsiderate Practisers of Physicke in England* (1612) reflected the commonly held views of learned physicians and so followed many of the themes in Dunk's *Letter*. Cotta reiterated the point that personal experience (what was to be a key to knowledge for the new science of the seventeenth century) was inadequate for reaching a true and full knowledge of medicine. Only a true method and habit or disposition aided by books could do this:

The defect in the Empericke hence appeareth to be want of true methode and the habit of right operation and practise according to reason, (which is art) through which defect his actions must needs oft be reasonlesse, and by consequent as blind in their intention, so likely to be foolish in their issue and execution. For there must needs be in all actions want of much more neccessary knowledge then sense and experience can advance unto: and experience must

166

needes witnesse against it selfe, that the longest age of experience doth nothing so fully furnish and instruct in many things, as much more speedily doth prudent invention; which though occasioned and helped by bookes and reading which are both keys unto all knowledge, and also rich storehouse of experiences ... yet do they [books] only glut the sense with stories of experiences past, but reason and judgement truly enrich the mind and give daily new increase and light before untried and unexperienced truths.[22]

So, maybe there was no epistemology of a serious sort in early modern learned medicine, apart from the odd disagreement over some qualitative, subjective, interpretation of the type noted earlier. Or, perhaps our use of the terms 'teaching' and 'epistemology' have to be altered. If the discovery of new knowledge by experience was precluded then it may be apposite to talk equally of the discovery, teaching or learning of medical knowledge through books. For if Paracelsus, Galileo and Harvey wanted to learn from the book of nature rather than from the books of the ancients they still retained from the latter the sense of personally learning. Such a sense of personal learning, which we now take for granted, forms a natural association with experience (that is, 'personal experience'). But if the distinction between discovery and teaching is blurred, as perhaps it has to be in any well-established medical learned tradition (are there comparative views on this?), then it may be easier to talk of epistemology in the context of how one learns, discovers or empathizes with a body of pre-established knowledge and acquires the Art and true 'reason and judgement'. Either that or we have to conclude that to talk of epistemology is not appropriate to learned medicine at this time, at least in relation to its basic theories and rules.

The second question as to why English Galenic physicians stressed learning so much does give rise to epistemological issues. As well as their general opposition to empirics, they were concerned with the rise of an ethnocentric medicine, that is an English medicine written in English books which sometimes claimed that there were specifically English remedies for English diseases. Classical medicine was Greek, but it was applied in the early modern period not only to other areas in the Mediterranean but also to countries north of the Alps. The question arose as to the universal applicability of this medicine. Clearly, Mediterranean and North European medicinal herbs were different.

But more fundamental differences were pointed out. As the Hippocratic text *Airs, Waters, Places* had indicated, the place in which someone was born and lived influences their constitution, their physical and psychological characteristics. The view then developed that the place where one was born was most natural to be in and the

[22] John Cotta (note 19), p. 11.

healthiest. Christianity, from the early Church Fathers, also emphasized how God had put remedies on earth for man's use. This was
repeated by writers such as Timothie Bright in his *A Treatise Wherein
is Declared the Sufficiencie of English Medicines* (1580) and William
Harrison in his *Description of England* (1586–7) to mean that God gave
to each nation remedies specific for the diseases prevalent in it.

The claims of learned medicine to universality were thus curtailed and
on this view some of the details of learned medicine if not its basic
theories had to be modified. (Here the comparative dimension of, for
instance, the applicability of Indian or Chinese medicine across large
geographical areas would be interesting.) It tended to be opponents of
learned medicine who argued for the ethnocentric approach, men such
as Nicholas Culpeper (who repeated Bright's *Treatise* in his *School of
Physick* (1659)) and who were concerned to prescribe to the poor cheap
English herbal remedies that could be picked from English fields rather
than expensive drugs from the Middle East, the Indies or America.

For Bright these latter remedies were 'things rather of superfluous
pleasure than necessary reliefs and serving rather for a certain pomp
than for maintenance of life'.[23] More specifically and pragmatically,
Bright wrote that the English should not be dependent on supplies of
drugs from 'heathen and barbarous nations' who, in any case, often
corrupt or counterfeit them (pp. 8–9).

Bright also found theoretical reasons for dismissing foreign medicines.
Not only did individuals have different temperaments or complexions
(balance of humours) but so did nations. As the diet of Indians and
Egyptians was different from that of the English, argued Bright, so
would their humours and excrements also be different – which meant
that the remedies to balance the humours in turn had to be different (pp.
19–20).

The universalism of classical medicine was also founded on its use of
the universal scholarly language, Latin. Motivated by a Christian
charitable desire to make their work available to all, to avoid obscurity
and perhaps spurred on by a sense of nationalism and the example of the
use of English in the Protestant religion, English medical writers began
to write in their own tongue. Thomas Phayre in *The Book of Children*
(1553) justified the practice, by stating that in the past 'Galen the Prince
of this art being a Grecian wrote in Greek' and Avicenna, an Arab, in
Arabic. Medicine in England, which was 'a thing that was made to be
common to all', should not therefore be kept amongst a few.[24] A

---

[23] Timothie Bright, *A Treatise Wherein is Declared the Sufficiencie of English Medicines for
Cure of all Diseases, Cured with Medicine* (London, 1580), p. 8.
[24] Thomas Phayre, *The Book of Children* (London, 1591), pp. a2r–a2v.

nationalistic local view of medicine could equally lead to the use of the vernacular and to locally produced remedies.

Language, of course, figured large in the claims of learned medicine to apply across all of Europe. If few students of learned medicine or their professors in the universities of North or South Europe knew Greek, the language of the *prisca medicina*, at least they were united by a shared knowledge of the next best, Latin. The use of Latin perhaps blurred geographical and national distinctions. It was a distinguishing mark of the learned physician as it helped to establish that he was learned.[25] It was also claimed that Latin gave a better type of medical knowledge, and also of philosophy, the basis of learned medicine. English books just were not good enough; with Latin one gained access to the best knowledge available.

The Salisbury physician John Securis, who had studied with the conservative Galenist Sylvius in Paris, defended learned medicine in his *A Detection and Querimonie of the Daily Enormities and Abuses Committed in Physick* (1566). To the objection that 'we have Englishe bokes enough to teach us divers medicins for diverse purposes',[26] Securis replied at length. Medicine could be understood only when placed in its philosophical context (which was expressed in Latin):

I answer that the englishe bookes teacheth nothinge of the trewe foundation of Phisike. For if there be any that doo it, howe can it be well understanded without logike and naturall philosophie. For Aristotle saith *Ubi desinit Physicus, ibi incipit medicus*. A man must first peruse naturall Philosophie, before he entre into phisycke. (pp. B1r–v)

Securis conceded that: 'to have some bokes of phisike in englyshe specially of the Simples, well and cunnyingly set foorthe for Surgeons, Apothicaries, yea and for sober and wyse men, that delyte to reade in suche thynges, and know not the Latine tongue, is not unmete nor hurtefull' (p. B1v). But Securis went to his main attack:

doo you thynke to have in youre Englyshe Bookes, all the perfecte knowledge that is required in Physicke? ... If Englyshe Bookes could make men cunnying Physitions, then pouchemakers, threshers, ploughmen and cobblers mought be Physitions as well as the best yf they can reade.

Then wer it a great foly for us to bestow so much labour and study all our lyfe tyme in the scholes and universities to breake our braynes in readynge so many authours, to be at the lectures of so many learned menne, yea and the greatest follye of all were, to procede in any degree in the Universities with our great coste and charges, when a syr Johne Lacke Latin, a pedler, a weaver and

---

[25] A learned physician by definition had gone to university. There were no women at universities in England in this period.

[26] Securis (note 19), p. Aviii verso.

oftentymes a presumptous woman, shall take uppon them (yea and are permytted) to mynister Medicine to all menne, in every place, and at all tymes. *O tempora O mores, O Deum immortalem.* (pp. Biiv–r)

Latin (and its associations with the universities and learned culture) helped to mark out proper medicine. And in Latin there was to be had more medical knowledge than in English. Epistemologically, if I can use the word in a strained way, in Latin lay the key to finding the best and the most certain knowledge in medicine.

This was certainly the view of Dunk. In his *Letter* he wrote that a reason 'brought in defence of Empiriks is, That they reade English books sufficient to instruct them in their practise' (p. 35). His reply recognized that language could be a bar to the profession, but he emphasized that only if one knew Greek and Latin could medicine be grasped in a holistic sense. His reasons were pragmatic. Too little was written in English books, but also there is the sense that medicine is integrated into the whole corpus of learning, ignorance of which affects the proper understanding of medicine:

All the large volumes of Hipp[ocrates] Gal[en], Avicen[na], and all other famous Physicians both new and olde, were first written in the Greeke or Latine tongues, or afterward translated into one of them; the ignorance whereof hath in all ages beene accounted a strong barre to exclude all men from the profession of that Arte. That which is written in English is very littel and light in respect of the whole: neither can it be perfectly understood without the helpe of Grammer and Logicke, as every meane scholar will confesse. (p. 35)

Dunk was well aware of medicine as a learned profession and he compared it with the law and religion, both of which in his view required Latin at their highest levels. He noted that civil law (i.e., Roman law) depended on Latin (an obvious point!):

All nations Christian, wherein the civill is used, can not affoord one man of any meane account in that profession, that understands not the Latine tongue, wherein their large books are written. And I dare confidently affirme, that Physicke is as profound and intricate a study as the Civill law, and requireth as much reading and knowledge of tongues, as that doth. (p. 35)

Dunk also pointed to the example of religion as requiring a knowledge of Latin. Here, he was faced with a problem, for the Reformation had made the vernacular the norm. Dunk's answer is perhaps strained and shows how events were making his defence of Latin appear out of touch with the realities of early seventeenth-century England:

What though there be a profitable use of Ministers in our Church, that understand English books only, being yet able to execute their office in some commendable maner? yet this reason holdeth not in Empiriks: for first there is farre more Divinity than Physicke written in our vulgar idiome all the grounds and principles of religion are set forth at large in it; whereas no part of Hipp[ocrates], Gal[en] etc is translated into that tongue. Secondly, Ministers have farre greater help in hearing the learned of that profession, and in frequent conference with them: whereas Empirickes labour always to avoid the presence and company of learned Physicians ... As no Minister is able to confute a learned adversarie, that hath not skill at the least in the Latine tongue; so no Empirike is able to encounter with sicknesse, that great adversaire to nature, without weapons fetched from the Greek or Latine tongue. M. Latimer sayeth in one of his sermons, English Divinity will never be able to expell Popery out of this land and it may as truely be sayd; English Phyisicans can not cure English diseases. (pp. 35–6)

The learned professions in England were certainly changing and perhaps medicine too changed with them. Dunk forgot to mention that the civilians were being ousted from the English law, whilst Henry VIII had already abolished canon law. Moreover, English law in its attorneys provided practitioners akin to the empirics.[27] They used experience just as did the empirics (they were not allowed entry to the Inns of Court and their education), but this, argued Dunk, was no justification for the empirics or of experience. As one reads the learned physicians, whether Dunk, John Cotta or James Hart or even the great divine William Perkins who supported learned medicine, it is clear that the attack on experience is the counterpart to their support for learning. Their defence of learned medicine, although it echoed Galen's attack on empirics, also reflected the realities of the competitive medicine market place.

But by excluding experience, they confirmed that they were not interested in change. Or, at least this is how it appears in hindsight for change in medical knowledge was often to come from those who expressed a commitment to empiricism. On attorneys Dunk wrote:

This grand reason of experience is further urged of some by the example of Attorneys at the common law: most of these have nothing to direct them but experience and observation and yet sundry things passe thorow their hands as substantially and effectually performed, as by learned Councellers: therefore unlearned Physicians well instructed by experience, may do some cures as well as great scholars. The answer to this is easie: There are many things in law which belong merely to Attorneys, and require no learning: also they follow presidents and usuall formes, and many things which they doe, are plaine transcripts written out of books *verbatim*, wherein they cannot erre, if they folowe their paterne. But it is farre otherwise in Physicke: there is no usuall forme to follow in

27   See C.W. Brooks, *Pettyfoggers and Vipers of the Commonwealth. The 'Lower Branch' of the Legal Profession in Early Modern England* (Cambridge: Cambridge University Press, 1986). Also Ronald A. Marchant, *The Church Under the Law* (Cambridge: Cambridge University Press, 1969); R.H. Helmholz, *Roman Canon Law in Reformation England* (Cambridge: Cambridge University Press, 1990).

iudging or curing of disease; things seldome fall out after the same maner; the Physician must alter and change his course, as the disease and accidents require, wherein experience can not guide him, but the rules of the Arte. (p. 34)

Attorneys were at this time often considered the dregs of the legal profession, and many barristers and judges would have concurred with Dunk's view that as the attorneys in doubtful cases 'ask the opinion of learned Councillers' so they depend on learning. Learned civil law had been limited to the Admiralty and Church Courts and was under attack from the common law courts by means of prohibitions preventing particular cases being heard in the civil courts, and canon law did not run in England. Yet the common law, despite its lack of classical antiquity and its potential to be exposed to experience (changing precedents, and the experiential assessment of juries) could still be considered learned, even if it was a native form of learning. Sir Edward Coke, the great exponent of the common law, supported learned medicine when in Bonham's case (1608–9) he judged that the College of Physicians of London could not convict someone of malpractice if they were unlicensed.[28] Coke felt that in this case the learning of a university graduate was sufficient to guarantee good practice. (He also condemned 'Mountebanks and cheating Quacksalvers' in his exposition of the witchcraft statutes.)[29] There certainly was a learned culture beyond medicine which shared some of its values, but it was also a culture which was not as static as the defenders of learned medicine might have hoped.

In the end, learned medicine precluded real change – that was precisely why it was learned, for the past supplied it with its learning (and its attack on its competitors made the orthodoxy more rigid). John Cotta described the 'True Artist' (the true physician), and stressed the constant and unchanging nature of learned knowledge in a way which echoes later ideas of unchanging laws of nature. Cotta wrote that the more studious men were the more they would know nature,[30] and of the latter he stated:

The order of nature in all her works is constant, full of wonder and unchanged truth in the continuall cohesion, sequence and fatall necessitie of all things, their causes and effects: wherein therefore how the Almigthie Dietie hath commanded all things by an unchangeable law to be ordered, is both true and necessarie wisdom to understand, and the true patterne, rule, and square of everie discrete, sober and wise designe and consultation. Hence upon the principles of nature stand everlastingly founded all arts and sciences ... And all true arts thus

---

28 See Harold J. Cook, 'Against Common Right and Reason: the College of Physicians versus Dr Thomas Bonham', *American Journal of Legal History*, 29 (1985), 301–22.
29 Sir Edward Coke, *The Third Part of the Institutes of the Laws of England* (London, 1797), p. 46 (1st edition, 1644).
30 Cotta (note 19), p. 117.

founded upon the undeceiving grounds of nature, in themselves are ever certtain and infallible, whose rules although discretion according to circumstance may continually diversly vary, yet can no time nor circumstance ever or at any time abrogate. (p. 118)

Medicine, in Cotta's view, was such a 'true art'.

Conclusion

This has been a paper about how knowledge was perceived in a fully developed tradition of learned medicine in a country where it was faced with significant competition. It may be that in this case we cannot talk of epistemology, or that learning is its own epistemology.

It might have been useful to explore how in reports of their cases learned physicians put their learning into practice. Did they practise what they preached and take into account the age, constitution, life-style etc. of the individual patient? But this has not much to do with epistemology; it is merely a question of whether the rules of learned medicine were properly applied or not. The data are, in any case, inconclusive. The case notes, for instance, of John Hall, Shakespeare's son-in-law, vary widely from the brief recitation of a disease and its remedy (in almost empirical fashion) to a consideration of a patient's constitution and diet.

As it turns out there is very little that is or can be new about the epistemology of the mature learned medicine of sixteenth- and early seventeenth-century England. Some of the pressures leading to change have been mentioned in the paper, and perhaps the very orthodoxy of learned medicine was a pressure in its own right.

Other reasons for changes in the epistemology of medicine in the seventeenth century are well known – Paracelsianism, the calls for medical reform during the Civil War and Interregnum, the mechanical and chemical approach of the new science, the associated emphasis on observation. But learned medicine itself did not change fundamentally, though it did accept chemical remedies, and by the end of the seventeenth century much of it had died out. Some structures remained, for instance, the six non-naturals (air, diet, exercise and rest, sleep and waking, the evacuations including sexual activity, and the passions of the soul or mind) which helped to pattern advice on regimen and the prevention of disease. Much of therapeutics (bleeding, purging, emetics, some drugs) also remained the same. But what was no longer held even amongst eighteenth-century 'regular' physicians was the view that theirs was an unchanging learned profession – there were too many systems and schools of medicine quickly succeeding each other for that to have happened, and, in any case, the moderns with their view of progress had won.

Yet the very survival of much of traditional learned therapeutics raises an epistemological question. In a sense, there was an epistemological void in therapeutics. It was impossible to know with certainty if a treatment was effective or not in a particular case. This was something which was not resolved until the nineteenth century and the use of statistical trials. This uncertainty allowed the fight between the learned physicians and empirics to be undecided and it also allowed old and new therapies to co-exist in the eighteenth century. As Henry Edmundson put it in his *Comes Facundus in Via, The Fellow Traveller* (1658):

> It is a great Question what does the cure, the Vulgar will tell you the last thing they took did the cure, as the last thing they did caused the disease; Some physicians will ascribe it to the rarity and dearnesse, others to the variety and composition, others to the fitnesse and order etc. others think it is not the Physick or Physicians but Nature being disburthened returns to her functions by degrees, and men from weakness to a more cheerful condition, from a long hunger to a more greedy appetite etc. And some adde, that it is not Nature but the God of Nature which heals us, and as the Proverb is, God heals, and the Physician hath the thanks. It is Gods compassion on the poor man who contemneth no means but is without any. It is the reward of his patience. It is God's seeing his teares, or hearing his or the Churches prayers for him . . .[31]

In the eighteenth century the providential God was less conspicuous, but the uncertainty remained. So, at least, did one clear epistemological issue.

[31] Henry Edmundson, *Comes Facundus in Via, The Fellow Traveller* (1658), pp. 111–12, cited in A. Wear, 'Interfaces: Perceptions of Health and Illness in Early Modern England', in R. Porter and A. Wear, *Problems and Methods in the History of Medicine* (London: Croom Helm, 1987), pp. 240–1.

INDEX

INDEX

Printed and bound by CPI Group (UK) Ltd, Croydon, CR0 4YY

17/10/2024

01775690-0001